Art and Science of
Breastfeeding & Beyond

Art and Science of Breastfeeding & Beyond

Editors

Durgappa H MD
Professor and Head
Department of Pediatrics
Vijayanagar Institute of Medical Sciences
Ballari, Karnataka, India

Anita Nyamagoudar MD (Ped) DNB (Neonatology)
Assistant Professor
Department of Neonatology
SDM Medical College and Research
Dharwad, Karnataka, India

CR Banapurmath MD DCH MNAMS FIAP
Former Professor and Head
Department of Pediatrics
JJM Medical College
Davanagere, Karnataka, India
Former Director Bapuji Child Health
Institute and Research Centre, Davanagere
Chairperson, IYCF Chapter of IAP 2018–2020

Foreword

VD Patil

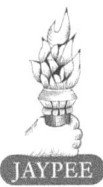

JAYPEE BROTHERS MEDICAL PUBLISHERS
The Health Sciences Publisher
New Delhi | London

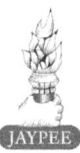 **Jaypee Brothers Medical Publishers (P) Ltd**

Headquarters
Jaypee Brothers Medical Publishers (P) Ltd
EMCA House, 23/23-B
Ansari Road, Daryaganj
New Delhi 110 002, India
Landline: +91-11-23272143, +91-11-23272703
+91-11-23282021, +91-11-23245672
Email: jaypee@jaypeebrothers.com

Corporate Office
Jaypee Brothers Medical Publishers (P) Ltd
4838/24, Ansari Road, Daryaganj
New Delhi 110 002, India
Phone: +91-11-43574357
Fax: +91-11-43574314
Email: jaypee@jaypeebrothers.com

Overseas Office
JP Medical Ltd.
83, Victoria Street, London
SW1H 0HW (UK)
Phone: +44 20 3170 8910
Email: info@jpmedpub.com

EU GPSR Authorised Representative
Logos Europe, 9 rue Nicolas Poussin
17000, La Rochelle, France
Phone: +33 (0) 6 67 93 73 78
E-mail: Contact@logoseurope.eu

Website: www.jaypeebrothers.com
Website: www.jaypeedigital.com

© 2024, Jaypee Brothers Medical Publishers

The views and opinions expressed in this book are solely those of the original contributor(s)/author(s) and do not necessarily represent those of editor(s) or publisher of the book.

All rights reserved. No part of this publication may be reproduced, stored or transmitted in any form or by any means, electronic, mechanical, photo copying, recording or otherwise, without the prior permission in writing of the publishers.

All brand names and product names used in this book are trade names, service marks, trademarks or registered trademarks of their respective owners. The publisher is not associated with any product or vendor mentioned in this book.

Medical knowledge and practice change constantly. This book is designed to provide accurate, authoritative information about the subject matter in question. However, readers are advised to check the most current information available on procedures included and check information from the manufacturer of each product to be administered, to verify the recommended dose, formula, method and duration of administration, adverse effects and contra indications. It is the responsibility of the practitioner to take all appropriate safety precautions. Neither the publisher nor the author(s)/editor(s) assume any liability for any injury and/or damage to persons or property arising from or related to use of material in this book.

This book is sold on the understanding that the publisher is not engaged in providing professional medical services. If such advice or services are required, the services of a competent medical professional should be sought.

Every effort has been made where necessary to contact holders of copyright to obtain permission to reproduce copyright material. If any have been inadvertently overlooked, the publisher will be pleased to make the necessary arrangements at the first opportunity.

Inquiries for bulk sales may be solicited at: jaypee@jaypeebrothers.com

Art and Science of Breastfeeding & Beyond

First Edition: **2024**

ISBN: 978-93-5696-990-2

Dedicated to

All Mothers and Children

Supported by

E Srinivas
(s/o EGSV Ramana)
(Managing Director, Shirdi Sai Steels Pvt Ltd, Bellary, Karnataka, India)

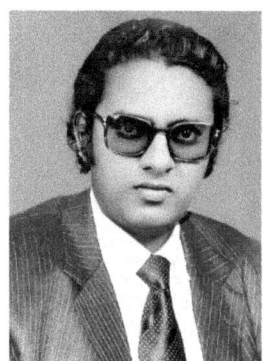

Shri EGSV Ramana

Contributors

Abhishek S Aradhya MD
Consultant
Ovum Woman and Child Specialty Hospital
Bengaluru, Karnataka, India

Adhisivam B DCH DNB PhD
Professor
Department of Neonatology
Jawaharlal Institute of Postgraduate Medical
Education and Research
Puducherry, India

Afshan Nazneen MD
Resident
Department of Pediatrics
Vijayanagar Institute of Medical Sciences
Ballari, Karnataka, India

Anish B Samaga MD
Resident
Department of Pediatrics
Vijayanagar Institute of Medical Sciences
Ballari, Karnataka, India

Anita Nyamagoudar
MD (Ped) DNB (Neonatology)
Assistant Professor
Department of Neonatology
SDM Medical College and Research
Dharwad, Karnataka, India

Anu Sachdeva MD DM (Neonatology)
Associate Professor
Department of Pediatrics
All India Institute of Medical Sciences
New Delhi, India

Arpita JS MD DNB
Consultant Pediatrician
Shri Raghavendra Hospital
Jagalur, Karnataka, India

Asha Doddamane Benakappa MD
Professor and Head
Department of Pediatrics
Dr Chandramma Dayananda Sagar Institute of
Medical Education and Research
Harohalli, Karnataka, India

Ashok R Datar MBBS DCH
Consultant Pediatrician
General and Developmental Pediatrics
Bijoy Child Guidance Centre
Bengaluru, Karnataka, India

B Shantharam Baliga MD DCH
Emeritus Professor
Department of Pediatrics
Kasturba Medical College
Mangaluru, Karnataka, India

Basavanthappa SP MD
Professor and Head
Department of Pediatrics
Basaveshwara Medical College and Hospital
Chitradurga, Karnataka, India

Bharathi Balachander MD DM
Associate Professor
Department of Neonatology
St John's Medical College
Bengaluru, Karnataka, India

Chaitali Raghoji
DCH Fellowship in Perinatal Medicine
Consultant Neonatologist and Pediatrician
Chigateri Government Hospital
Davangere, Karnataka, India

CR Banapurmath MD DCH MNAMS FIAP
Former Professor and Head
Department of Pediatrics, JJM Medical College
Davanagere, Karnataka, India
Former Director
Bapuji Child Health Institute, Davanagere
Chairperson, IYCF Chapter of IAP 2018-2020

Dhyanesh DK MD LLB
Professor
Department of Pediatrics
KAHER's JN Medical College
Belagavi, Karnataka, India

Durgappa H MD
Professor and Head
Department of Pediatrics
Vijayanagar Institute of Medical Sciences
Ballari, Karnataka, India

G Guruprasad MD DM FNNF
Professor and Head
Department of Neonatology
Bapuji Child Health Institute
JJM Medical College
Davanagere, Karnataka, India

Ganashree B MBBS MD
Assistant Professor
Department of Pediatrics
Shridevi Institute of Medical Sciences
Tumkur, Karnataka, India

Hari Dattatreya M MBBS
Senior Resident
Department of Pediatrics
Vijayanagar Institute of Medical Sciences
Ballari, Karnataka, India

Jayashree K MD PGDAP
Associate Professor
Department of Pediatrics
Kasturba Medical College
Mangaluru, Karnataka, India

Jayashree Purkayastha MD
Professor
Department of Pediatrics
Kasturba Medical College
Manipal, Karnataka, India

K Nagaraj MD
Assistant Professor
Department of Pediatrics
Vijayanagar Institute of Medical Sciences
Ballari, Karnataka, India

Kanya Mukhopadhyay MD DNB DM FNFF
Professor of Neonatology
Department of Pediatrics
Postgraduate Institute of Medical Education and Research
Chandigarh, India

KV Raghunath MBBS DCH
Senior Consultant Pediatrician
Madhavi Mother and Child Clinic
Adoni, Andhra Pradesh, India

Latha GS MD DCH
Professor
Department of Pediatrics
SS Institute of Medical Sciences and Research Centre
Davanagere, Karnataka, India

Leslie Lewis MD
Professor and Head
Department of Pediatrics
Kasturba Medical College
Manipal, Karnataka, India

Madhu B Jagalasar MD DM
Assistant Professor
Department of Neonatology
Jawaharlal Nehru Medical College
Belagavi, Karnataka, India

Madhu Pujar MD
Professor
Department of Pediatrics
JJM Medical College
Davanagere, Karnataka, India

Mahesh Kamate MD DNB DM (Ped Neuro)
Professor and Head
Department of Pediatric Neurology
KAHER's JN Medical College
Belagavi, Karnataka, India

Mallanagouda M Patil MD
Professor
Department of Pediatrics
BLDE University Shri BM Patil
Medical College Hospital
Vijayapur, Karnataka, India

Mallesh Gowda GS DCh FIAP
Consultant Pediatrician
New Amrutha Hospital
Raichur, Karnataka, India

Mallikarjuna Honnali Bannajji
MD DCH FIAP IYCF
Professor and Head
Department of Pediatrics
The Oxford Medical College Hospital
Bengaluru, Karnataka, India

Mallikarjuna R Patil MD DCH DrNB
(Med Genetics) PDCC (PICU)
Senior Consultant and Medical Geneticist
Med Genome Labs Pvt Ltd
Bengaluru, Karnataka, India

Manisha Bhandankar MD MRCPCH PhD
Professor
Department of Neonatology
KAHER's JN Medical College
Belagavi, Karnataka, India

Maria Pais MD
Assistant Professor
Department of Obstetrics and Gynecology
Manipal College of Nursing (MAHE)
Manipal, Karnataka, India

Medha Goyal MD
Consultant Neonatologist
King Edward Memorial (KEM) Hospital
Mumbai, Maharashtra, India

Megha Pai Pediatics MBBS MD (Pediatrics)
Senior Resident
Department of Pediatrics
Kasturba Medical College
Manipal, Karnataka, India

Mudka Suchit MD
Resident
Department of Pediatrics
Vijayanagar Institute of Medical Sciences
Ballari, Karnataka, India

Neelamma Patil MS (Obs & Gyne) DNB
Professor
Department of Obstetrics and Gynecology
BLDE University Shri BM Patil
Medical College Hospital
Vijayapur, Karnataka, India

NS Mahanthashetti MD
Professor
Department of Pediatrics
KAHER's JN Medical College
Belagavi, Karnataka, India

Padmashri S Kudachi MD
Professor and Head
Department of Physiology
KAHER's JN Medical College
Belagavi, Karnataka, India

Prakash M Kabbur MD DCH (UK) MRCPCH (UK)
FAAP (USA)
Neonatologist
Medical City Arlington
Texas, USA

Pramod Jog MD MNAMS FIAP FICMCH
Professor and Head
Department of Family Medicine
DY Patil Medical College
Pune, Maharashtra, India

Pranam GM MD
Professor
Department of Pediatrics
Navodaya Medical College
Raichur, Karnataka, India

Prathibha Rao MBBS DCh (London) FRCPCH (UK)
Consultant Pediatrician
Kettering General Hospital
Kettering, UK

Prathik Bandiya MD DM
Associate Professor
Department of Neonatology
Indira Gandhi Institute of Child Health
Bengaluru, Karnataka, India

Ramaraju HE MS
Associate Professor
Department of Obstetrics and Gynecology
Vijayanagar Institute of Medical Sciences
Ballari, Karnataka, India

Ramesh R Pol MD
Professor
Department of Pediatrics
S Nijalingappa Medical College
Bagalakote, Karnataka, India

Roopa Bellad MD
Professor
Department of Pediatrics
KAHER's JN Medical College
Belagavi, Karnataka, India

Ruchi Nanavathi MD DM
Professor
Department of Neonatology
King Edward Memorial (KEM) Hospital
Mumbai, Maharashtra, India

Sandeep R MD DM
Consultant Neonatologist
Rainbow Children's Hospital
Bengaluru, India

Sangappa M Dhaded MD DM
Professor and Head
Department of Neonatology
KAHER's JN Medical College
Belagavi, Karnataka, India

Satishkumar D MD
Professor
Department of Biochemistry
ESIC Medical College
Kalaburagi, Karnataka, India

Shashidhar A
MD DM (Neonatology) PGDMLE (NLSIU) MBA
Associate Professor
Department of Neonatology
St John's Medical College
Bengaluru, Karnataka, India

Shilpa C MD PGDAP
Senior Resident
Department of Pediatrics
SDM Medical College and Research
Dharwad, Karnataka, India

Shivanand I MBBS MD
Professor
Department of Pediatrics
Karnataka Institute of Medical Sciences
Hubli, Karnataka, India

Shivananda R MD DCH
Former Director, Professor and Head
Department of Pediatrics
Indira Gandhi Institute of Child Health
Bengaluru, Karnataka, India

Shobha C Banapurmath MD DCh
Senior Consulting Pediatrician
Department of Pediatrics
Banapurmath Children's Clinic
Davanagere, Karnataka, India

Shradha Salunke MBBS DNB PHD PGDDN
Professor
Department of Pediatrics
DY Patil Medical College
Pune, Maharashtra, India

Shrikanth Kulkarni MD DM
Consultant Neonatologist
Rainbow Children Hospital
Bengaluru, Karnataka, India

Sneha J Andrade MD
Assistant Professor
Department of Pediatrics
Kasturba Medical College
Manipal, Karnataka, India

Sowmya D MBBS MS (Obs & Gyne)
Associate Professor
Department of Obstetrics and Gynecology
Kodagu Institute of Medical Sciences
Madikeri, Karnataka, India

Srikanth BK MD MRCPCH (UK)
Associate Professor
Department of Pediatrics
Vijayanagar Institute of Medical Sciences
Ballari, Karnataka, India

Srilaxmi AN MBBS MS (OBG)
Assistant Professor
Department of Obstetrics and Gynecology
Basweshwara Medical College and Hospital
Chitradurga, Karnataka, India

Suchetha S Rao MD
Additional Professor
Department of Pediatrics
Kasturba Medical College
Mangaluru, Karnataka, India

Sudhakar Hegade MD
Associate Professor
Department of Pediatrics
Vijayanagar Institute of Medical Sciences
Ballari, Karnataka, India

Sudhindrashayana R Fattepur
MD Fellow in Neonatology
Associate Professor
Department of Pediatrics
Karnataka Institute of Medical Sciences
Hubli, Karnataka, India

Suman Rao PN MD DM
Professor
Department of Neonatology
St John's Medical College Hospital
Bengaluru, Karnataka, India

Sumana Nanjundachar
MBBS MPH-TM (Tulane University), USA
Vice-President
Train and Help Babies Organization, USA

Sumitha Nayak MD DNB FIAP Int Cert in Vaccinology PGDMLS PGDGC
Consultant Pediatrician
Shishu—The Children's Clinic
Bengaluru, Karnataka, India

Suvarna P Reddy MD
Assistant Professor
Department of Pediatrics
Vijayanagar Institute of Medical Sciences
Ballari, Karnataka, India

Swarna Rekha Bhat MD
Former Professor and Head
Department of Pediatrics and Neonatology
St John's Medical College Hospital
Bengaluru, Karnataka, India

Tanmaya Metgud MD
Professor
Department of Pediatrics
KAHER's JN Medical College
Belagavi, Karnataka, India

Udaykumar B MD
Senior Resident
Department of Pediatrics
Vijayanagar Institute of Medical Sciences
Ballari, Karnataka, India

Vani KT MD
Assistant Professor
Department of Pediatrics
Vijayanagara Institute of Medical Sciences
Ballari, Karnataka, India

Varsha CR MD
Assistant Professor
Department of Pediatrics
S Nijalingappa Medical College
Bagalakote, Karnataka, India

Veerendra Kumar MS DNB
Professor and Head
Department of Obstetrics and Gynecology
Vijayanagar Institute of Medical Sciences
Ballari, Karnataka, India

Venkatasheshan DCH DNB
Professor
Department of Neonatology
Jawaharlal Institute of Postgraduate Medical Education and Research
Puducherry, India

Vijay Venkataiah MD PhD
Associate Professor
Department of Biochemistry
Vijayanagar Institute of Medical Sciences
Ballari, Karnataka, India

Vikas Patil MD
Assistant Professor
Department of Pediatrics
KAHER's JN Medical College
Belagavi, Karnataka, India

Vinod H Ratageri MD DCEH
Professor
Department of Pediatrics
Karnataka Institute of Medical Sciences
Hubli, Karnataka, India

Vishwanath B MD DNB
Professor
Department of Pediatrics
Vijayanagar Institute of Medical Sciences
Ballari, Karnataka, India

Foreword

I have a great sense of pride in penning the foreword to the book *"Art and Science of Breastfeeding & Beyond"* by Dr Durgappa H, Dr Anita Nyamagoudar and Dr CR Banapurmath.

Though the importance of breastfeeding is well known since immemorial time, we the human race have been struggling to improve breastfeeding rates beyond 50% below 6 months of age across the globe. Various organizations such as WHO, UNICEF, WABA, IAP, BPNI, and NHM are also striving hard at various levels to improve breastfeeding practices.

Successful breastfeeding needs an active involvement of stakeholders, healthcare workers, healthcare professionals, volunteers, breastfeeding women, and caretakers. The optimal knowledge of IYCF is essential for the promotion of breastfeeding.

In this book, the authors have put forth the most relevant and practical aspects of IYCF in a lucid way.

Moreover, I know Dr Durgappa H for a long time. He is dedicated and passionate in the field of Infant and Young Child Feeding (IYCF) and has put his heart soul into and over a decade of experience in the simplest way in this book.

The chapters like the composition of breast milk, breast milk and genetics, breastfeeding benefits, breastfeeding technique, breastfeeding difficulties, feeding in infants with cleft lip and palate, functional gastrointestinal disorders (FGIDs), nursing strikes and bottle-feeding are dealt with in a great way.

This is a comprehensive book with the state-of-the-art information. I am sure this book will be most useful for the healthcare workers (HCWs), healthcare professionals (HCPs) and volunteers to understand optimal methods of IYCF.

I congratulate all the contributing authors for their excellent contribution to the book.

I appreciate Dr Anita Nyamagoudar for her contribution and active involvement in the promotion of infant and young child feeding and for sharing her all-practical experience in the book.

I immensely appreciate the most benevolent Teacher–Professor Dr CR Banapurmath for invaluable guidance and support to Dr Durgappa H and Dr Anita Nyamagoudar in bringing out this book in a great way.

VD Patil
Professor of Pediatrics
Former Principal
JN Medical College
Pediatrician
KLE Dr Prabhakar Kore Hospital
Former Registrar
KLE Academy of Higher Education and Research (Deemed to be University)
Belagavi, Karnataka, India

Preface

I consider it as an honor to be writing the preface to this unique, *Art and Science of Breastfeeding & Beyond*.

Our interest in the topic dates back to three decades of passionate interest and work, in the field of Breastfeeding. The journey into Human Lactation Management was deeply founded by Professor RK Anand and (Late) Dr Nirmala Kesaree. Dr Durgappa H, a passionate soldier and co-worker in the pathway to the fascinating journey of helping mothers to successfully breastfeed has been remarkable.

This book comprises of 5 sections and 41 chapters, to cover all aspects of breastfeeding, has been a herculean effort stewarded by Dr Durgappa H and the editorial team. A total of nearly 82 contributors dedicated to this field bring to the reader up-to-date information stressing on practical help and tips to the person navigating in the field of Human Lactation along with Infant and Young Child Feeding.

The contributors of this book have provided state-of-the-art information with the latest references. Each article ends with key points apart from providing latest developments related to the topic. The reader would find the flow in simple English presented in a reader-friendly manner.

Happy reading.

CR Banapurmath MD DCH MNAMS FIAP
Former Professor and Head
Department of Pediatrics
JJM Medical College
Davangere, Karnataka, India

Acknowledgments

My heartfelt gratitude to Dr CR Banapurmath for his constant invaluable guidance and encouragement throughout the endeavor and for having added soul to the book.

I thank Dr Anita Nyamagoudar for her valuable input and support. I sincerely thank my teachers; Drs VD Patil, and (Mrs) NS Mahantashetti, Roopa Bellad, Sangappa M Dhaded, Arun Desai, Sujata Jali, MS Kaddi, BK Hukkeri, Kavita Mugale, Manisha Bhandankar, and RM Wali, for their wishes and blessings. I would like to acknowledge the efforts of the contributing authors for their time, patience, and knowledge sharing and for helping fulfil the project.

My profound thanks to Kanekal S Gautham, USA, for the insightful guidance on the content of the book.

My special thanks to Dr Vijay VA for the technical help and support. I also thank Dr Padmashri Kudachi for the support and suggestions. I am grateful to my colleagues, postgraduates, undergraduates, and nursing officers for their great input and suggestions.

I extend my regards to Drs Shivanand R, Latha GS, GV Basavaraj, Vinod H Ratageri, Gnanamurthy N, Jagadish Chinnappa, Santosh Soan, B Shantharam Baliga, RT Patil, Vijay Kulkarni, KB Rangaswamy, Dinkar More, Mallikarjun HB, KV Raghunath, Leslie Lewis, Veerashankar M, Venkatasheshan, Kanya M, Ruchi N, Anu S, K Kesavulu, and Somasekar for their valuable suggestions.

I am honored to thank Shri Srinivas Sanganakallu, a philanthropist, for appreciating our work and providing financial assistance for the book publication.

I would like to express my special appreciation to Shri Pavan Kumar Malapati IAS, Dr Mohana Y for their great support and encouragement.

I would also like to thank Shri Prashant Kumar Mishra IAS and Shri Rahul Sankanur IAS for their encouragement and support.

I also would like to extend my regards to Drs T Gangadhar Goud, Krishnaswami D, Bala Bhaskar, Indumathi V and Shri MG Goud, for their good wishes and encouragement. I also want to thank Drs Mahesh Kamate, Jayaraj Sindhur, Mallikarjun R Patil, Sunil Patil, and Mahantesh Patil, for their valuable feedback.

I thank the mother-infant dyad who helped us realize our dream of writing a book on the most essential topic for pediatricians.

I want to offer a tribute of love, admiration and respect for my wife Dr Parimala, son Tanush, daughter Tanvi and maternal uncle Shri Anthoneppa, for their cooperation and encouragement during the endeavor.

Last but not least I would like to express my special gratitude to Shri Jitendar P Vij (Group Chairman), Mr Ankit Vij (Managing Director), Mr MS Mani (Group President), Ms Chetna Malhotra (Senior Director—Professional Publishing, Marketing, and Business Development), Ms Pooja Bhandari (Director—Production), Ms Asmi Bharati (Development Editor) and Priyansh Saxena (Development Editor), M/s Jaypee Brothers Medical Publishers (P) Ltd, New Delhi, India, for the much required technical support in all the possible way to publish this book.

Durgappa H

Contents

SECTION 1: Basics of Human Lactation and Pediatric Nutrition

1. **Introduction to Breastfeeding** 3
   Durgappa H

2. **History of Breastfeeding** 6
   Durgappa H, Afshan Nazneen, Mudka Suchit

3. **Anatomy and Physiology of Breast** 11
   Padmashri S Kudachi

4. **Composition of Human Milk** 22
   Vijay Venkataiah, K Nagaraj, Durgappa H

5. **Breast Milk and Genetics** 33
   Pramod Jog, Mallikarjuna R Patil, Shradha Salunke

6. **Benefits of Breastfeeding** 42
   Durgappa H, Anita Nyamagoudar, Vijay Venkataiah

7. **Harms from Delayed Initiation of Breastfeeding** 53
   Latha GS, Durgappa H, Megha Pai

8. **Maternal Nutrition and Quality of Breast Milk** 57
   Padmashri S Kudachi

9. **Micronutrients in Infants and Children** 64
   Sumitha Nayak, Sangappa M Dhaded, Satishkumar D, Durgappa H

SECTION 2: Methods of Infant and Young Child Feeding

10. **Mother–Baby-Friendly Environment** 75
    Ramesh R Pol, Shivanand I, Ganashree B, Durgappa H

11. **Kangaroo Mother Care** 78
    Abhishek S Aradhya, Kanya Mukhopadhyay

12. **Breastfeeding Technique** 85
    Suman Rao PN, Durgappa H

13. **Feeding in Preterm and Low Birthweight Infants** 92
    Manisha Bhandankar, Tanmaya Metgud, Durgappa H

14. **Breastfeeding and Working Mother** 98
    Shrikanth Kulkarni, Anu Sachdeva

15. **Breastfeeding and Maternal Medications** 106
    Sandeep R, Madhu B Jagalasar

16. **Complementary Feeding** 112
    KV Raghunath, Vishwanath B, Durgappa H

17. **Functional Gastrointestinal Disorders in Infants and Toddlers** 117
    B Shantharam Baliga, Jayashree K, Durgappa H

SECTION 3: Problems of Infant and Young Child Feeding Practices

18. **Anatomical Problems of Breast and Nipple** 127
    Veerendra Kumar, Srilaxmi AN, Ramaraju HE

19. **Barriers of Breastfeeding** 131
    Basavanthappa SP, Anita Nyamagoudar, Sudhakar Hegade

20. **Breastfeeding Difficulties** 135
    Madhu Pujar, Sowmya D, Durgappa H

21. **Practical Problems of Lactation** 142
    Swarna Rekha Bhat, Durgappa H

22. **"Not Enough Milk"** 147
    Ruchi Nanavathi, Medha Goyal, Durgappa H

23. **Breastfeeding Myths** 154
    Varsha CR, Ashok R Datar, Durgappa H, Anita Nyamagoudar

24. **Feeding During and After Illnesses** 158
    Sudhindrashayana R Fattepur, Shilpa C, Vinod H Ratageri

25. **Hypernatremic Dehydration in Infants** 165
    Sumana Nanjundachar, Prakash M Kabbur, Anita Nyamagoudar, Durgappa H

26. **Infant Milk Substitutes** 172
    Prathibha Rao, Srikanth BK, Pranam GM

27. **Bottle-feeding** 178
    Vikas Patil, Durgappa H, Vani KT, Arpita JS

28. **Feeding and Eating Disorders in Children** 184
    Suchetha S Rao, B Shantharam Baliga

SECTION 4: Breastfeeding in Special Circumstances

29. Feeding in Infants with Cleft Lip and Palate 195
    Mallikarjuna Honnali Bannajji, Suvarna P Reddy, Durgappa H

30. Breastfeeding and Maternal Infections 200
    Mallanagouda M Patil, Neelamma Patil, Durgappa H

31. Breastfeeding and Metabolic Disorders 206
    Prathik Bandiya, Mahesh Kamate

32. Breastfeeding during Emergency 217
    G Guruprasad, Chaitali Raghoji, Durgappa H

33. Nursing Strike 224
    Shashidhar A, Durgappa H, Anish B Samaga

34. Relactation and Induced Lactation 226
    Shobha C Banapurmath, CR Banapurmath

SECTION 5: Promotion of Infant and Young Child Feeding Practices

35. Global Networking and Promotion of Breastfeeding 241
    Anita Nyamagoudar, Venkatasheshan, Mallesh Gowda, Bharathi Balachander

36. Mothers Support Group and Breastfeeding 248
    NS Mahanthashetti, Durgappa H, Roopa Bellad

37. Infant Milk Substitute Act 254
    Dhyanesh DK, Asha Doddamane Benakappa, Hari Dattatreya M

38. Human Milk Banking 260
    Adhisivam B, Roopa Bellad, Durgappa H

39. Policy Making at the National Level for the Promotion of Breastfeeding 266
    Shivananda R, Durgappa H

40. Role of Research in Lactation: Present and Future 271
    Sneha J Andrade, Jayashree Purkayastha, Leslie Lewis, Maria Pais

41. Counseling in Breastfeeding 277
    Anita Nyamagoudar, Udaykumar B, Durgappa H

Index *281*

Abbreviations

AFASS: Acceptable, Feasible, Affordable, Sustainable, and Safe
AOM: Acute Otitis Media
ASPEN: American Society for Parenteral and Enteral Nutrition
BFHI: Baby Friendly Hospital Initiative
BPNI: Breastfeeding Promotion Network of India
CF: Complementary Feeding
CL: Cleft Lip
CP: Cleft Palate
CDC: Centers of Disease Control and Prevention
CMV: Cytomegalovirus
CVS: Cyclical Vomiting Syndrome
DHA: Docosahexaenoic acid
EBF: Exclusive Breastfeeding
EGF: Epidermal Growth Factors
FGIDs: Functional Gastrointestinal Disorders
ESPGHN: European Society of Pediatric Gastroenterology, Hepatology, and Nutrition
FAO: Fatty Acid Oxidation
GBC: Global Breastfeeding Collective
GALT: Gut-associated Lymphoid Tissue
GDP: Gross Domestic Product
HMB: Human Milk Banking
HMO: Human Milk Oligosaccharide
HAMLET: Human alpha-lactalbumin Made Lethal to Tumor Cells
HACCP: Hazard Analysis Critical Control Point
HB-EGF: Heparin Binding-Epidermal Growth Factor
IBD: Inflammatory Bowel Disease
IBFAN: International Baby Food Action Network
IF: Interferon
IGF: Insulin-like Growth Factor
IMS: Infant Milk Substitute
IYCF: Infant and Young Child Feeding

IL: Interleukin
iKMC: Immediate Kangaroo Mother Care
LBW: Low Birth Weight
LCFAOD: Long Chain Fatty Acid Oxidation Disorders
LCPUFA: Long Chain Polyunsaturated Fatty Acids
MOM: Mother's Own Milk
mRNA: micro-RNA
MTCT: Mother-To-Child Transmission
MAA: Mothers Absolute Affection
NGF: Nerve Growth Factor
NIN: National Institute of Nutrition
PIMS: Perception of Insufficient Milk Secretion
PKU: Phenylketonuria
PDSA: Plan-Do-Study-Act
PROBIT: Promotion of Breastfeeding Intervention Trial
QII: Quality Improvement Initiative
SIDS: Sudden Infant Death Syndrome
SST: Supplementary Suckling Technique
STAMP: Screening Tool for Assessment of Malnutrition in Pediatrics
SDGs: Sustainable Developmental Goals
SVN: Small Vulnerable Newborn
TF: Tube Feeding
TNF: Tumor Necrosis Factor
UNICEF: United Nations International Children's Emergency Fund
VEGF: Vascular Endothelial Growth Factor
WABA: World Alliance for Breastfeeding Action
WHA: World Health Assembly

SECTION 1: Basics of Human Lactation and Pediatric Nutrition

1. **Introduction to Breastfeeding**
   Durgappa H

2. **History of Breastfeeding**
   Durgappa H, Afshan Nazneen, Mudka Suchit

3. **Anatomy and Physiology of Breast**
   Padmashri S Kudachi

4. **Composition of Human Milk**
   Vijay Venkataiah, K Nagaraj, Durgappa H

5. **Breast Milk and Genetics**
   Pramod Jog, Mallikarjuna R Patil, Shradha Salunke

6. **Benefits of Breastfeeding**
   Durgappa H, Anita Nyamagoudar, Vijay Venkataiah

7. **Harms from Delayed Initiation of Breastfeeding**
   Latha GS, Durgappa H, Megha Pai

8. **Maternal Nutrition and Quality of Breast Milk**
   Padmashri S Kudachi

9. **Micronutrients in Infants and Children**
   Sumitha Nayak, Sangappa M Dhaded, Satishkumar D, Durgappa H

CHAPTER 1

Introduction to Breastfeeding

Durgappa H

"Breastfeeding is a universal solution"
—**World Health Organization (WHO)**

Breastfeeding is an indispensable infant-feeding method for the optimal growth, development, and health of infants and young children. On recognizing the incredible benefits of breastfeeding, the World Health Organization (WHO) and the United Nations International Children's Emergency Fund (UNICEF) have jointly recommended early initiation of breastfeeding, preferably within 1 hour of delivery, exclusive breastfeeding for 6 months, continued breastfeeding for up to 2 years or beyond, and appropriate adequate and safe complementary feeding at 6 months of age.

Despite the efforts of various national and international organizations in protecting, promoting, and supporting breastfeeding practices, the desired goal is not achieved. According to recent reports, globally, only 37% of infants are exclusively breastfed for below 6 months of age in low-to-middle income countries and 20% of infants are never breastfed. In India, the recent "National Family Health Survey-5"(NFHS-5) also showed that only 63.7% of infants below 6 months are exclusively breastfed and 11% of infants between 6–23 months of age are receiving adequate diet across the country.

The optimal breastfeeding practice has positive impacts on the health of the baby and mother. Recent studies have shown that improving breastfeeding practices to a universal level could prevent 823,000 under 5 years and 40,000 maternal deaths annually across the globe.

However, there are various challenges for mothers and healthcare professionals in optimizing breastfeeding practices, such as myths of no milk secretion in the first few days of delivery, delayed initiation of breastfeeding, breastfeeding difficulties, feeding in premature infants, maternal infections, the infant with craniofacial anomalies, working mothers, perception of insufficient milk, and influence of advertisement of infant milk substitutes (IMS).

WAYS TO OVERCOME

Early initiation of breastfeeding has positive impacts on the survival of infants. Antenatal education on the benefits of breastfeeding and timely skilled practical assistance and support is important in optimizing feeding practices.

Breastfeeding difficulties are commonly encountered among mothers in the postpartum period. Most problems of breastfeeding are due to improper techniques of breastfeeding. Hence, timely optimization of the technique of breastfeeding is important in preventing breastfeeding difficulties.

Feeding in preterm is challenging. Early initiation of breastfeeding or breast milk feeding is crucial in preventing neonatal morbidity and mortality due to sepsis and necrotizing enterocolitis. Breast milk has an analgesic property which is known to be reducing pain during minor procedures such as heel prick and intravenous (IV) lines.

Returning to the job is one of the common barriers to breastfeeding among working mothers. Mothers need to be provided with a workplace-friendly environment, support from coworkers, flexibility in working hours, and paid maternity leaves. They can express breast milk and keep it at room temperature for 6 hours and caretakers can feed the baby. Mothers can also maintain breastfeeding by feeding the baby before going to the job and after coming from the job, feeding at night hours, and increasing feeding frequencies at weekends.

The perception of insufficient milk secretion (PIMS) is one of the common reasons for premature cessation of breastfeeding. In most cases, it is simply due to a false PIMS. In such situations, it is important to assess the adequacy of breast milk secretion in the mother. The frequent and efficient emptying of the breast is most important in maintaining sufficient milk flow.

Maternal infections are one of the barriers to breastfeeding. However, recent studies have shown that breastfeeding can safely be practiced in most maternal infections under appropriate preventive measures as the risk of transmission of infections through breast milk is minimal.

Infants with craniofacial anomalies often have feeding difficulties. These babies need some modifications in the feeding strategies such as feeding in the straddle position and dancer's hand position. In severe cases, specially designed feeding devices can be utilized to feed the infants. Mothers also need to be counseled regarding the surgical repair of cleft lip and palate at appropriate time.

Infant milk substitute usage is widely prevalent across the globe. Infant formula has negative impacts on the health of babies. Recognizing this, in 1981, the International Code of Infant Milk Substitute was adopted at the 34th World Health Assembly, held in Geneva. In the same year, the Government of India also adopted and implemented the Infant Milk Substitute Act for protecting, promoting, and supporting breastfeeding practices.

PROMOTION OF BREASTFEEDING

Though the most mothers are enthusiastic to breastfeed their babies, they often face difficulties at early initiation and maintenance of breastfeeding. The reasons for suboptimal breastfeeding practices could be due to a lack of education, a mother–baby-friendly environment, and timely assistance and support. Hence, the WHO and UNICEF have jointly recommended 10 steps of the Baby-Friendly Hospital Initiative to protect, promote, and support breastfeeding across the world. In India also, the Breastfeeding Promotion Network of India (BPNI) has taken active initiatives in the promotion of breastfeeding. It has also recommended to the Government of India to implement a stringent IMS law to protect, promote, and support breastfeeding across the country. In addition, other various programs such as

Mothers Absolute Affection (MAA) Program and mothers support groups are involved in the promotion of breastfeeding.

Healthcare professionals play an important role in the promotion of breastfeeding practices. They need to undergo periodic training on optimal infant and young child feeding (IYCF) practices. The healthcare professionals involved in the care of the baby and mother need to change their attitude toward lactation. In addition to this, there is a need to involve civil society and create awareness among them by conducting the breastfeeding sensitization programs such as the breastfeeding week celebration. Overall, collective societal responsibility is important in the promotion of breastfeeding.

It is also important to sensitize the medical graduates by incorporating the optimal infant and young child feeding practices into the medical education curriculum. In addition, it is also important to undertake research projects to uncover the unknown facts about breastfeeding. To strengthen the initiative, the policy makers at national levels need to take concrete innovative decisions to protect, promote and support breastfeeding practices across the country.

CHAPTER 2

History of Breastfeeding

Durgappa H, Afshan Nazneen, Mudka Suchit

"Breastfeeding is nature's health plan"

INTRODUCTION

Breastfeeding has been a natural norm among mammalian species. Since time immemorial, breastfeeding has been an integral part of human life and helps in establishing a perennial and everlasting bond between the newborn and the mother. Over time, different types of feeding practices have been started ranging from wet nursing to bottle-feeding and formula feeds.

Throughout time, ancient scriptures have referred to the importance of breastfeeding. However, the use of artificial food was attempted throughout the entire course of history but without much success. In periods of declining ethical and social standards, the rate of breastfeeding historically declines as well, whereas in times of social stability, the breastfeeding rate increases. Recent data shows that health in childhood, adolescence, and adulthood is strongly associated with the diet at beginning of life.[1] Adequate and optimal breastfeeding is required for the survival of the infant, and thus discussing the change in practices and review of history becomes important.

Dating back to the era of the first humanoids, Neanderthals, hunter-gatherers, and stone age people, it is believed that they fed their offspring like other primates, i.e., feeding on demand for several years till they can hunt on their own. Little to no evidence is present regarding the weaning period during these times.[2]

However, Arora and coworkers attempted to accurately detect when babies were weaned by analyzing the prehistoric tooth. They postulated that weaning time can be detected from the amount of barium in the growing teeth. They conducted the study on the molars of a 100–1,000-year-old Neanderthal child found at Scladina Cave in Belgium and concluded that the barium levels were particularly high immediately after birth due to exclusive breastfeeding and gradually decreased to intermediate levels at around 7 months and subsequently fell to very low levels by 1–2 years of life.[3]

In Babylonian, Egyptian, and Roman cultures, breast milk was considered sacred and essential for the survival of the infant. If maternal breast milk is insufficient, then wet nurses were employed to feed the infants.[4]

In 950 BC Greece, there was an increased demand for wet nurses, especially in higher socioeconomic background families and often, they used to appoint paid wet to nurses to feed their infants and hold a higher status over the other slaves.[5]

Breastfeeding was universally considered sacred in every religion and was often considered a religious obligation. In 536 BC Talmudic, a central text of Rabbinic Judaism recommended newborn to be placed immediately on the mother's breast and breastfed for about 2 years.[5]

Aristotle (384-322 BC) considered breastfeeding a maternal duty and opposed the use of wet nurses. He was the first one to conceptualize breastfeeding as a contraceptive method. Plutarch (46-120 AD) famously quoted that "Mothers must breastfeed their children because they will indulge them with more love and kindness".[6,7]

Even though the practice of wet nurses was prevalent and well acknowledged at that time, many eminent personalities criticized the use of wet nurses for feeding. Cicero (106-43 BC) and Tacitus (56 BC to 117 AD) believed that breastfeeding was the first family bond of love that would turn into love for the motherland.[7]

The first Indian scripture, the Veda (1800 BC) stated that the milk and the breast are symbols of longevity and have the sweetness of nectarine. Sushruta Samhita indicated the introduction of solid foods at the age of 6 months when teething starts. Other ancient ayurvedic texts such as Charak Samhita and Kashyap Samhita considered breast milk to have vivifying power.[8,9]

The importance of breastfeeding in Islam can be assessed by the Hadith stating that the mother received a reward for every drop of breast milk given to her child. The physician IbnSina (980-1037 AD) described breast milk as "White Blood". The holy Quran recommends, if possible, the mother should breastfeed her offspring for 2 years and that every newborn infant had the right to breastfeed.[10,11]

During Middle Ages, breast milk was considered to have magical properties and it was thought that breast milk could transmit both physical and psychological characteristics of the women. This led to objections against the use of wet nurses. During the Renaissance period, there was a surge of printed work on pediatrics. Physicians such as Paul Bagellardu (1492), Thomas Phayer (1510-1560), Thomas Muffett (1553-1604), and Simon de Vallambert wrote various books on breastfeeding and wet nurses.[5,12,13]

In 1419, an influential silk worker Guild established a global research center by the name Ospedale degli Innocenti in Florence, Italy to house and care for city's orphans and abandoned children.[14]

In the 16th century, M Etmuller was the first to advocate that babies should be put on their mother's breast during the colostrum period, a practice that was usually forbidden in the preceding era.[15]

In the 17th century, Jacques Guillemeau also advocated for breastfeeding. However, he had four major objections against wet nursing. The first objection was the possibility of the child being exchanged for another child, the second was that the love between mother and child might be reduced, the third was the possibility of the child adopting an undesirable trait from the nurse, and finally, the child might inherit the wet nurse's bad physique.[16]

In the mid-18th century, Jacque Rousseau objected to wet nursing as the concurrent; growing popularity of maternal breastfeeding was associated with a significant decline in infant mortality. By the end of the 18th century, the dilemma "mother versus wet nurse" was bypassed by the new controversy that emerged "bottle versus the breast".[4]

Another method for breastfeeding that was gaining popularity was Pap and Panada. Pap consisted of hot water and flour or bread soaked in water or milk and egg, whereas Panada was cereals that were cooked in broth. At the end of the 18th century, four methods of infant feeding were available, breastfeeding by the mother, wet nurse, with animal milk, and with pap and panada.[17]

During the industrial revolution in the 19th century, breastfeeding was becoming impossible due to women being separated from their infants for several hours daily. Hence, artificial nutrition became the first choice. To cope with the demand for breast milk, breast milk banks were established all over Europe, where breast milk from several women was pooled and pasteurized before distribution.[18]

It was in the 19th century when glass bottles were first manufactured and the concept of the modern feeding bottle evolved. The first step toward the production of dehydrated milk was made by Newton in 1835 and it was put in tin boxes for the first time in 1866. Professor von Leibig devised a formula in 1863 for the perfect infant food consisting of cow's milk, flour, potassium bicarbonate, and malt.[19,20]

It was during this period, Pasteur and Koch drew attention to the dangers of microorganisms in milk and for this reason, it was preferred that they use sterilized undiluted cow's milk when breast milk was not available. Unfortunately, these dried milk and starchy foods became the first nutrition for infants, which led to an increased incidence of scurvy and rickets due to insufficient vitamins.[18]

A steady reduction in infant mortality was noticed in the 20th century, which was attributed to welfare clinics, education of the mothers regarding breastfeeding, and the right use of dried milk. Pierre Bud was the first person who found a welfare clinic where breastfeeding was encouraged and sterilized cow's milk was provided in a sealed bottle.[15] But due to extensive advertising, a high percentage of babies were fed formula feeds during this century as large companies were able to convince parents that artificial feeding was the safest option for the babies.

During the 1950s and 1960s, breastfeeding steadily decreased and by the early 1970s, only about 25% of infants were breastfed at the age of 1 week and only 14% at 2–3 months of age. With time, robust evidence started accumulating and the importance of breastfeeding for babies was realized. On August 1st, 1989, a convention was held at Innocenti, Florence, Italy, inviting 30 representatives of different countries across the world to discuss and form a consensus with global ambitions of protecting, promoting, and supporting breastfeeding practices across the world and after extensive discussions and debates over 2 days, the document called the "Innocenti Declaration" was prepared.[21,22]

Ever since, to sensitize the importance of breastfeeding in the public, the first week of August is being celebrated as world breastfeeding week. This was endorsed at the 45th World Health Assembly (WHA) by the World Health Organization (WHO), United Nations International Children's Emergency Fund (UNICEF), and various government representatives of different countries. Following this, WHO and UNICEF jointly recommended 10 steps of Baby-Friendly Hospital Initiative (BFHI) in the year 1991.[23] India adopted the BFHI in 1991 the same year Breastfeeding Promotion Network Of India (BPNI) was founded in Wardha, Maharashtra to protect, promote, and support breastfeeding.

In 1981, the 34th WHA took the initiative of formulating an international code regarding infant feeding and based on the recommendations of WHA, the Indian government enacted "The infant milk substitutes, feeding bottles, and infant foods" Act, 1992, which came into force on August 1st, 1993, and was subsequently amended in 2003 and enacted on June 2nd, 2003. In 2019, the Taj Mahal became the first Indian monument to get a breastfeeding room.[24-26]

With the dawn of the 21st century, there was a surge in mothers opting for breastfeeding rather than artificial feeds. This was possible because of the healthcare workers and clinics educating mothers about the advantages of breastfeeding. It is widely accepted now that breast milk is the best nutrition for the baby. Furthermore, it decreases the risk of various infections and is associated with higher intelligence quotient (IQ) in children. The great impact of breastfeeding is obvious for world health and the economy, as the rates of hospitalization and morbidity had decreased over time.

Though most mothers wish to breastfeed their infants, they often encounter the difficulties at the start and maintenance of breastfeeding. This implies that there is a need for innovative interventions to promote breastfeeding practices.

KEY MESSAGES

- Breastfeeding is a natural instinct of mother and baby.
- The importance of breastfeeding has been known since ancient time.
- Ongoing efforts are on to protect to promote and support breastfeeding practice across the globe.
- Lays a good foundation for the long quality of life which in turn helps in Nation building.

REFERENCES

1. Papastavrou M, Genitsaridi SM, Komodiki E, Paliatsou S, Midw R, Kontogeorgou A, et al. Breastfeeding in the Course of History. J Pediatr Neonatal Care. 2015;2(6):00096.
2. Palmer B. (2012). Breast-Feeding in Prehistoric Times. Did cave-babies have attachment parents? [online] Available from: https://slate.com/news-and-politics/2012/05/time-magazine-breast-feeding-cover-how-nursing-worked-in-prehistoric-times.html [Last accessed November, 2023].
3. Science NOW. (2013). Neanderthal Breastfeeding Habits Revealed By Analysis Of Prehistoric Tooth. How Long Did Neanderthals Nurse? Old Tooth Yields Answer. [online] Available from: https://www.huffpost.com/entry/neanderthal-breastfeeding-prehistoric-tooth_n_3321809 [Last accessed November, 2023].
4. Fildes V (Ed). Breasts, bottles, and babies: a history of infant feeding. Edinburgh: Edinburgh University Press; 1986. p. 462.
5. Wickes IG. A history of infant feeding. Part I. Primitive peoples: ancient works: renaissance writers. Arch Dis Child. 1953;28(138):151-8.
6. Minchin, M. (2018). Infant Feeding in History: an Outline. In Breastfeeding and Breast Milk – from Biochemistry to Impact, (Ed, Family Larson- Rosenquist Foundation) Georg Thieme Verlag KG. The Global Health Network.
7. Colon AR, Colon PA (Eds). Nurturing Children: A History of Pediatrics. Westport: Greenwood Press; 1999. p. 329.
8. Khanal V, Sauer K. Determinants of the introduction of prelacteal feeds in rural Nepal: a cross-sectional community-based study. Breastfeed Med. 2013;8(3):336-9.
9. Gartner LM, Stone C. Two thousand years of medical advice on breastfeeding: comparison of Chinese and western texts. Semin Perinatol. 1994;18(6):532-6.
10. IbnSina, Abu Ali al-Husaynibn Abd Allah (Eds). The Canon of Medicine (al-Qānūn Fī'l-ṭibb). Chicago: Great Books of the Islamic World, Inc.; 2000. pp. 710.

11. Doolan P. (2008). Nursing Times. [online] Available from: https://www.historytoday.com/archive/nursing-times [Last accessed November, 2023].
12. Osborn ML. The rent breasts: a brief history of wet-nursing. Midwife Health Visit Community Nurse. 1979;15(8):302-6.
13. Ruhrah J. Pediatrics of the Past. JSTOR. 1926;8(2):386-8.
14. UNICEF. (2015). Children and Research at Innocenti: 25 Years of UNICEF Commitment. [online] Available from: https://www.unicef-irc.org/publications/773-children-and-research-at-innocenti-25-years-of-unicef-commitment.html [Last accessed November, 2023].
15. Wickes IG. A history of infant feeding. Part III: eighteenth and nineteenth-century writers. Arch Dis Child. 1953;28(140):332-40.
16. Wickes IG. A history of infant feeding. Part II. Seventeenth and eighteenth centuries. Archives of Disease in Childhood. 1953;28: 232-40.
17. Von Strandmann S. (2013). A brief history of infant feeding. [online] Available from: https://www.womensviewsonnews.org/2013/08/a-brief-history-of-infant-feeding/ [Last accessed November, 2023].
18. Swan P. Infant nutrition. The kind biomedical library historical collection of Vanderbilt university medical center. 1866–1966.
19. Radbill S. Infant feeding through the ages. Clin Pediatr (Phila). 1981;20(10):613-21.
20. Fomon S. Infant Feeding in the 20th century; formula and beikost. J Nutr. 2001;131(2):409S-20S.
21. SNS. (2019). World Breastfeeding Week. What is Innocenti Declaration? [online] Available from: https://www.thestatesman.com/world/world-breastfeeding-week-innocenti-declaration-1502667464.html [Last accessed November, 2023].
22. UNICEF. 1990–2005 Celebrating the Innocenti Declaration on the Protection, Promotion, And Support of Breastfeeding. New York, USA: UNICEF; 2013. p. 38.
23. World Health Organization. (2009). Baby-friendly hospital initiative: revised, updated, and expanded for integrated care. [online] Available from: https://www.who.int/publications/i/item/9789241594950 [Last accessed November, 2023].
24. Tiwari SK, Chaturvedi P. The IMS Act 1992: need for more amendments and publicity. Indian Pediatr. 2003;40(8):743-6.
25. Mishra D, Chikitsalaya CN. Infant Milk Substitutes (IMS) Act 2003-Surrogate Promotion Continues. Indian Pediatr. 2005;42(1):88.
26. Dewan A. Important milestones in breastfeeding history and unique facts you should know. [online] Available from: https://www.parentcircle.com/important-milestones-of-breastfeeding-history-and-breast-milk-facts/article [Last accessed November, 2023].

CHAPTER 3

Anatomy and Physiology of Breast

Padmashri S Kudachi

"Breastfeeding is the priceless gift of the mother to the baby"

INTRODUCTION

The mammary gland is a unique feature of humans and all mammals which produce milk for the nourishment of offspring. It consists of glandular and fat tissue supported by connective tissue. The breast undergoes significant morphological and functional changes during various phases of a woman's life. This chapter describes the dramatic developmental changes of the breast observed during the fetal stage, puberty, pregnancy, lactation, and involution. Further the role of hormones, lactation, and recent updates related to this topic are discussed.

MAMMARY GLAND DEVELOPMENT

Embryology (Fetal stage)

The two compartments of breast include epithelial component originating from ectoderm and surrounding stromal part from mesoderm.[1] The ectoderm forms the ducts and alveoli, whereas the mesenchyme forms the connective tissue and its vessels. Early development of human mammary gland gets initiated at 4th week of intrauterine life as a localized thickening of the ectoderm.[2] The mammary band is identified at 5-6th week of intrauterine life as milk line (thickened ectoderm), also known as galactic band seen extending from axilla to groin. The mammary band involutes during 6-7th week, except for the thoracic region which presents as four-to-six cell wide thickening representing the future breast location. Mesenchymal cells around epithelial bud differentiate into mammary mesenchyme. During 7-8th week, the mammary bud invades into the mesenchyme beneath and starts branching as it reaches the fat pad. Between 10-12th weeks of gestation, mammary epithelial buds form and start showing different differentiation stages[3] **(Figs. 1A to E)**. By 13-20th week, 15-25 epithelial cords which later with multiple openings (galactophores) join at each nipple; among them, 8-15 ducts are patent. These cords branch and canalize, leading to formation of primary milk (lactiferous) ducts by 32 weeks of gestation.[2,3] The term branching morphogenesis refers to the tree-like ductal branches extending from epithelial bud.[4] In 80-90% of newborn infants, the ducts may contain milk-like secretion called the "witch's milk"; due to influence of maternal hormones circulating in fetal circulation, fetal pituitary prolactin (PRL) gradually reaches its peak levels at term pregnancy.[2,5] Around a

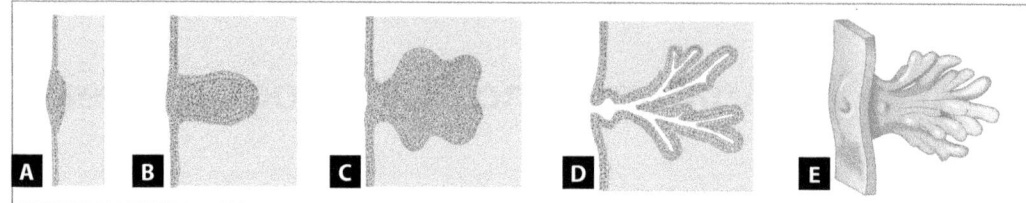

Figs. 1A to E: Various embryonic stages of mammary tissue development. [A: Mammary bud (5th week of gestation); B: Downward growth of mammary bud; C: Secondary bud formation (5–12th week); D: Mammary lobules development (12 week); E: Further growth of lobules, branching of duct) converging at inverted nipple (>12 weeks)]
Source: Adapted from Jesinger RA. Breast anatomy for the interventionalist. Tech Vasc Interv Radiol. 2014;17(1):3-9.

month after birth, the newborn's mammary gland regresses with low PRL levels.[3]

At birth, the ducts open on the outer surface of the skin as a small pit. The nipple everts during proliferation of underlying mesenchyme and the skin surrounding the nipple forms the areola after proliferation. Duct branching and terminal lobule development is seen till the age 2, later the lobules involute and breast remains dormant until pubertal hormonal influence but grows in proportion to the other tissues till puberty.[6,7] The embryonic development of mammary gland is hormone independent, while later stages are influenced by multiple hormones.[8] At birth the gland consists of number of blind-ended tubes and terminal duct lobular units (TDLU).[9-11]

The areola around the breast nodule is formed by the ectoderm during the 5th month of intrauterine life. The infants born before term fail to develop the breast nodules, which indicates the importance of the intrauterine environment for breast development.[11]

Terminal duct lobular unit is a group of acini originating from one terminal duct **(Fig. 2)**, which is the functional unit of the breast. On the basis of differentiation, four types of TDLU are recognized. Type I lobules are most primitive, seen among adult nulliparous breast (18–20 years of age), and have great number of receptors of estrogen and progesterone with complete ductal and stromal maturation. Type II and III show terminal duct with many branches, forming more number of acini, characterized by less proliferative index. Type IV lobules are present only in lactating women. Postmenopause, breast shows Type I TDLU.[8]

Pubertal Stage

Thelarche, the phase where adult breast development begins is the indicator of the onset of puberty, observed between 8–13 years of age, about 2 years before menarche[12,13] **(Table 1)**. During initial anovulatory cycles after the menarche, the breast tissue is exposed to uninhibited action of estrogen known as estrogen window[14] which causes ductal epithelial thickening elongation of existing ducts, formation of secondary ducts by branching, and clusters of alveolar budding, forming lobules.

With the onset of ovarian cycle at puberty, in follicular phase of menstrual cycle, the ducts in the mammary gland have little or no lumen, while in midcycle, the lumen epithelium becomes taller due to the effect of estrogen. The vascularity of the breast is known to increase during the ovulation

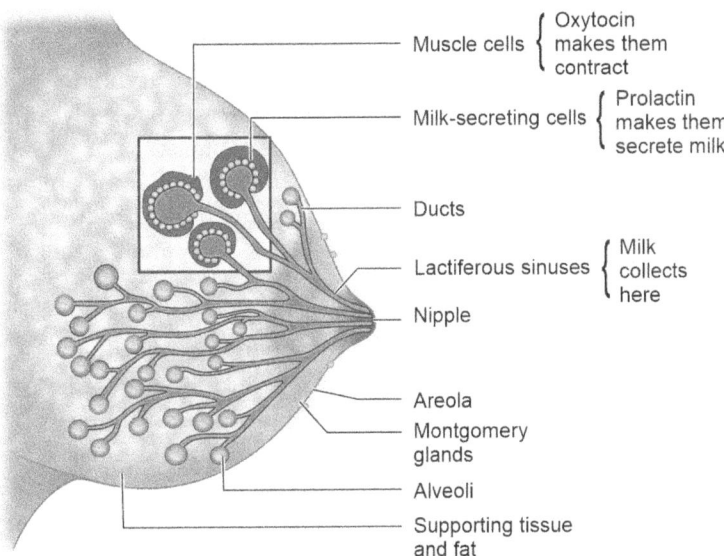

Fig. 2: Schematic diagram indicating terminal duct lobular unit (TDLU).

Stages	Age (years)	Features in the breast
		TABLE 1: The developmental stages of breast described by Tanner.[18]
1	10 or <10	Slight elevation of only papilla, no palpable glandular tissue (preadolescent)
2	10–11.5	Breast and papilla both elevated, palpable breast bud (first pubertal sign)
3	11.5–13	Enlargement of the breast beyond areolar region
4	13–15	Further enlargement of areola and papilla form a secondary mound above the breast
5	15 and above	Adult breast, areolar mound recession to the general contour of the breast, nipple protrusion

phase of menstrual cycle.[15] The luteal phase shows second phase of mammary gland growth under the influence of progesterone secreted by corpus luteum which is termed lobuloalveolar growth, which attains full growth during pregnancy.

In luteal phase, duct cells differentiate to be able to secrete; blood flow in the stromal tissue increases, leading to discomfort caused by edema and hyperemia of the breast experienced during premenstrual period. The lobules with alveoli reach maximum size and number in secretory phase, during 21–27 days of menstrual cycle, correlated with serum progesterone levels.[5,12] The breast lobules which show greater proliferation rate exhibit more receptors for both estrogen and progesterone.[5] The lobuloalveolar structure undergoes regression with the hormonal withdrawal with the onset of menstrual bleeding and regains growth during luteal phase dominated by progesterone.[16] These cyclical changes continue and contribute to the new development and new budding in lobule with each menstrual cycle till the age of 35 years.[5,17]

Role of Hormones

Secretion of gonadotropin-releasing hormone (GnRH) from the hypothalamus during puberty stimulates follicle-stimulating hormone (FSH) and luteinizing hormone (LH). Key regulator of pubertal breast before menses is estrogen, secreted by ovary, which acts on estrogen receptor-alpha (ERα). Estrogen action depends on the growth hormone and in turn on insulin-like growth factor-1 (IGF-I) in the mammary gland.[19] Estrogen also favors the action of FSH and LH for normal breast growth.[2,20]

Hence, the hormones, estrogen, growth hormone, IGF-I, and epidermal growth factor are known to cause ductal elongation. Progesterone, PRL, and thyroid hormone favor duct branching and more alveolar formation.[2] PRL increases progesterone secretion from the corpus luteum and acts indirectly by facilitating progesterone's actions on the breast. Insulin by acting on IGF-I receptors may also contribute to ductal or lobuloalveolar development, but it is not essential.[12,16] Triiodothyronine, glucocorticoids, and vitamin D3 are the other hormones involved in breast development during puberty.[5,11]

Breast Changes in Pregnancy

Mammary gland undergoes dramatic changes and full development in pregnancy. First trimester of pregnancy shows increased distal duct proliferation to form TDLU-4 with more lobules and alveoli. In second trimester of pregnancy, the mammary gland prepares itself for milk synthesis called lactogenesis I, characterized by increased cell organelles and cytoplasmic lipid droplets. During pregnancy, high PRL levels will not cause milk production due to the suppression by progesterone.[21] In the last trimester, fat droplets will get collected in the epithelial cells and the acini gets filled with colostrum. More of glandular tissue replaces the connective tissue and fat in the breast. Vascularity of the mammary tissue increases markedly, attributing to large volume of breast.[12,13]

The breast size in pregnancy does not determine milk production of lactation, neither the preconception of breast size is related to the magnitude of increase in size during pregnancy.[8,22] The changes during pregnancy are influenced by estrogen, progesterone, adrenal corticoids along with protein hormones of the PRL, and glycoside hydrolases (GH) family.[23,24] During midpregnancy, insulin increases secretory differentiation of mammary gland and decreases its proliferation.[16,25]

Breast Changes During Lactation Phase

Metabolic demand increases significantly in lactation with need of 25% of daily energy intake for milk synthesis.[3] The important changes seen from pregnancy to lactation are increase in alveoli with secretory capacity and peak levels of gene expression for the synthesis of lipid, enzymes, lactose, and milk protein seen during 3-4 days postpartum.[23,24]

Metabolic hormones including insulin and thyroxin prepare the myoepithelial cells to synthesize mature milk composed of fat, lactose, and protein in 30-40 hours postpartum phase.[26] The onset of milk secretion around parturition is because of fall in levels of progesterone and further maintained by PRL and glucocorticoid.

Key hormone in regulating lactogenesis is PRL which has receptors on the alveolar basal membrane and secreted in response to infant suckling or stimulation. However, serum PRL levels do not control milk production but infant suckling and nipple stimulation do, which explains the basis of skin-to-skin (S2S) theory. The feedback inhibitor of lactation (FIL) is a whey protein identified in breast milk that acts as the local negative feedback mechanism for milk synthesis.[22] Insulin, thyroid hormone, estrogen, and GH are known to enhance the action of PRL. Other hormones involved in regulation of lactation are estrogen and oxytocin.

The hormones also increase the mammary blood flow. There are also increased stromal lymph vessels to help clearance of particles and fluid from breast.[27]

The phases of lactation[28] are as follows:
1. *Mammogenesis:* Development and proliferation of the mammary tissue under the influence of estrogen and progesterone to stimulate mammogenesis and simultaneously inhibit PRL.
2. *Lactogenesis:* The proliferative state of breast in pregnancy gains secretory function during lactation is called lactogenesis.[29]
3. *Galactopoiesis:* Further maintenance of milk secretion[28]
4. Involution.[30]

Lactogenesis I is observed at 15–20 weeks of gestation with the ability to produce milk. Colostrum secretion begins and collects in the alveolar lumen at this phase. This colostrum contains no fat unlike milk secreted in postpartum period.[31,32] After child birth, removal of placenta causes rapid fall of progesterone, resulting in lactogenesis II (L-II).

Large amount of milk secreted during first 3–4 days after parturition known as "milk coming in" in the first 40 hours,[16] which is accompanied with great rise in blood flow. The oxygen and glucose uptake also increases in breast tissue. Milk volume increases from 100 mL/day—an initial value to approximately 600 mL/day by 4–5 days.[21,33] The maximum amount of storage of milk in breast ranges from 80–600 mL.[22] The normal, healthy, lactating woman can produce up to 1 liter of milk in a day.[12]

The relation of blood flow and outcome of milk is observed and the ratio[3] is described as 500:1.

Lactogenesis I and II occur irrespective of initiation of breastfeeding, independent of any stimulus, such as suckling or pumping of milk.[34] Further, the lactation is sustained by the epithelial cells following the L-II phase known as galactopoiesis (lactogenesis-III). Both lactogenesis I and II are controlled by hormones, while the galactopoiesis is regulated, mainly maintained by regular milk removal (autocrine control).[22,35]

Important pathways by which milk components are secreted in the lumen are exocytosis for proteins, fat by forming milk fat globule, transcytosis for immunoglobulins, and secretion for water and ions.[16]

Involution

Infrequent breastfeeding after the start of weaning, apoptosis of epithelial cells sets in and the gland regains nonlactating form; however, the breast structure is not similar to the nulliparous state.

Low levels of PRL, GH, and IGF-I are observed in this stage.[30,36] The secretory parts in the breast undergo regression, lobules decrease in size with decreased alveoli without involving ducts, unlike the involution of menopause, where both alveoli and ducts reduce in number (**Fig. 3**). The first phase of involution is reversible, as suckling will restart the milk flow, while in the second phase, women experience loss of lactation secondary to absent suckling for more than 48 hours.[12,37]

Milk Ejection

Release of stored milk is called milk let down or milk ejection reflex.[12]

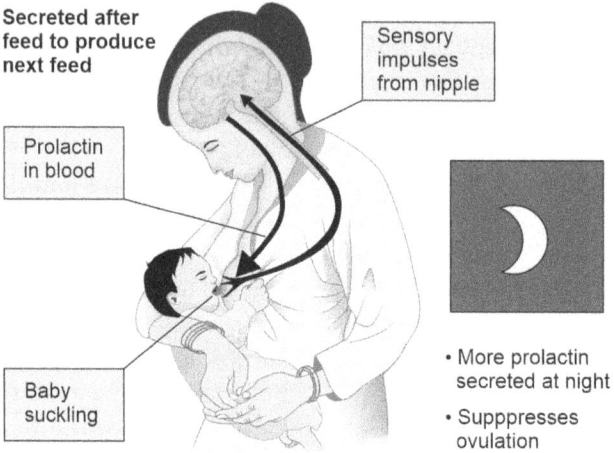

Fig. 3: Prolactin reflex.

Oxytocin is the main hormone regulating this reflex, which is released from the maternal neurohypophyseal-posterior pituitary axis by neuroendocrine mechanism. Physical stimulation of the nipple areolar complex causes activation of somatosensory afferent neurons (T4, T5, and T6 nerve roots).[38] Oxytocin acts on receptors of myoepithelial cells causing expulsion of milk in the ducts, leading to increased intraductal pressure[39] dilation of duct and increased milk flow rate **(Fig. 4)**.[40] Such multiple milk ejections may occur during feeding the infant. Milk secretion is influenced by emotions; stimulated with hearing a cry of baby, preparing to breastfeed and inhibited by factors such as anxiety, embarrassment, and pain.[22,41] Neuropeptide Y secreted from sympathetic fibers as a result of stress may inhibit this reflex, causing less milk outcome.[42]

Menopause

Between the age of 45–55 years, breast shows moderate reduction of glandular tissue followed by the regression of breast stroma which is replaced by fat and apoptosis of glandular epithelium. Both ducts and lobules decrease in the mammary gland, showing more of lobule type I and reduced number of lobule type 2 and 3 in menopause.

Menopause is associated with low levels of estrogen and progesterone and rise in ovarian androgens, testosterone androstenedione, and dehydroepiandrosterone.[12]

■ BREAST—GROSS ANATOMY

This section includes the structure of breast, originally described by Cooper in 1840,[43] along with the newer findings observed by few studies in later years.

Breast is hemispherical or teardrop-shaped structure composed of glands (secretory) and adipose tissue held by connective tissue, located on the chest between the 2nd and 6th ribs, lateral to sternum and medial to the anterior axillary line. It lies anterior to the deep pectoral fascia with the superior pectoral fascia covering it ventrally. The muscles pectoralis major, serratus anterior, and inferiorly, external oblique situated underneath the deep pectoral fascia. The suspensory ligaments of Cooper provide structural support to the breast parenchyma by connecting both superficial and deep pectoral fascia.[44]

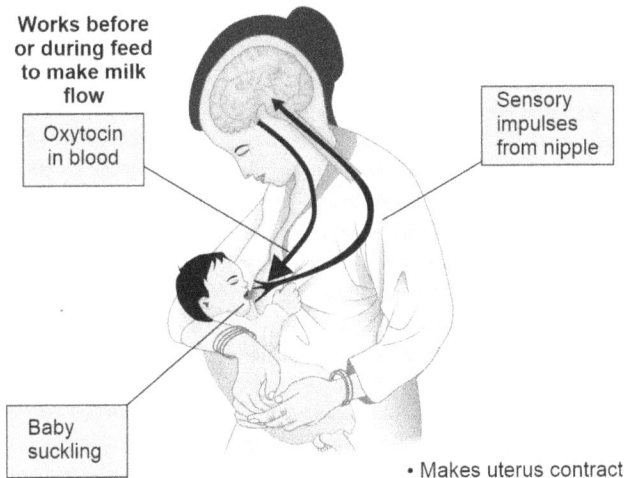

Fig. 4: Oxytocin reflex.

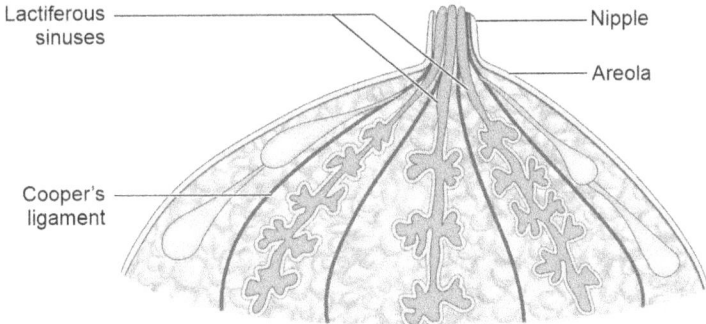

Fig. 5: Cooper's ligament and division of lobes.

Retromammary space, which separates the breast with the underlying deep pectoral fascia, allows the mobility of the breast tissue.[45] Cooper's suspensory ligaments divide the mammary gland into 15-20 sections, also called as lobes[46,47] composed of lobules containing 10-100 alveoli of approximately 0.12 mm in diameter[3,48] **(Figs. 5 and 6)**. The alveoli are lined by secretory epithelial cells and connected to very small ducts that join to form larger ducts which drain the lobules. These larger ducts finally join together to a single duct coming out from each lobe. Such 15-20 ducts converge toward the nipple, terminating at its orifice on the surface of the nipple, out of which only 7-12 ducts appear to be generally patent. Adipose tissue in the breast is present more between lobes than within lobules.[48] Recent ultrasound study has shown that the dilation of the duct located near alveolar area known as "lactiferous sinuses" are not seen, which were believed to store milk before milk ejection. Instead, it is found that the ducts only distend during milk ejection, indicating that the ducts transport milk rather than store it.[49]

Two layers of epithelial cells form the lining for each duct—cuboidal cells capable of differentiating into milk secretory cells during lactation, while the outer contractile

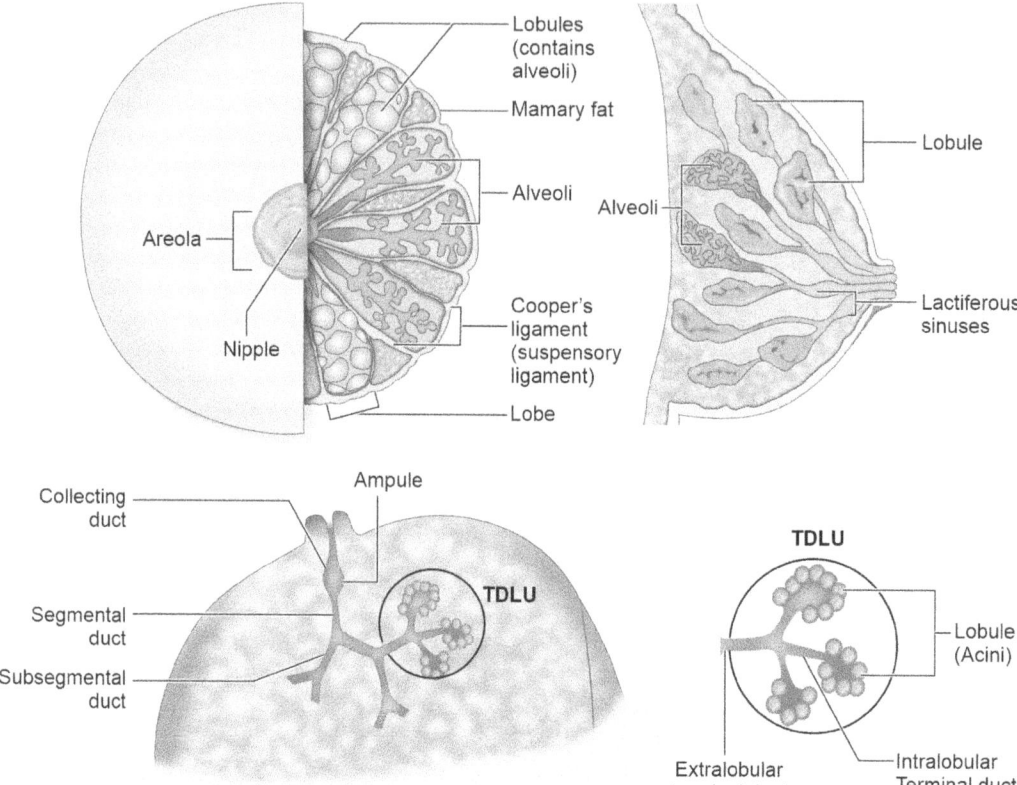

Fig. 6: Structure of mammary tissue. (TDLU: terminal duct lobular units)

myoepithelial cells surrounding the lumen have properties of smooth muscle cells.[3] Basement membrane is adjacent of myoepithelial layer on the outer side[45] **(Fig. 7)**. Luminal cell function is to generate milk-secreting cells during lactation and myoepithelial cells help in expulsion of milk.[50]

The periphery of the areola has Morgagni tubercles, the elevations formed by the duct openings of the modified accessory glands known as Montgomery glands which are capable of producing milk.[51]

Blood Supply

Major vascular supply (60%) of the mammary tissue is by internal thoracic artery (internal mammary artery), lateral thoracic artery supplies 30% and minor 10% of the blood supply is contributed by the thoracoacromial, intercostals, subscapular, and thoracodorsal arteries.[22,44] The venous drainage is to the intercostal, axillary, and internal thoracic veins.[44]

Innervation

The nerve supply to the breast is by anterior and lateral cutaneous branches of intercostal nerves IV, V, and VI. The nipple is mainly innervated by fourth intercostal nerve.[46,52]

The areola and the nipple area are very sensitive because of the cutaneous nerve plexus which is located underneath the areola.[45,51] Sympathetic fibers innervate the circular muscles of the nipple and the smooth muscle around the ducts and blood vessels. There is no parasympathetic supply to the breast as

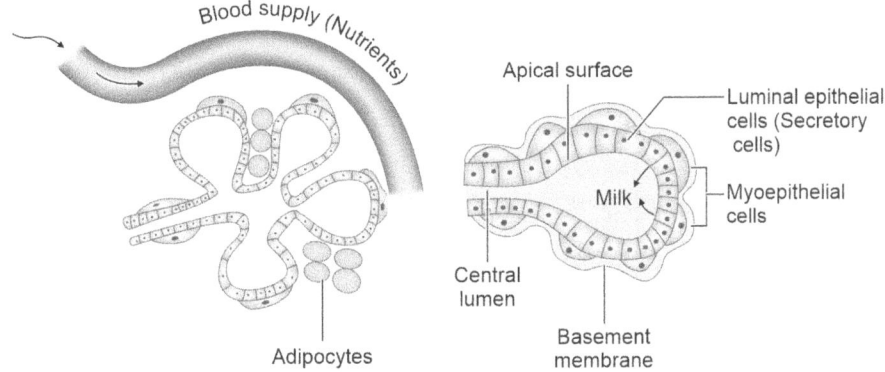

Fig. 7: The alveolar structure.

the mammary gland secretion is regulated by hormones.

Lymphatic Drainage

Approximately, 75% of the lymph from the mammary gland (medial and lateral portions) is received by axillary lymph nodes. The internal mammary nodes drain largely from the deeper region of the breast.[53] Lymphatic vessels may cross the central plane and connect with the contralateral breast.[3] Densely arranged lymphatic vessels are located underneath the areola in the subcutaneous layer, also known as Sappey's subareolar plexus.[51,54]

RECENT UPDATES

Recent studies have not found the presence of dilated duct (lactiferous sinuses), the function of which is to transfer and not storage of milk as believed in the past.[55] Milk flows out by the vacuum created in the infant's mouth rather than duct peristalsis. These ducts are few in number, branch near the nipple, are superficially located, and easily compressible.[56,57]

KEY MESSAGES

- Positive state of mind is critical for the efficient lactation.
- Prolactin and oxytocin are the main hormones involved in synthesis and ejection of breast milk respectively.

REFERENCES

1. Macias H, Hinck L. Mammary gland development. Wiley Interdiscip Rev Dev Biol. 2012;1(4):533-57.
2. Hovey RC, Trott JF, Vonderhaar BK. Establishing the framework for the functional mammary gland: from endocrinology to morphology. J Mammary Gland Biol Neoplasia. 2002;7(1):17-38.
3. Hassiotou F, Geddes D. Anatomy of the human mammary gland: Current status of knowledge. Clin Anat. 2013;26(1):29-48.
4. Naccarato AG, Viacava P, Vignati S, Fanelli G, Bonadio AG, Montruccoli G, et al. Bio-morphological events in the development of the human female mammary gland from fetal age to puberty. Virchows Arch. 2000;436(5):431-8.
5. Johnson MC. Anatomy and physiology of the breast. Management of Breast Diseases. Berlin, Heidelberg: Springer; 2010. pp. 1-36.
6. Russo J RI. Mammary gland development. In: Knobil E, Neill JD (Eds). Encyclopedia of Reproduction. San Diego: Academic Press; 1999.
7. Kaufmann M. Management of breast diseases. In: Jatoi I (Ed). Heidelberg: Springer; 2010.
8. Howard BA, Gusterson BA. Human breast development. J Mammary Gland Biol Neoplasia. 2000;5:119-37.

9. Gusterson BA, Stein T. Human breast development. Semin Cell Dev Biol. 2012;23(5):567-73.
10. Sternlicht MD. Key stages in mammary gland development: the cues that regulate ductal branching morphogenesis. Breast Cancer Res. 2005;8(1):201.
11. Javed A, Lteif A. Development of the human breast. Semin Plast Surg. 2013;27(1):5.
12. Sun SX, Bostanci Z, Kass RB, Mancino AT, Rosenbloom AL, Klimberg VS, et al. Breast physiology: normal and abnormal development and function. In: Bland KI, Copeland III EM, Klimberg VS, Gradishar WJ. The Breast: Comprehensive Management of Benign and Malignant Diseases, 5th edition. USA: Elsevier; 2018. pp. 37-56.
13. Sadovnikova A, Wysolmerski JJ, Hovey RC. The onset and maintenance of human lactation and its endocrine regulation. In: Kovacs CS, Deal CL (Eds). Maternal-Fetal and Neonatal Endocrinology. UK: Academic Press; 2020. pp. 189-205.
14. Korenman SG. The endocrinology of breast cancer. Cancer. 1980;46(suppl 4):874-8.
15. Weinstein SP, Conant EF, Sehgal CM, Woo IP, Patton JA. Hormonal variations in the vascularity of breast tissue. J Ultrasound Med. 2005;24(1):67-72.
16. Neville MC. Anatomy and physiology of lactation. Pediatr Clin North Am. 2001;48(1):13-34.
17. Russo J RI. Development of human mammary glands. In: Neville MC, Daniel CW (Eds). The Mammary Gland: Development, Regulation, and Function. New York: Plenum Press; 1987.
18. Marshall WA, Tanner JM. Variations in pattern of pubertal changes in girls. Arch Dis Child. 1969;44(235):291-303.
19. Kleinberg DL, Ruan W. IGF-I, GH, and sex steroid effects in normal mammary gland development. J Mammary Gland Biol Neoplasia. 2008;13(4):353-60.
20. Delouis C, Djiane J, Houdebine LM, Terqui M. Relation between hormones and mammary gland function. J Dairy Sci. 1980;63(9):1492-513.
21. Berens PD. Applied physiology in the peripartum management of lactation. Clin Obstet Gynecol. 2004;47(3):643-55.
22. Sriraman NK. The nuts and bolts of breastfeeding: anatomy and physiology of lactation. Curr Probl Pediatr Adolesc Health Care. 2017;47(12):305-10.
23. Forsyth IA. Variation among species in the endocrine control of mammary growth and function: the roles of prolactin, growth hormone, and placental lactogen. J Dairy Sci. 1986;69(3):886-903.
24. Houdebine LM, Djiane J, Dusanter-Fourt I, Martel P, Kelly PA, Devinoy E, et al. Hormonal action controlling mammary activity. J Dairy Sci. 1985;68(2):489-500.
25. Neville MC, Webb P, Ramanathan P, Mannino MP, Pecorini C, Monks J, et al. The insulin receptor plays an important role in secretory differentiation in the mammary gland. Am J Physiol Endocrinol Metab. 2013;305(9):E1103-14.
26. Yu JH, Kim MJ, Cho H, Liu HJ, Han SJ, Ahn TG. Breast diseases during pregnancy and lactation. Obstet Gynecol Sci. 2013;56(3):143-59.
27. Hartmann P, Sherriff J, Kent J. Maternal nutrition and the regulation of milk synthesis. Proc Nutr Soc. 1995;54(2):379-89.
28. Hooley RD, Findlay JK. The hormonal control of lactation. In: Pethes G, Frenyó VL (Eds). Advances in Animal and Comparative Physiology. UK: Pergamon; 1981. pp. 165-72.
29. Canoy JM, Mitchell GS, Unold D, Miller V. A radiologic review of common breast disorders in pregnancy and the perinatal period. Semin Ultrasound CT MR. 2012;33: 78-85.
30. Svennersten-Sjaunja K, Olsson K. Endocrinology of milk production. Domest Anim Endocrinol. 2005;29(2):241-58.
31. Guyton AC, Hall JE. Guyton and Hall Textbook of Medical Physiology. Philadelphia, PA: Saunders Elsevier; 2011. p. 107.
32. Vashi R, Hooley R, Butler R, Geisel J, Philpotts L. Breast imaging of the pregnant and lactating patient: physiologic changes and common benign entities. Am J Roentgenol. 2013;200(2):329-36.
33. Neville MC, Keller R, Seacat J, Lutes V, Neifert M, Casey C, et al. Studies in human lactation: milk volumes in lactating women during the onset of lactation and full lactation. Am J Clin Nutr. 1988;48(6):1375-86.

34. Hale TW, Hale HP. Hartmann's Textbook of Human Lactation. Amarillo: Hale; 2007. pp. 215-53.
35. Tucker HA. Symposium: hormonal regulation and milk synthesis-Hormones, Mammary Growth, and Lactation: A 41-Year Perspective. J Dairy Sci. 2000;83(4):874-84.
36. Neville MC. Lactation and its hormonal control. In: Neill JD (Ed). Knobil and Neill's Physiology of Reproduction, 3rd edition. Academic Press; 2006. pp. 2993-3054.
37. Lund LR, Rømer J, Thomasset N, Solberg H, Pyke C, Bissell MJ, et al. Two distinct phases of apoptosis in mammary gland involution: proteinase-independent and -dependent pathways. Development. 1996;122:181-93.
38. Uvnas-Moberg K, Eriksson M. Breastfeeding: physiological, endocrine and behavioural adaptations caused by oxytocin and local neurogenic activity in the nipple and mammary gland. Acta Paediatr. 1996;85:525-30.
39. Alekseev NP, Omel'ianuk EV, Talalaeva NE. Dynamics of milk ejection reflex during continuous rhythmic stimulation of areola-nipple complex of the mammary gland. Ross Fiziol Zh Im I M Sechenova. 2000;86(6):711-9. [Russian].
40. Ramsay DT, Mitoulas LR, Kent JC, Cregan MD, Doherty DA, Larsson M, et al. Milk flow rates can be used to identify and investigate milk ejection in women expressing breast milk using an electric breast pump. Breastfeeding Med. 2006;1:14-23.
41. Bland KI, Copeland III EM. The Breast: Comprehensive Management of Benign and Malignant Diseases. Plast Reconstr Surg. 1993;92(5):973-4.
42. Eriksson M, Lindh B, Uvnäs-Moberg K, Hökfelt T. Distribution and origin of peptide-containing nerve fibres in the rat and human mammary gland. Neuroscience. 1996;70(1):227-45.
43. Cooper A. On the Anatomy of the Breast. London: Longman, Orme, Green, Brown, and Longmans; 1840.
44. Bistoni G, Farhadi J. Anatomy and physiology of the breast. In: Farhadieh RD, Bulstrode NW, Cugno S (Eds). Plastic and Reconstructive Surgery (Approaches and techniques). UK: Wiley Blackwell; 2015. pp. 477-85.
45. Johnson MC, Cutler ML. Anatomy and Physiology of the Breast. In: Jatoi I, Rody A (Eds). Management of Breast Diseases. Switzerland: Springer, Cham; 2016. pp. 1-39.
46. Sarhadi NS, Shaw-Dunn J, Soutar DS. Nerve supply of the breast with special reference to the nipple and areola: Sir Astley Cooper revisited. Clin Anat. 1997;10(4):283-8.
47. Nelson CM, Bissell MJ. Modeling dynamic reciprocity: engineering three-dimensional culture models of breast architecture, function, and neoplastic transformation. Semin Cancer Biol. 2005;15(5):342-52.
48. Zucca-Matthes G, Urban C, Vallejo A. Anatomy of the nipple and breast ducts. Gland Surg. 2016;5(1):32.
49. Jones E, Spencer S. The physiology of lactation. Paediatr Child Health (Oxford). 2007;17(6):244-8.
50. Fu NY, Nolan E, Lindeman GJ, Visvader JE. Stem cells and the differentiation hierarchy in mammary gland development. Physiol Rev. 2020;100(2):489-523.
51. Palhazi P. Gross anatomy of the breast and axilla. In: Wyld L, Markopoulos C, Leidenius M, Senkus-Konefka E (Eds). Breast Cancer Management for Surgeons: A European Multidisciplinary Textbook. Switzerland: Springer, Cham; 2018. pp. 3-10.
52. Schlenz I, Kuzbari R, Gruber H, Holle J. The sensitivity of the nipple-areola complex: an anatomic study. Plast Reconstr Surg. 2000;105(3):905-9.
53. Sabel MS. Essentials of Breast Surgery: A Volume in the Surgical Foundations Series. USA: Elsevier Health Sciences; 2009.
54. Tanis PJ, Nieweg OE, Valdés Olmos RA, Kroon BB. Anatomy and physiology of lymphatic drainage of the breast from the perspective of sentinel node biopsy. J Am Coll Surg. 2001;192(3):399-409.
55. Ramsay DT, Kent JC, Owens RA, Hartmann PE. Ultrasound imaging of milk ejection in the breast of lactating women. Pediatrics. 2004;113:361-7.
56. Geddes DT. Inside the Lactating Breast: The Latest Anatomy Research. J Midwifery Women's Health. 2007;52(6):556-63.
57. Geddes DT. The anatomy of the lactating breast: latest research and clinical implications. Infant. 2007;3(2):59-63.

CHAPTER 4

Composition of Human Milk

Vijay Venkataiah, K Nagaraj, Durgappa H

"If a new vaccine became available that could prevent one million or more child deaths a year, and that was moreover cheap, safe, administered orally, and required no cold chain, it would become an immediate public health imperative. Breastfeeding can do all of this".

—**Lancet, A Warm Chain For Breastfeeding**

INTRODUCTION

Breastmilk is an ideal infant food and is the complete source of nutrition up to 6 months of age and continues to contribute major nutrients and calories throughout the duration of breastfeeding. Breast milk is a "dynamic living fluid that is baby-specific, species-specific, and tailor-made".[1] The quantity of breast milk secretion varies among mothers with the time of the day and frequency of emptying of the breast.

BREAST MILK SECRETION

The first milk, colostrum, secreted during the first 5 days of delivery (40–50 mL/day), which is rich in nutrients and bioactive factors, plays an important role in immune functions (*natural vaccine*) and is critical for the survival of infants (*liquid gold*). Thereafter, the amount of breast milk secretion during the first 6 months is 600–800 mL/day, between 6 and 12 months is 400–600 mL/day, and in the second year of life is around 400 mL/day. However, the amount of breast milk secretion will be influenced by the efficiency and frequency of breast milk removal.[2]

VARIATIONS IN THE COMPOSITION OF BREAST MILK

Colostrum

Colostrum is thick, yellowish milk produced during the first few days of childbirth, which is nutrient-dense, rich in bioactive factors, and critical for providing immunity to infants. It has a high amount of immune cells (lymphocytes), antibodies [immunoglobulin A (IgA), IgG, and IgM], antimicrobial agents, (lactoferrin, lysozyme, and lactoperoxidase) various complements, and proline-rich polypeptides. The concentration of human milk oligosaccharides (HMOs) is highest in colostrum (20-25 g/L) and the whey-casein ratio in the colostrum is 90:10, whereas in mature milk, it is 60:40. Several immunomodulators and growth factors are found in higher concentration in colostrum. All these bioactive components in colostrum provide passive immunity to the newborn. Colostrum also acts as a mild *laxative* that enhances the elimination of the bilirubin-rich meconium from the gut, thus favoring the newborn's digestive system to grow and function properly.[3]

The breast milk which is secreted between 7 days and 2 weeks of the postpartum period is called *transitional milk* and the milk that is produced beyond 2 weeks of the postpartum period is called *mature milk*. The breast milk secreted at the beginning of feeding is called *foremilk,* which is bluish, watery, and rich in proteins and satisfies the thirst of an infant. The breast milk secreted toward the end of breastfeeding is called *hind milk,* which is yellowish, thick, and rich in fat, satisfying the hunger of an infant.[4]

Preterm Milk

Preterm milk is the milk secreted in the mother who had preterm labor that furnishes all the necessary nutrients for the preterm baby, thus tailored for preterm babies. It contains a higher concentration of protein, free amino acids, and lipids compared to term milk. Calcium is lower in preterm milk, while copper and zinc are in higher concentration. Lactose is relatively low in preterm milk and glycosaminoglycans (GAGs—antiadhesive agents against harmful microbes on the infants' intestinal wall) are in higher concentration compared to term milk.[1,5]

Human milk contains macronutrients, micronutrients, minerals, several bioactive factors, and genetic materials.

Macronutrients in Human Milk

Macronutrients in human milk; proteins, carbohydrates, and fats.
- *Protein components in human milk:* They include whey proteins, caseins, and mucins.
  - *Whey proteins:* They include lactalbumin, lactoferrin, secretory IgA, lysozyme, haptocorrin, and amylase which are water soluble. Generally, these whey proteins are responsible for the development of the immune system. Alpha-lactalbumin comprises 10–20% of the total protein in human milk. It provides all essential amino acids to the infant and increases the absorption of calcium, zinc, and iron. It also has antimicrobial activity.[6] Lactoferrin is a glycoprotein that facilitates the uptake of iron in enterocytes by binding with two ferric ions present in breast milk. Lactoferrin binds to an iron molecule (iron chelation), and thus making iron unavailable to iron-dependent microorganisms, namely *Escherichia coli* (*E. coli*), thereby decreasing the risk of infection. Lactoferrin has antiviral activity [against human immunodeficiency virus (HIV), herpes simplex virus (HSV), cytomegalovirus (CMV)]. It is also anti-adhesive for *E coli* and anti-invasive for *Shigella*. In addition it also has Immuno-modulating and anti tumor activity[6] and favours the intestinal cell growth.[7-9]
  - *Secretory IgA (sIgA):* This is the most abundant immunoglobulin present in breast milk, which is resistant to digestion and aids in boosting an infant's immature immune system.
  - *Lysozyme in breast milk:* It helps in the degradation of the outer cell wall of gram-positive bacteria and inactivates gram-negative bacteria in the presence of lactoferrin. It is also known to exhibit antiamoebic and anti-HIV activity.
  - *Haptocorrin:* Haptocorrin helps in absorption of vitamin B_{12} in early life by binding with it. It resists digestion and has antimicrobial activity.

- *Amylase:* It aids in the digestion of oligosaccharides and polysaccharides in breast milk. It may also have an antibacterial function by breaking down the polysaccharides of the bacterial cell wall.[6,7]
- *Casein:* It is a phosphoprotein and is present in milk as a complex molecule, along with calcium and phosphate called casein micelles. Casein in human milk is easily digestible and helps in the growth and development of the child.[10,11]
- *Human milk mucins:* They are glycoproteins and the majority of them are present in the milk fat globular membrane. They inhibit pathogens binding to the host cell surface (specifically rotaviruses and binding of S-fimbriated *E. coli* to buccal epithelial), also involved in the inhibition of viral replication, thus offering protection against infections.[12,13]
- *Carbohydrate components of breast milk:* They include lactose and HMOs. The lactose content of breast milk is 7 g/dL, and is the major source of energy. Lactose provides galactose which acts as a substrate for gangliosides and cerebrosides synthesis in the brain. HMOs are the natural prebiotics in the breast milk and play an important role in the protection of infants against infections. HMOs prevent adhesion and invasion of microorganisms across the intestinal wall. In addition, HMOs also provide sialic acid which is an important constituent of gangliosides and plays an important role in neurodevelopment.[14-17]
- *Fat components of human milk:* They are mainly triglycerides, free fatty acids, and cholesterol. *Triacylglycerol* is the major component of fat in breast milk (98–99%) and is another major source of energy. Human milk is a rich source of essential *fatty acids* such as linoleic acid, linolenic acid, and their long-chain derivatives [long-chain polyunsaturated fatty acids (LCPUFAs)], namely docosahexaenoic acid (DHA) and arachidonic acid (AA), which play an important role in the development of retinal and neural tissue. The preformed *cholesterol* in breast milk helps in delivering the fatty acids to membranes and target organs of the infant.[18]

Micronutrients

Breast milk contains vitamins (both water and fat-soluble) and minerals. Breast milk is rich in water-soluble vitamins, namely thiamin, riboflavin, vitamins B_6 and B_{12}, and fat-soluble vitamin A. Minerals and a multitude of trace elements are present in breast milk (copper, zinc, barium, cadmium, chromium, cobalt, cerium, lanthanum, manganese, molybdenum, nickel, lead, rubidium, tin, and strontium), which have high bioavailability. Vitamin D and K are found in very low concentrations in human milk.[6,7]

Vitamin A in human milk is present mainly as retinyl palmitate, whose primary function is in cell differentiation, epithelium formation, retinal tissue development, and antioxidant action.[6,7] Carotenoids in human milk are mainly lutein, lycopene, and zeaxanthin, which help in neural and retinal tissue synthesis and play an important role in an infant's cognition and early memory.[19]

Vitamin D is essential for calcium absorption, bone and teeth mineralization, neurodevelopment, and immune function,[6] which needs to be supplemented (400 IU/day from birth) as its concentration in human milk is very low.[20]

Colostrum contains a high concentration of vitamin E, an antioxidant that plays an important role in immune function. The concentration of vitamin E decreases as the maturation of milk advances and gets stabilized after 4 weeks of the postpartum period.[6]

Human milk is deficient in vitamin K and therefore, newborns are at higher risk for hemorrhagic diseases. Hence, every newborn child should receive a prophylactic dose of vitamin K at birth.[6]

Vitamin B_{12} is essential for folate metabolism and deoxyribonucleic acid (DNA) synthesis. In human milk, vitamin B_{12} is tightly bound to apo-haptocorrin, a cobalamin-binding protein. Folic acid is necessary for protein and DNA and ribonucleic acid (RNA) biosynthesis and its requirement is greatest in the phase of growth and development.[6]

Choline is an important nutrient present in human milk; it plays a crucial role in fetal and infant development. Total choline concentrations in breast milk increase rapidly between the 7- and 22-day postpartum period and remain relatively stable in mature milk.[20] This serves as a precursor for the synthesis of acetylcholine, phospholipids (critical for cell membrane), surfactants (important in lung maturity), and bile formation. Choline also has a significant role in brain development, along with DHA and lutein; further, it can influence infant memory.[21-23]

Vitamin C in human milk functions as an antioxidant and immune modulator. It stimulates leukocytes, augments antibody production, and enhances the synthesis of interferons.[6]

The iron content in human milk is relatively low but has high bioavailability. Iron plays an important role in the synthesis of hemoglobin, the formation of new tissue, immune function, and cognitive and neurodevelopment.[18] In preterm babies, since the iron reservoir is not sufficient, it has been recommended to supplement iron in the dose of 2–4 mg/kg/day starting at 2 weeks and continuing until 6 months of age.[24]

In human milk, copper is bound with ceruloplasmin and it plays an important role in cellular respiration, iron metabolism, and connective tissue synthesis.[6] Breast milk is relatively deficient in zinc, but it is absorbed efficiently (high bioavailability). It takes part in cell differentiation, especially in tissues that are characterized by rapid turnover and proliferation such as the immune cellular network and the gastrointestinal system.[18] Zinc deficiency in infants results in stunted growth and compromised immune functions, resulting in high morbidity and mortality associated with diarrhea and respiratory infections.[6]

The iodine in breast milk is essential for thyroid hormone synthesis, neurodevelopment, infant growth, and survival. Similarly, selenium in human milk is a component of a potent antioxidant glutathione peroxidase.[6,18]

Minerals

Predominant minerals present in human milk include calcium, phosphorus, sodium, potassium, chloride, and magnesium.

Both calcium and phosphorus are essential for bone and teeth mineralization. Magnesium plays a structural role in bone and is involved in more than 300 essential metabolic reactions.[6] Other major minerals such as sodium, potassium, and chlorides are adequate in human breast milk **(Table 1)**.

Bioactive Factors[27]

Varieties of *cytokines* [tumor necrosis factor (TNF), interleukin 1 (IL-1), IL-6, and

TABLE 1: Composition of human milk.[25,26]

Macronutrients	Per deciliter
Proteins	0.9 g
Carbohydrates	7 g
Fats/lipids	3.5 g
Micronutrients	
Vitamin A	61 µg
Vitamin D	0.1 g
Vitamin E	0.08 mg
Vitamin K	0.3 µg
Vitamin B_1	0.01 mg
Vitamin B_2	0.04 mg
Vitamin B_3	0.18 mg
Vitamin B_5	0.22 mg
Vitamin B_6	0 mg
Vitamin B_{12}	0.05 µg
Folate	5 µg
Choline	15.76 mg
Iron	0.03 mg
Zinc	0.16 mg
Copper	0.04 mg
Selenium	1.76 µg
Manganese	0.04 mg
Minerals	
Calcium	31.6 mg
Phosphorus	13.6 mg
Magnesium	3 mg
Sodium	16.8 mg
Potassium	50 mg
Chloride	43 mg

IL-8, interferon-gamma (IFN), and transforming growth factor beta (TGF-β)], *adipokines* (leptin, adiponectin, resistin, ghrelin, obestatin, nesfatin, and apelin), immunoglobulins (sIgA), *antioxidants* (beta-carotenes, tocopherols, lycopene, glutathione, melatonin, superoxide dismutase, catalases, and glutathione peroxidases), and *growth factors (GF)* (epidermal GF, neuronal GF, insulin-like GF (IGF), vascular endothelial GF, etc.) are found in human breast milk **(Tables 2 and 3)**.

Human Milk Cells

Breast milk contains white cells, stem cells, and mesenchymal cells, which are involved in the development of immune cells that help in tissue repair.[33] Stem cells have the potential to reprogram into multiple tissue types.[34]

Micro-RNAs

Human milk is particularly rich in micro-RNAs, which are potentially involved in the development and maturation of a child's immature immune system.[35] Micro-RNAs are small noncoding RNA molecules that regulate gene expression at the post-transcriptional level, modulating several cell functions such as cell cycle, proliferation, differentiation, apoptosis, immune response, and neurodevelopment.[11,36]

Exosomes: They are extracellular microvesicles derived from mammary glands that contain micro-RNAs with the size of around 22 nucleotides. These exosomes combine with micro-RNAs and prevent their digestion in infants' gut, thus allowing the micro-RNAs to exert their function. Human milk exosomes can be protective against the development of intestinal injuries, such as necrotizing enterocolitis (NEC).[37]

HAMLET

Human alpha-lactalbumin made lethal to tumor cells (HAMLET) in human milk is a complex made up of alpha-lactalbumin and oleic acid that induces cell death in tumor cells but not in normal cells. HAMLET kills a wide range of malignant cells, which

TABLE 2: Major constituents in human colostrum and transitional and mature milk[28] (average per 100 mL).

	Colostrum	Transitional milk	Mature milk
Energy (kcal)	58	74	71
Lactose (g)	5.3	6.6	7.0
Casein (g)	1.2	0.7	0.4
Fat (g)	2.9	3.6	3.8
Minerals			
Calcium	31	34	33
Magnesium	4	4	4
Potassium	74	64	55
Sodium	48	29	15
Iron	0.09	0.04	0.15

TABLE 3: Bioactive components.[29]

Bioactive components	Functions
Antimicrobial: • Lactoferrin • Lactadherin • Lysozymes • Casein	• Acute phase protein, chelates iron, antibacterial, antioxidant • Antiviral enhances phagocytosis of apoptotic cells • Bacterial lysis, immunomodulating activity, and binding to bacterial lipopolysaccharide—reduce the endotoxic effect[6,7] • Antiadhesive for H pylori, H influenza, and S pneumonia • The strong growth-promoting factor for B bifidium[11]
Immunoglobulins: • sIgA • IgG • IgM	• Pathogen-binding inhibition • Phagocytosis, anti-inflammatory, antimicrobial, etc. • Agglutination, complement activation

Immunomodulators:
• Cytokines
  – IL-1
  – IL-6
  – IL-7
  – IL-8
  – IL-10
  – INF-γ
  – TNF-β
  – TNF-α
• Chemokines
• Cytokine inhibitors
	
	• Production of defense agents in mammary glands
	• Acute phase response, B-cell activation
	• Increased thymic size and output
	• Recruitment of neutrophils and proinflammatory
	• Repressing inflammation, antibody production
	• Proinflammatory
	• Anti-inflammatory, stimulation of T cell
	• Inflammatory immune activation
	• Prevents macrophage movement
	• Inhibition of TNF-alpha, anti-inflammatory

Growth factors: • EGF • HB-EGF • VEGF • NGF • IGF • Erythropoietin	• Stimulates cell proliferation and maturation • Protection against hypoxia and ischemia • Promotion of angiogenesis and tissue repair • Promotion of neuron growth and maturation • Stimulation of growth and development, RBCs, and Hb • Erythropoiesis, intestinal development

Contd...

Contd...

Bioactive components	Functions
Hormones: • Calcitonin • Somatostatin • Cortisol • Insulin • Thyroid hormone	 • Development of enteric neurons • Regulation of gastric epithelial growth • Physiological stress response, immunity, metabolism[30] • Gut maturation in the infant[31] • Regulate breathing, heart rate, BMR, growth, and development[32]
Metabolic hormones: • Adiponectin • Leptin • Ghrelin	 • Reduction of baby's BMI and weight, anti-inflammatory • Regulation of energy conversion and appetite • Regulation of energy conversion and appetite
Oligosaccharides: • HMOs • Gangliosides • Glycosaminoglycans	 • Prebiotics, stimulate beneficial colonization • Anti-inflammatory • Brain development, anti-infective/antiadhesive
Mucins	Blocks infections by viruses and bacteria
Cells: • Macrophages • Stem cells • Probiotic bacteria • HAMLET cells	 • Protection against infection, T-Cell activation • Regeneration and repair • Probiotic • Anticancer cells
Genetic materials: • Micro-RNAs • Exosomes	 • Infant protection and development • Modulates cell cycle, proliferation, differentiation, apoptosis, and immune response and neurodevelopment[11,36] • Protects against the development of intestinal injury such as that seen in NEC[37]

(BMI: body mass index; BMR: basal metabolic rate; EGF: epidermal growth factor; HAMLET: human alpha-lactalbumin made lethal to tumor cells; Hb: hemoglobin; HB-EGF: heparin-binding EGF; HMOs: human milk oligosaccharides; IgG: immunoglobulin G; IGF: insulin-like growth factor; IL: interleukin; INF-γ: interferon gamma; NEC: necrotizing enterocolitis; NGF: neuronal growth factor; RBCs: red blood cells; RNAs: ribonucleic acid; sIgA: secretory IgA; TNF: tumor necrosis factor; VEGF: vascular endothelial growth factor)

explains why no tumors are seen in breast milk-fed babies.[38]

Human Milk Microbiota

Breast milk is a natural source of prebiotic (HMOs) and probiotic (microbiota) such as *Bifidobacterium breve (B. breve), B. adolescentis, B. longum, B. bifidum,* and *B. dentium*) which play a major role in the gut priming, thus offering protection.[39,40]

UNIQUE FEATURES OF HUMAN MILK[41]

Human milk contains alpha-lactalbumin, whereas cow's milk contains more β-lactoglobulin.

The casein component of human milk is easily digestible as compared to cow's milk. The ratio between casein to whey protein in human milk is 40:60, whereas it is 80:20 in cow's milk.

Human milk has high polyunsaturated fatty acid (PUFA) content compared to cow's milk. The fatty acids namely AA and DHA are high in human milk, both of which are essential for brain development and functioning, whereas cow's milk does not contain these fatty acids.

Human milk oligosaccharides (10-20 g/L) are specific to the baby, whereas cow milk oligosaccharides (1 g/L) are nonspecific.

Although iron and zinc levels are relatively low in human milk, they have good bioavailability. Human milk has a relatively low concentration of vitamins D and K.

Infants of other mammals need to grow quickly; hence, more protein is in their milk than in human milk. Human infants need to develop their brains and nerves quickly, therefore providing less protein and more fat in human milk.[42] The detailed nutritional composition of other animals' milk is compared with human milk in **Table 4**.

TABLE 4: Nutritional composition of different types of milk of animal origin.

	Composition in 100 g								
	Human	Cow	Buffalo	Goat	Sheep	Yak	Horse	Donkey	Camel
Energy (kcal)	70	62	99	66	100	100	48	37	76
Water (g)	87.5	87.7	83.2	87.7	82.1	82.6	89.8	90.8	84.8
Total protein (g)	1.0	3.3	4	3.4	5.6	5.2	2	1.6	3.9
Total fat (g)	4.4	3.3	7.5	3.9	6.4	6.8	1.6	0.7	5
Lactose (g)	6.9	4.7	4.4	4.4	5.1	4.8	6.6	6.4	4.2
Minerals:									
Calcium (mg)	32	112	191	118	190	129	95	91	154
Iron (mg)	0.1	0.2	0.3	0.1	0.6	0.1			
Magnesium (mg)	3	11	12	14	18	10	7	4	8
Phosphorus (mg)	14	91	185	100	144	106	58	61	132
Potassium (mg)	51	145	112	202	148	95	51	50	186
Sodium (mg)	17	42	47	44	39	29	16	22	66
Zinc (mg)	0.2	0.4	0.5	0.3	0.6	0.9	0.2	0	0.7
Copper (mg)	0.1				0.1	0.1	0.1	0	
Selenium (g)	1.8	1.8		1.1	1.7	11			
Manganese (g)		8		18	18				
Vitamins:									
Retinol (g)	60	35	69	45	64				
Carotene (g)	7	16		13					
Vitamin A (gRE)	61	37	69	48	64				97
Vitamin E (mg)	0.08	0.08	0.19	0.05	0.11				0.15
Thiamine (mg)	0.01	0.04	0.05	0.06	0.07		0.03	0.06	0.01

Contd...

Contd...

	Composition in 100 g								
	Human	Cow	Buffalo	Goat	Sheep	Yak	Horse	Donkey	Camel
Riboflavin (mg)	0.04	0.2	0.11	0.13	0.34		0.02	0.03	0.12
Niacin (mg)	0.18	0.13	0.17	0.24	0.41		0.07	0.09	
Vitamin B_5 (mg)	0.22	0.43	0.15	0.3	0.43				
Vitamin B_6 (mg)		0.04	0.33	0.05	0.07				0.05
Folate (g)	5	8.5	0.6	16					
Biotin (g)		2	13	2.5	2.5				
Vitamin B_{12} (g)	0.05	0.51	0.4	0.07	0.66				
Vitamin C (mg)	5	1	2.5	1.1	4.6		4.3		3
Vitamin D (g)	0.1	0.2		0.1	0.2				1.6

Source: Food and Agriculture Organization (FAO) of the United Nations.[25]

KEY MESSAGES

- Breast milk contains macronutrients, micronutrients, minerals, and bioactive substances.
- Breast milk is a dynamic living fluid, species-specific, baby-specific, and tailor-made.
- The colostrum, in addition to nutritional superiority, also has bioactive substances which play an important role in the prevention of infections in infants and hence is called natural vaccine.
- Breast milk has genetic materials which play an important role in inheritance and immune and tissue maturation.
- Breast milk has two components—foremilk which is white, watery, and rich in proteins that satisfies thirst and hindmilk which is yellowish, thick, and rich in fats satisfies hunger.
- Breast milk secretion is influenced by the gestational age, time of the day, frequency and efficacy of extraction, and psychological status of the mother.

REFERENCES

1. Gross SJ, Geller J, Tomarelli RM. Composition of breast milk from mothers of preterm infants. Pediatrics. 1981;68(4):490-3.
2. Park K. Preventive medicine in Obstetrics, Pediatrics, and geriatrics: Feeding of infants. Park's Textbook of Preventive and Social Medicine, 25th edition. Pune: M/s Banarsidas Bhanot Publishers; 2019. pp. 590-2.
3. Palmeira P, Carneiro-Sampaio M. Immunology of breast milk. Rev Assoc Med Bras. 2016;62(6):584-93.
4. World Health Organization, UNICEF. Breastfeeding counseling. A training course. Participants' manual. Part one. Sessions 1-9.
5. Underwood MA. Human milk for the premature infant. Pediatr Clin North Am. 2013;60(1):189-207.
6. Geddes D, Hassiotou F, Wise M, Hartmann P. Human Milk Composition and Function in the Infant. In: Polin RA, Abman SH, Rowitch DH, Benitz WE, Fox WW (Eds). Fetal and Neonatal Physiology, 5th edition. Philadelphia: Elsevier; 2017. pp. 273-80.e3.
7. Dror DK, Allen LH. Overview of Nutrients in Human Milk. Adv Nutr. 2018;9:278S-94S.
8. Niaz B, Saeed F, Ahmed A, Imran M, Maan AA, Khan MKI, et al. Lactoferrin (LF):

8. a natural antimicrobial protein. Int J Food Prop. 2019;22(1);1626-41.
9. Kell DB, Heyden EL, Pretorius E. The Biology of Lactoferrin, an Iron-Binding Protein That Can Help Defend Against Viruses and Bacteria. Front Immunol. 2020;11:1221.
10. Basdeki AM, Fatouros DG, Biliaderis CG, Moschakis T. Physicochemical properties of human breast milk during the second year of lactation. Curr Res Food Sci. 2021;4:565-76.
11. Kim SY, Yi DY. Components of human breast milk: from macronutrient to microbiome and micro-RNA. Clin Exp Pediatr. 2020; 63(8):301-9.
12. Yolken RH, Peterson JA, Vonderfecht SL, Fouts ET, Midthun K, Newburg DS. Human Milk Mucin Inhibits Rotavirus Replication and Prevents Experimental Gastroenteritis. J Clin Invest. 1992;90:1984-91.
13. Schroten H, Hanisch FG, Plogmann R, Hacker J, Uhlenbruck G, Nobis-Bosch R, et al. Inhibition of adhesion of S-fimbriated Escherichia coli to buccal epithelial cells by human milk fat globule membrane components: a novel aspect of the protective function of mucins in the non-immunoglobulin fraction. Infect Immun. 1992;60(7):2893-9.
14. Romero-Velarde E, Delgado-Franco D, García-Gutiérrez M, Gurrola-Díaz C, Larrosa-Haro A, Montijo-Barrios E, et al. The Importance of Lactose in the Human Diet: Outcomes of a Mexican Consensus Meeting. Nutrients. 2019;11:2737-57.
15. Marcobal A, Sonnenburg JL. Human milk oligosaccharide consumption by intestinal microbiota. Clin Microbiol Infect. 2012;18(Suppl 4):12-5.
16. Hobbs M, Jahan M, Ghorashi SA, Wang B. Current Perspective of Sialylated Milk Oligosaccharides in Mammalian Milk: Implications for Brain and Gut Health of Newborns. Foods. 2021;10:473.
17. Andreas NJ, Kampmann B, Le-Doare KM. Human breast milk: a review on its composition and bioactivity. Early Hum Dev. 2015:1-7.
18. Savarino G, Corsello A, Corsello G. Macronutrient balance and micronutrient amount through growth and development. Ital J Pediatr. 2021;47:109.
19. Conboy SR, Ross RP, Stanton C. Carotenoids in Milk and the Potential for Dairy-Based Functional Foods. Foods. 2021;10:1263-86.
20. Wagner CL, Greer FR; American Academy of Pediatrics Section on Breastfeeding; American Academy of Pediatrics Committee on Nutrition. Prevention of Rickets and Vitamin D Deficiency in Infants, Children, and Adolescents. Pediatrics. 2008;122: 1142-52.
21. Zeisel SH. The fetal origins of memory: The role of dietary choline in optimal brain development. J Pediatr. 2006;149:S131-6.
22. Cheatham CL, Sheppard KW. Synergistic Effects of Human Milk Nutrients in the Support of Infant Recognition Memory: An Observational Study. Nutrients. 2015;7(11): 9079-95.
23. Chiurazzi M, Cozzolino M, Reinelt T, Nguyen TD, Elke Chie S, Natalucci G, et al. Human Milk and Brain Development in Infants. Reprod Med. 2021;2:107-17.
24. World Health Organization. Guidelines on optimal feeding of low birth-weight infants in low- and middle-income countries. Geneva: World Health Organization; 2011.
25. Muehlho E, Bennet A, McMahon D; Food and Agriculture Organization of the United Nations. Milk and Dairy Products in Human Nutrition (2013). Dairy Technol. 2014;67:303-4.
26. Ann Prentice. Constituents of human milk. Food Nutr Bulletin. 1996;17(4):1-10.
27. Gila-Diaz A, Arribas SM, Algara A, Martín-Cabrejas MA, López de Pablo AL, Sáenz de Pipaón M, et al. A Review of Bioactive Factors in Human Breast milk: A Focus on Prematurity. Nutrients. 2019;11:1307.
28. Ballard O, Morrow AL. Breastfeeding updates for the pediatrician. Morrow and Chantry. Pediatr Clin North Am. 2013;60(1):1-10.
29. Ballard O, Morrow AL. Human Milk Composition: Nutrients and Bioactive Factors. Pediatr Clin North Am. 2013;60(1): 49-74.
30. Pundir S, Gridneva Z, Pillai A, Thorstensen EB, Wall CR, Geddes DT, et al. Human Milk

Glucocorticoid Levels Are Associated With Infant Adiposity and Head Circumference Over the First Year of Life. Front Nutr. 2020;7:166.
31. Shehadeh N, Khaesh-Goldberg E, Shamir R, Perlman R, Sujov P, Tamir A, et al. Insulin in human milk: postpartum changes and effect of gestational age. Arch Dis Child Fetal Neonatal Ed. 2003;88:F214-6.
32. van Wassenaer AG, Stulp MR, Valianpour F, Tamminga P, Ris Stalpers C, de Randamie JS, et al. The quantity of thyroid hormone in human milk is too low to influence plasma thyroid hormone levels in the very preterm infant. Clin Endocrinol (Oxf). 2002;56:621-7.
33. Witkowska-Zimny M, Kaminska-El Hassan E. Cells of human breast milk. Cell Mol Biol Lett. 2017;22:1-11.
34. Patki S, Kadam S, Chandra V, Bhonde R. Human breast milk is a rich source of multipotent mesenchymal stem cells. Hum cell. 2010;23:35-40.
35. Yi DY, Kim SY. Human Breast Milk Composition and Function in Human Health: From Nutritional Components to Microbiome and MicroRNAs. Nutrients. 2021;13:3094.
36. Mosca F, Giannì M. Human milk: composition and health benefits. Pediatr Med Chir. 2017;39(2):155.
37. Gao R, Zhang R, Qian T, Peng X, He W, Zheng S, et al. A comparison of exosomes derived from different periods of breast milk on protecting against intestinal organoid injury. Pediatr Surg Int. 2019;35(12):1363-8.
38. Ho CSJ, Rydström A, Trulsson M, Bålfors J, Storm P, Puthia M, et al. HAMLET: functional properties and therapeutic potential. Future Oncol. 2012;8(10):1301-13.
39. McGuire MK, McGuire MA. Human Milk: Mother Nature's Prototypical Probiotic Food? Adv Nutr. 2015;6(1):112-23.
40. Moossavi S, Atakora F, Miliku K, Sepehri S, Robertson B, Duan QL, et al. Integrative Analysis of Human Milk Microbiota With Oligosaccharides and Fatty Acids in the CHILD Cohort. Front Nutr. 2019;6:58.
41. Verduci E, D'Elios S, Cerrato L, Comberiati P, Calvani M, Palazzo S, et al. Cow's Milk Substitutes for Children: Nutritional Aspects of Milk from Different Mammalian Species, Special Formula, and Plant-Based Beverages. Nutrients. 2019;11(8):1739.
42. Luyt D, Ball H, Makwana N, Green MR, Bravin K, Nasser SM, et al.; Standard of Care Committee (SOCC) of the British Society for Allergy and Clinical Immunology (BSACI). BSACI guideline for the diagnosis and management of cow's milk allergy. Clin Exp Allergy. 2014;44:642-72.

CHAPTER 5

Breast Milk and Genetics

Pramod Jog, Mallikarjuna R Patil, Shradha Salunke

"The breastmilk is another inherited genetic material"

INTRODUCTION

Breast milk is a dynamic living fluid. Its composition is influenced by various factors such as period of gestation, twins or multiple pregnancies, maternal infections, maternal obesity, maternal diet, and postnatal period and genetic factors.

Breast milk is a true biological fluid which has both nutritional and functional components. It is a complex mixture which includes macronutrients, micronutrients, and a wide range of non-nutritive bioactive factors such as hormones, growth factors, micro-ribonucleic acid (miRNAs), cells, as well as prebiotics. All of them have significant impact on infant's growth and development. Many of the health benefits of breast milk are mediated through epigenetic mechanisms. The genetic information that is inherited from the parents is called genome. Epigenetic mechanism is a heritable change in the genetic material without change in sequence variation. Epigenome is what directs the genome and is influenced by an individual's internal and external environment. The external environmental influences are nutrition, chemicals, toxins, etc. The internal factors are neuropeptides (emotional molecules) and stress hormones.

We are all unique, yet related to our ancestors by genetic information that can potentially change throughout our lifetime. Most critical developmental period which can influence our growth, individual personalities, and long-term health is the period from conception to 2 years of life (first 1,000 days of life). At this time, our deoxyribonucleic acid (DNA) is most receptive to epigenetic modifications which mark our DNA and change the way our organs develop and our susceptibility to certain diseases. Epigenetic modifications influence genes related to human metabolism, hormone production, and tissue sensitivity. Nutritional and environmental factors through epigenetic modification may permanently affect individual's biological, metabolic, and psychosocial development, which in turn make adaptive pathophysiological alterations later in childhood and or at adulthood, leading to noncommunicable diseases such as diabetes mellitus, cardiovascular diseases, cancers, anxiety, and depressive disorders.

Plastic interaction between inherited genes and environmental or exogenous factors during crucial stages of life leading to developmental adaptation is known as "programming". Impaired quality and quantity of nutritional support including not breastfeeding in early developmental periods may be responsible for an increased risk for morbidity and severe chronic diseases in later life.[1] Epigenetic processes determine when and where specific genes are to be expressed. Any change in epigenetic regulation of genes may modify the phenotype significantly. Various epigenetic mechanisms are—methylation, acetylation, phosphorylation, ubiquitylation, histone modification, and through miRNA. These epigenetic mechanisms are responsible for either expression or suppression of particular genes, thereby regulating gene expression and hence their effects. Epigenetic mechanisms bring changes in breast milk composition, which in turn modify various disease processes such as diabetes mellitus, obesity, cholesterol disorders, nonalcoholic fatty liver, and cancers. Breastfeeding practices and breast milk bring down the cancer risk in genetically susceptible individuals.

Breastfeeding through epigenetic mechanisms influences neurocognitive development, neuronal multiplication, dendritic arborization,[2] and autoimmune dysregulation or allergic diseases. Formula feeding in early postnatal life may lead to obesity through altered development of organ structure or persistent alteration at cellular level and altered gene expression through epigenetic pathways. Epigenetic changes are not just related to breast milk itself but also related to the act of breastfeeding practice also. Animal studies have observed that babies of mother rats who lick, groom, and arch their back during breastfeeding and allow more skin-to-skin contact have been shown to have moderate stress response due to epigenetic process that influences hippocampus and glucocorticoids receptor expression.[3] These studies indicate that how we touch, hold, and practice skin-to-skin contact with our babies can change epigenome as well. Epigenome is also responsible for priming the breast tissue between pregnancies. Epigenetic memory of mammary gland helps to prime the breast tissue to hormonal changes in subsequent pregnancies.[4]

The World Health Organization (WHO) considers noncommunicable diseases as "The world's biggest killers" and they can affect all people irrespective of age and geographic area.[5] Endocrine or nutritional interventions during early postnatal life can reverse epigenetic and phenotypic changes.[6] A study in the past showed that breastfeeding is similar to consanguinity between individuals even with no blood relations.[7] Breastfeeding is the only other way of transmitting genetic material other than sexual transmission. The possible reasons for this transmission of genetic information through breast milk are—exosomes, miRNA, and stem cells.

EXOSOMES

Exosomes are tiny particles that are excreted by every cell including mammary cells and they play a role in cell-to-cell talking and alter the behavior of neighboring cells. This communication via exosomes is genetically based. Breastfeeding or breast milk sharing to a baby other than their own will transfer mother's genetic exosomes (material) which influence the behavior of that baby similar to genetic influence on any individual.

STEM CELLS

There is a constant exchange of stem cells between mother and baby during pregnancy. Breastfeeding also contributes to this sharing, and hence is similar to chimerism. Mothers are protected immunologically for long period of time so that they can take care of their growing baby. Nearly, 1,000 to millions of stem cells are ingested during breastfeeding that are unique to mother.

MICRO-RNA

Breast milk is rich in miRNA and its levels are high in breast milk in the first 6 months of lactation. A baby receives approximately 1.3×10^7 copies/liter/day of miRNA which can modulate immune system.[8] miRNAs are small, noncoding RNA molecules with approximately 22 nucleotides, which play a role in post-transcriptional regulation of gene expression and have protective functions. They are synthesized by enzyme RNA-polymerase-II and undergo maturation by RNAase III family.[9] It is estimated that approximately 1,400 different miRNA are present in breast milk.[10] They are found in either free or packaged vesicles.

The composition and expression of miRNA varies depending on the process of feeding, lactation progress, maternal stress, immune dysfunction, or mastitis. Similar to miRNA, other small RNA species secreted in breast milk are—circular RNA, transfer RNA, small nuclear RNA, small nucleolar RNA, long noncoding RNA, and Piwi-interacting RNA at different profiles.[11,12]

Potential Effects of Micro-RNA

Micro-RNA has diverse roles. miRNA-148 suppresses DNA methyltransferase (DNMT), leading to hypomethylation and alter gene functions. The important implications of miRNA are related to the genes involving metabolism [insulin (*INS*), *insulin-like growth factor 1* (*IGF-1*), and *Caveolin-1* (*Cav-1*)], immunity (*FOXP3* and *NRA-4*), adipogenesis [*fat mass and obesity associated* (*FTO*), *fatty acid-binding protein 4* (*FABP-4*), *Cav-1*, *peroxisome proliferator-activated receptor gamma 2* (*PPARG-2*), *sterol regulatory element-binding protein 1* (*SREBP-1*), and *lipoprotein lipase* (*LPL*)], myogenic programming (*NR4A3*), osteogenesis (*NRF2*), and epidermis (*NRF2*).[13]

EPIGENETIC EFFECTS OF BREAST MILK

Breast milk has a beneficial effect on gene expression related to noncommunicable diseases such as obesity, type-II diabetes mellitus, and cholesterol metabolic disorders through epigenetic mechanisms, either directly or by hormonal activity. Through nutrigenomics, it is possible to tailor individualized nutritional care to improve the pathological conditions to which they are predisposed and prevent them from occurring. Nutrition and genes are in constant interaction which determines when and where specific genes are to be expressed or suppressed. Any change in epigenetic regulation of genes may lead to significant phenotypic change.

Obesity

Obesity is one of the best examples of epigenetic regulation through breast milk. Leptin is produced by fat cells and is responsible for food intake. Breastfeeding reduces the methylation of leptin gene and increased expression, leading to satiety and reduced food intake and weight gain.[14] In formula-fed babies, the leptin gene is dampened and they are at increased risk of developing obesity. Gut dysbiosis is associated with necrotizing enterocolitis (NEC) and secretary immunoglobulin A (IgA) from breast milk has a protective role. Apart from this, lactoferrin in breast milk also modulates the immune function of lymphoid follicles in small intestine.

One of the most important health benefits of breast milk is prevention of infections such as otitis media and gut infections. Some of the proinflammatory polymorphisms such as tumor necrosis factor alpha-308 (TNF-α-308) and interleukin-174 (IL-174) have been associated with increased risk of otitis media due to their genetic susceptibility and they are protected by breastfeeding.[15] Breastfeeding also reduces the risk of other disorders such as inflammatory bowel disease (IBD), celiac disease due to interaction of immunomodulatory effects of human milk, and the underlying genetic susceptibility of the infant.[16] The programming of immune function is modulated by gut microbiota indirectly through expression pattern of proinflammatory cytokine genes.

Obesity risk depends upon the interaction between the genotype, fetal environment, and individual lifestyle and nutrition in early stages of life. Breastfeeding has beneficial effects on genetically predisposed obesity risk conditions such as *PPARG-2* gene polymorphism. It also reduces the risk of nonalcoholic fatty liver diseases such as fatty steatosis and liver fibrosis. Long-chain polyunsaturated fatty acids (LCPUFAs), especially docosahexaenoic acid (DHA), are implicated in protection against liver disease.

Cancer

Breastfeeding has beneficial effects on mother as well. Breast milk through epigenetic modulation of gene expression might positively modify phenotype and the outcome, even if there is a genetic predisposition for the development of diseases. Women carrying deleterious *BRCA1 (BReast CAncer gene 1)* mutation who fed their babies for more than 1 year have statistically significant reduction in risk of breast cancer than those who did not breastfeed their children.[17] DHA is a natural ligand for PPAR that is able to modulate PPAR-beta-mRNA expression, inhibiting breast cancer cell growth and mammary tumor growth.

Gut Microbiota

Gut microbiota is another factor which influences the epigenetic modifications. The methyl and acetyl groups which are created by fermentation of proteins and polysaccharides in breast milk affect DNA and gene expression by turning on and off certain genes. Various microbials like bacteria, viruses, fungi, and archaea, inhabiting in gut, constitute nearly 50% of the total human body cell and play vital role in host's health.[18] Close interaction with microbial world is crucial for normal development in early life. They have a significant contribution in maintaining homeostasis, metabolic, immunologic, and neuronal and psychological functions. Any change in gut microbiota composition, abundance, diversity, and functions are associated with disorders such as neuro-degenerative diseases, type-2 diabetes, obesity, and low-grade inflammatory disorders,[19-28] atopy, IBD, NEC in preterm infants, obesity, and neurological conditions ranging from autism spectrum disorders to Parkinson's disease.[29,30]

FACTORS AFFECTING MICROBIOME

The milk microbiome varies with each individual. A variety of factors such as genetic background, ethnicity, milk sampling, geographical location, circadian rhythm, maternal age, diet and body mass index (BMI), delivery mode, gestational age, therapies and food supplements, infant and maternal health status, and others have been under evaluation in recent times **(Fig. 1)**.

CHAPTER 5: Breast Milk and Genetics

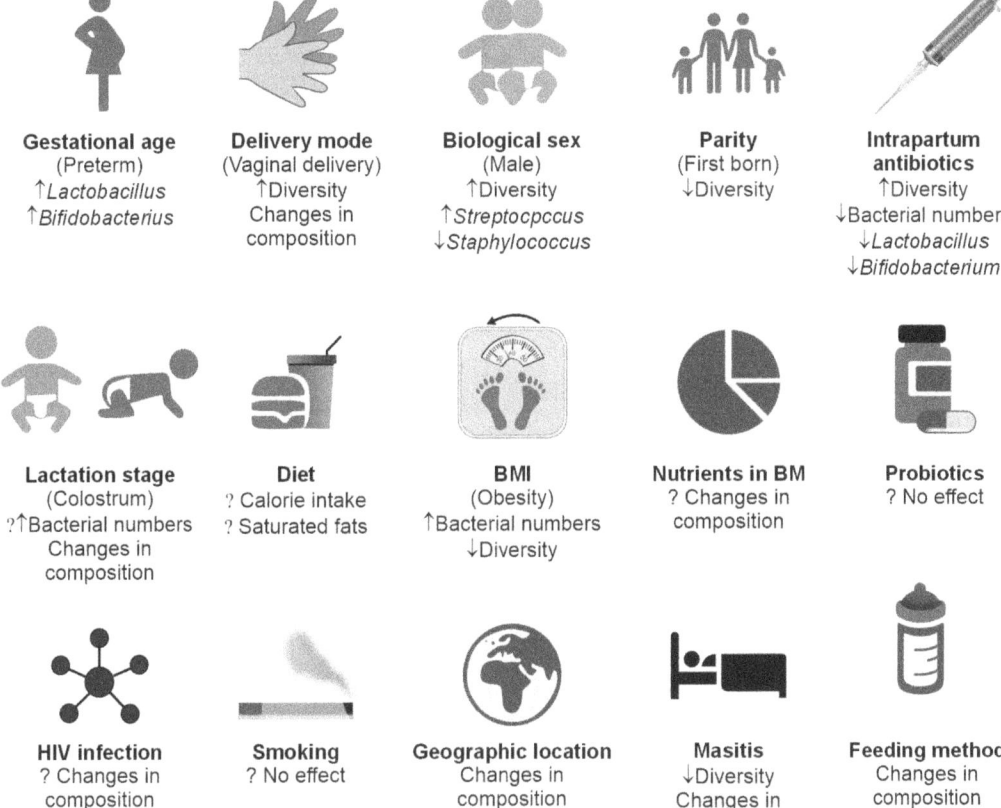

Fig. 1: Factors that influence the composition of the intestinal microbiota.[31] (BM: breast milk; BMI: body mass index; HIV: human immunodeficiency virus)

Mode of delivery is important in establishing the bacterial colonization. Vaginal delivery leads to colonization of *Lactobacillus* and *Bifidobacterium* in newborn infants,[32] whereas in cesarean section (C-section), colonization of skin bacteria is common and is associated with a higher incidence of staphylococcal diseases in adulthood.[33,34] The type of infant-feeding practice plays a vital role in the development of an infant's gut microbiota.[35] Exclusive breastfeeding up to 6 months is recommended by the WHO as mothers' own milk (MOM) provides all probiotics and macro- and micronutrients necessary for the infant.[36] MOM is rich in nucleotides, fatty acids, immunoglobulins, cytokines, immune cells, lysozyme, lactoferrin, and commensal bacteria (109 bacteria per liter).[37,38] Early antibiotic exposure in early neonatal period is associated with NEC and late onset sepsis.[39,40]

The origin of bacteria in breast milk is probably through two mechanisms:
1. Enteromammary pathway
2. Oro-mammary pathway.

In enteromammary pathway, the bacteria, assisted by dendritic cells, translocate across the maternal intestinal mucosa and are delivered to the lactating mammary gland for neonatal immune response.

The retrograde backflow during nursing or suckling may cause bacterial establishment in the mammary ducts that is known as oromammary pathway. Multiple factors such as maternal BMI, weight gain, hormones, lactation stage, gestational age, and mode of delivery are associated with the bacterial composition of human milk. Most predominant bacteria in breast milk are *Lactobacillus, Enterococcus, Streptococcus*, and the abundance of *Bifidobacterium* and *Enterococcus* species, which increase throughout the lactation period.

Human milk oligosaccharides (HMOs) are complex carbohydrates, which are synthesized in mammary gland. They directly or indirectly modulate the physiological systems of infants by regulating microbial composition and preventing adhesion of pathogenic microbes, invasion, and intestinal epithelial cell response. They interact with various pathogenic organisms and protect against bacterial infections, viral infections (rotavirus, norovirus, influenza, other respiratory viruses), protozoal infections such as *Entamoeba histolytica* (*E. histolytica*), and fungal infections such as *Candida albicans* (*C. albicans*).[41] More than 200 HMOs have been identified.[42] There is a negative correlation between HMOs and infant adiposity,[43,44] which shows that HMOs could play a role in obesity protection.

Twenty percent of all carbohydrates in colostrum milk are HMOs.[45,46] In addition, HMOs can cross intestine and influence other physiological functions through G protein-coupled receptors such as olfaction, taste, hormone signaling, neurotransmission, and regulation of heart rate.[47,48] After ingestion, nearly 45% of them are fermented by intestinal microbiota, 1–4% are excreted in urine, 40–50% are excreted in feces,[49,50] and 1% of them are absorbed. The plasma concentration of HMOs may range from 0.01 to 0.1 mg/L.[51-53] The various epigenetic mechanism of human breast milk components on child's health outcome is summarized in **Table 1**.

TABLE 1: Possible epigenetic mechanisms of human breast milk components on child's health outcome.[54]

Breast milk component	Gene expression	Prevention
Lactoferrin	NF-κβ (suppression)	NEC, disorders of immune system
Prostaglandin-J	PPAR-γ (expression)	Obesity
LCPUFA(n-3)	Liver lipogenic and cholesterol biosynthetic enzyme (suppression)	NAFLD
	PPAR-α and γ (expression)	Progression of NAFLD
Cholesterol content of breast milk	HMG-CoA reductase (suppression)	High blood cholesterol in adulthood
Indigestible HMOs	Act on expression of different genes (NF-κβ)	Gut dysbiosis and related activation (NEC, infections, immunosuppression, and obesity-linked disorders)

(HMG: hydroxymethylglutaryl; HMOs: human milk oligosaccharides; NAFLD: nonalcoholic fatty liver disease; NEC: necrotizing enterocolitis; NF-κB: nuclear factor kappa B; *PPAR*: *peroxisome proliferator-activated receptor*)

KEY MESSAGES

- Many of the health benefits of breastfeeding are mediated through epigenetic mechanisms. Epigenetics are heritable changes in genomic material without nucleotide sequence variations.
- Developmental adaptation occurring due to interaction between genes and environmental factors during the early stages of development is known as "programming".
- Epigenetic mechanisms bring changes in breast milk composition, which can modify various disease processes.
- Breastfeeding practices help in priming of mammary gland and also bring down the cancer risk in genetically susceptible individuals (*BRCA1*).
- Gut microbiota has significant contribution in maintaining homeostasis of metabolic, immunologic, and neuronal and psychological functions through epigenetic mechanisms.
- Milk microbiome is influenced by various internal or external factors.
- Unwarranted antibiotic usage may lead to "dysbiosis" and is associated with complications such as NEC and IBD.
- HMOs are complex carbohydrates, which are secreted by mammary gland and they modulate directly or indirectly the physiological systems of infants.

REFERENCES

1. Langley-Evans SC. Nutrition in early life and the programming of adult disease: a review. J Hum Nutr Diet. 2014.
2. Waly M, Hornig M, Trivedi M, Hodgson N, Kini R, Ohta A, et al. Prenatal and Postnatal Epigenetic Programming: Implications for GI, Immune, and Neuronal Function in Autism. Autism Res Treat. 2012:190930.
3. Weaver IC, Cervoni N, Champagne FA, D'Alessio AC, Sharma S, Seckl JR, et al. Epigenetic programming by maternal behavior. Nat Neurosci. 2004;7(8):847-54.
4. Dos Santos CO, Dolzhenko E, Hodges E, Smith AD, Hannon GJ. An Epigenetic Memory of Pregnancy in the Mouse Mammary Gland. Cell Rep. 2015;11(7):1102-9.
5. United Nations. Political declaration of the High-level Meeting of the General Assembly on the Prevention and Control of Non-communicable Diseases 2011. New York: United Nations; 2011.
6. Hanson MA, Godfrey KM, Lillycrop KA, Burdge GC, Gluckman P. Developmental plasticity and developmental origins of non-communicable disease: theoretical considerations and epigenetic mechanisms. Prog Biophys Mol Biol. 2011;106:272-80.
7. Ozkan H, Tuzun F, Kumral A, Duman N. Milk kinship hypothesis in light of epigenetic knowledge. Clin Epigenetics. 2012;4(1):4-14.
8. Kosaka N, Izumi H, Sekine K, Ochiya T. microRNA as a new immune-regulatory agent in breast milk. Silence. 2010;1:7.
9. Król J, Loedige I, Filipowicz W. The Widespread Regulation of MicroRNA Biogenesis, Function, and Decay. Nat Rev Genet. 2010;11:597-610.
10. Tomé-Carneiro J, Fernández-Alonso N, Tomás-Zapico C, Visioli F, Iglesias-Gutierrez E, Dávalos A. Breast Milk MicroRNAs Harsh Journey Towards Potential Effects in Infant Development and Maturation. Lipid Encapsulation Can Help. Pharmacol Res. 2018;132:21-32.
11. Rubio M, Bustamante M, Hernandez-Ferrer C, Fernandez-Orth D, Pantano L, Sarria Y, et al. Circulating miRNAs, isomiRs and Small RNA Clusters in Human Plasma and Breast Milk. PLoS One. 2018;13:e0193527.
12. Zeng B, Chen T, Luo J, Xie M, Wei L, Xi Q, et al. Exploration of Long Non-coding RNAs and Circular RNAs in Porcine Milk Exosomes. Front Genet. 2020;11:652.
13. Carrillo-Lozano E, Sebastián-Valles F, Knott-Torcal C. Circulating microRNAs in Breast Milk and Their Potential Impact on the Infant. Nutrients. 2020;12:3066.

14. Ilcol YO, Hizli ZB, Ozkan T. Leptin concentration in breast milk and its relationship to duration of lactation and hormonal status. Int Breastfeed J. 2006;1:21.
15. Patel JA, Nair S, Revai K, Grady J, Saeed K, Matalon R, et al. Association of Proinflammatory Cytokines Gene Polymorphisms with Susceptibility to Otitis Media. Pediatrics. 2006;118:2273-9.
16. American Academy of Pediatrics. Breastfeeding and the use of human milk. Pediatrics. 2012;29:e827-41.
17. Jernström H, Lubinski J, Lynch HT, Ghadirian P, Neuhausen S, Isaacs C, et al. Breastfeeding and the risk of breast cancer in BRCA1 and BRCA2 mutation carriers. J Natl Cancer Inst. 2004;96:1094-8.
18. Sender R, Fuchs S, Milo R. Revised Estimates for the Number of Human and Bacteria Cells in the Body. PLoS Biol. 2016;14(8):e1002533.
19. Tremlett H, Bauer KC, Appel-Cresswell S, Finlay BB, Waubant E. The gut microbiome in human neurological disease: a review. Ann Neurol. 2017;81(3):369-82.
20. Alkasir R, Li J, Li X, Jin M, Zhu B. Human gut microbiota: the links with dementia development. Protein Cell. 2017;8(2):90-102.
21. Cani PD, Osto M, Geurts L, Everard A. Involvement of gut microbiota in the development of low-grade inflammation and type 2 diabetes associated with obesity. Gut Microbes. 2012;3(4):279-88.
22. Delzenne NM, Cani PD. Interaction between obesity and the gut microbiota: relevance in nutrition. Annu Rev Nutr. 2011;31(1):15-31.
23. Björkstén B, Sepp E, Julge K, Voor T, Mikelsaar M. Allergy development and the intestinal microflora during the first year of life. J Allergy Clin Immunol. 2001;108:516-20.
24. Schwiertz A, Jacobi M, Frick JS, Richter M, Rusch K, Köhler H. Microbiota in pediatric inflammatory bowel disease. J Pediatr. 2010;157:240-4.
25. Mshvildadze M, Neu J, Shuster J, Theriaque D, Li N, Mai V. Intestinal microbial ecology in premature infants assessed with non-culture-based techniques. J Pediatr. 2010;156:20-5.
26. Mai V, Young CM, Ukhanova M, Wang X, Sun Y, Casella G, et al. Fecal microbiota in premature infants prior to necrotizing enterocolitis. PLoS One. 2011;6:e20647.
27. Turnbaugh PJ, Hamady M, Yatsunenko T, Cantarel BL, Duncan A, Ley RE, et al. A core gut microbiome in obese and lean twins. Nature. 2009;457:480-4.
28. Kalliomäki M, Collado MC, Salminen S, Isolauri E. Early differences in fecal microbiota composition in children may predict overweight. Am J Clin Nutr. 2008;87:534-8.
29. De Angelis M, Piccolo M, Vannini L, Siragusa S, De Giacomo A, Serrazzanetti DI, et al. Fecal microbiota and metabolome of children with autism and pervasive developmental disorder not otherwise specified. PLoS One. 2013;8:e76993.
30. Scheperjans F, Aho V, Pereira PA, Koskinen K, Paulin L, Pekkonen E, et al. Gut microbiota are related to Parkinson's disease and clinical phenotype. Mov Disord. 2015;30:350-8.
31. Zimmermann P, Curtis N. Breast milk microbiota: a review of the factors that influence composition. J Infect. 2020;81:17-47.
32. Itani T, Ayoub Moubareck C, Melki I, Rousseau C, Mangin I, Butel MJ, et al. Establishment and development of the intestinal microbiota of preterm infants in a Lebanese tertiary hospital. Anaerobe. 2017;43:4-14.
33. Dominguez-Bello MG, De Jesus-Laboy KM, Shen N, Cox LM, Amir A, Gonzalez A, et al. Partial restoration of the microbiota of caesarean-born infants via vaginal microbial transfer. Nat Med. 2016;22(3):250-3.
34. Dominguez-Bello MG, Costello EK, Contreras M, Magris M, Hidalgo G, Fierer N, et al. Delivery mode shapes the acquisition and structure of the initial microbiota across multiple body habitats in newborns. Proc Natl Acad Sci USA. 2010;107(26):11971-5.
35. Korpela K, Blakstad EW, Moltu SJ, Strømmen K, Nakstad B, Rønnestad AE, et al. Intestinal microbiota development and gestational age in preterm neonates. Sci Rep. 2018;8(1):2453.
36. World Health Organization. (2001). The Optimal Duration of Exclusive Breastfeeding: Report of an Expert Consultation. [online] Available from https://www.who.int/

publications/i/item/WHO-NHD-01.09 [Last accessed November, 2023].
37. Cilieborg MS, Boye M, Sangild PT. Bacterial colonization and gut development in preterm neonates. Early Hum Dev. 2012;88 (Suppl 1):S41-9.
38. Jeurink PV, van Bergenhenegouwen J, Jiménez E, Knippels LM, Fernández L, Garssen J, et al. Human milk: a source of more life than we imagine. Benef Microbes. 2013;4(1):17-30.
39. Cotten CM, Taylor S, Stoll B, Goldberg RN, Hansen NI, Sánchez PJ, et al. Prolonged duration of initial empirical antibiotic treatment is associated with increased rates of necrotizing enterocolitis and death for extremely low birth weight infants. Pediatrics. 2009;123:58-66.
40. Shah P, Nathan E, Doherty D, Patole S. Prolonged exposure to antibiotics and its associations in extremely preterm neonates—the Western Australian experience. J Matern Fetal Neonatal Med. 2013;26:1710-4.
41. Zevgiti S, Zabala JG, Darji A, Dietrich U, Panou-Pomonis E, Sakarellos Daitsiotis M. Sialic acid and sialyl-lactose glyco-conjugates: design, synthesis and binding assays to lectins and swine influenza H1N1 virus. J Pept Sci. 2012;18(1):52-8.
42. Austin SC, De Castro A, Sprenger N, Binia A, Afolter M, Garcia-Rodenas CL, et al. Human milk oligosaccharides in the milk of mothers delivering term versus preterm infants. Nutrients. 2019;11(6):1282.
43. Alderete TL, Autran C, Brekke BE, Knight R, Bode L, Goran MI, et al. Associations between human milk oligosaccharides and infant body composition in the first 6 months of life. Am J Clin Nutr. 2015;102:1381-8.
44. Gridneva Z, Rea A, Tie WJ, Lai CT, Kugananthan S, Ward LC, et al. Carbohydrates in Human Milk and Body Composition of Term Infants during the First 12 Months of Lactation. Nutrients. 2019;11:1472.
45. Thurl S, Munzert M, Boehm G, Matthews C, Stahl B. Systematic review of the concentrations of oligosaccharides in human milk. Nutr Rev. 2017;75(11):920-33.
46. Xu G, Davis JC, Goonatilleke E, Smilowitz JT, German JB, Lebrilla CB. Absolute Quantitation of Human Milk Oligosaccharides Reveals Phenotypic Variations during Lactation. J Nutr. 2017;147(1):117-24.
47. Rudlof S, Pohlentz G, Borsch C, Lentze MJ, Kunz C. Urinary excretion of in vivo ^{13}C-labelled milk oligosaccharides in breastfed infants. Br J Nutr. 2012;107(7):957-63.
48. Wettschureck N, Ofermanns S. Mammalian G proteins and their cell type specific functions. Physiol Rev. 2005;85(4):1159-204.
49. Goehring KC, Kennedy AD, Prieto PA, Buck RH. Direct evidence for the presence of human milk oligosaccharides in the circulation of breastfed infants. PLoS One. 2014;9(7):e101692.
50. Dotz V, Rudlof S, Meyer C, Lochnit G, Kunz C. Metabolic fate of neutral human milk oligosaccharides in exclusively breast-fed infants. Mol Nutr Food Res. 2015;59(2):355-64.
51. Andreas NJ, Kampmann B, Mehring Le-Doare K. Human breast milk: a review on its composition and bioactivity. Early Hum Dev. 2015;91(11):629-35.
52. Kulinich A, Liu L. Human milk oligosaccharides: The role in the finetuning of innate immune responses. Carbohydr Res. 2016;432:62-70.
53. Vazquez E, Santos-Fandila A, Buck R, Rueda R, Ramirez M. Major human milk oligosaccharides are absorbed into the systemic circulation after oral administration in rats. Br J Nutr. 2017;117(2):237-47.
54. Verduci E, Banderali G, Barberi S, Radaelli G, Lops A, Betti F, et al. Epigenetic Effects of Human Breast Milk. Nutrients. 2014;6:1711-24.

CHAPTER 6

Benefits of Breastfeeding

Durgappa H, Anita Nyamagoudar, Vijay Venkataiah

"Breastfeeding is an essence of mother and baby"

INTRODUCTION

Breastfeeding is the best feeding for the optimal health of the mother and baby. In addition, it has positive impact on the environment and economy. Recent data has shown that exclusive breastfeeding for 6 months is associated with 13% reduced risk of under-five mortality. Breastfeeding provides short- and long-term benefits to baby and mother.

SHORT-TERM BENEFITS

Breastfeeding is the primary source of nutrition up to 6 months of age and continues to contribute 50% of nutrients and calories between 6 and 12 months and one third during second year of life.[1] Breastfeeding and breast milk feeding is vital in newborns, especially in premature and low-birth infants who are vulnerable for hypoglycemia, hypothermia, and infections.[2]

Necrotizing enterocolitis (NEC) is a serious problem in premature infants. Breastfeeding has protective effects against NEC. A recent systematic review and meta-analysis has shown that optimal breastfeeding is associated with 58% reduced risk of NEC in premature babies compared to non-breastfed premature babies.[3] The mechanisms that have been proposed to explain are the beneficial effect of prebiotic and probiotic in breast milk such as presence of certain biologically active substances, namely prebiotics (human milk oligosaccharide) and probiotics (microbiota), which are found to be playing an important role in maintaining the epithelial integrity of intestinal wall. Other factors found to be favoring are platelet-activating factor (PAF), acylhydrolase, interleukin 10 (IL-10), and polyunsaturated fatty acids.[4]

Jaundice is a common problem encountered in newborn infants. Colostrum administration has a beneficial effect in reducing bilirubin levels in the newborn. The colostrum, due to its laxative property, enhances the elimination of meconium from the gut, thus reducing the absorption of bilirubin through enterohepatic circulation.[5,6]

Human milk confers protection against sudden infant death syndrome (SIDS) in infants. A recent meta-analysis has shown that breastfeeding is associated with 36% reduced risk of SIDS.[7] The exact mechanism is not known; however, the following plausible mechanisms have been proposed: Some SIDS deaths are due to an uncontrolled inflammatory reaction to infectious agents, especially pyrogenic toxins of *Staphylococcus aureus* and possibly cigarette smoke. The proinflammatory cytokines induced by infections can cause respiratory and cardiac dysfunction, pyrexia, shock, hypoglycemia, and arousal defects. The anti-inflammatory agents present in breast milk attenuate this inflammatory reaction and thus prevent SIDS. Infant sleep studies have shown that breastfed infants are more easily arousable than formula-fed infants, which may be an alternative mechanism for the protective effect of breastfeeding against SIDS.[8]

Breast milk has an analgesic property, which has a beneficial effect in reducing pain during minor procedures such as heel prick, intravenous (IV) line, etc. in newborns. The analgesic effect has been explained by the presence of cortisol in breast milk along with the warmth and comfort provided by the mother during breastfeeding.[9] In addition, breastfeeding has been found to enhance the efficacy of vaccination during infancy.[10] The other supplementary advantages of breastfeeding include better audio–visual functions,[11,12] decreased child abuse, child neglect,[1] malocclusion of teeth,[13] and dental caries.[14]

Breastfeeding and Infections

Breastfeeding has protective effects against a wide range of infections in infants and young children, such as acute otitis media (AOM), respiratory infections, diarrheal diseases, urinary tract infections (UTIs), and sepsis.

- *AOM:* It is a common problem encountered in infants and young children. Breastfeeding has protective effects against AOM in children. A recent systematic review and meta-analysis has shown that exclusive breastfeeding for 6 months is associated with 43% reduced risk of AOM and this effect was particularly observed during the first 2 years of age and it had a dose-dependent response. The protective effect of breastfeeding is explained by the presence of secretory immunoglobulin A (IgA), prebiotics, and probiotics in the breast milk and negative pressure generated during breastfeeding, preventing the pooling of secretions and saliva into the eustachian tube, and thus reducing the risk of AOM in children.[15]

- *Respiratory infections:* Optimal breastfeeding is associated with significant reductions in respiratory infections and 70% lower risk of hospitalization due to bronchiolitis caused by respiratory syncytial virus. The presence of secretory IgA, prebiotics, probiotics, and lactoferrin in breast milk and good nutritional status of breastfed infants are claimed to be the tenable biological mechanisms in preventing nonspecific infections in general.[16,17]

- *Diarrheal diseases:* They are one of the leading causes of morbidity and mortality among children in low-middle-income countries. Current evidence shows that the scaling up of breastfeeding to a universal level could prevent 54% of diarrheal diseases and 72% of hospital admissions in children.

  The protective effect of breastfeeding against diarrhea diseases has been explained by the presence of the following:
  - Prebiotics (HMOs) in the breast milk which prevent attachment and

invasion of the microorganisms across the intestinal wall
- Secretary IgA which has inhibitory action on the growth of the microorganism
- Lactoferrin—one of the main protein present in the breast milk which can destroy the pathogens, reduce the inflammatory response, and increase the immune response.
- Non-breastfed babies are likely to have more exposure to pathogenic organisms.
- Breastfeeding prevents undernutrition and associated repeated infections with the use of overdiluted milk substitutes in low-income countries.[1,16]

- *UTI:* It is one of the common infections causing long-term morbidities such as hypertension and chronic renal diseases. Breastfeeding has protective effects against UTI in children and this is explained by the presence of bioactive factors—HMOs, lactoferrin, and secretary IgA in higher concentration in the urine.[18]
- *Sepsis:* Breastfed babies are at lower risk of sepsis. The protective effects of breastfeeding have been explained by the presence of several bioactive components in the breast milk such as immunomodulating agents, immunoglobulins, and antimicrobial agents.[19]
- *Allergic disorders:* Breastfed children are at lower risk of allergic conditions such as allergic rhinitis, atopic dermatitis, and bronchial asthma.[20,21] The lower risk of allergic conditions could be directly due to the presence of myriad of bioactive components, enzymes, hormones, growth factors, cytokines, immunological agents, and indirectly by prevention of early infections that are attributed to be the cause for allergies.[22]

LONG-TERM BENEFITS

Breastfeeding has dose-dependent response, i.e., longer the duration of breastfeeding, higher the protection against chronic illnesses.

- *Breastfeeding and neurodevelopment:* Breastfeeding has a positive impact on the neurodevelopment of children. Recent studies have shown that breastfeeding is associated with higher cognitive function, academic performance, intelligence quotient, learning capability, better social adjustments, and economic earning during adulthood. The mechanism proposed to explain is due to the presence of polyunsaturated fatty acids in breast milk which plays an important role in the neurodevelopment of the child.[23-26]
- *Breastfeeding and neuropsychiatric disorders:* Breastfed babies have a lower risk of neuropsychiatric disorders. Recent studies have shown that breastfed babies have a lower risk of autism[27] and attention deficit hyperactivity disorder[28] compared to non-breastfed babies.
- *Breastfeeding and chronic noncommunicable diseases:* Breastfeeding offers protection against chronic noncommunicable diseases in children. Recent studies have shown that breastfed babies have a lower risk of metabolic syndrome, overweight or obesity, type 2 diabetes mellitus, and hypertension compared to non-breastfed babies.[1,29,30] The plausible mechanism proposed to explain is—due to the presence of polyunsaturated fatty acids in higher concentration in the breast milk, which is an important constituent of the cell membrane. Other studies have also

shown that long-chain polyunsaturated fatty acid (LCPUFA) concentration in the cell membrane is inversely proportionate to fasting blood glucose level. Formula-fed infants have faster postnatal growth, a higher risk for metabolic cardiovascular disorders, and higher insulin levels eventually leading to the destruction of beta cells of Langerhans in the pancreas, thus increasing the risk of type 2 diabetes and other metabolic disorders.[31]

- *Autoimmune disorders:* Breastfeeding has protective effects against autoimmune disorders. Recent studies have revealed that breastfeeding is associated with a reduced risk of inflammatory bowel diseases,[32] Crohn's disease,[33] celiac disease,[34] multiple sclerosis,[35] Henoch-schooling purpura,[36] as compared to non-breastfed children. Breastfeeding protects infants against early infections and has anti-inflammatory properties, provides antigen-specific tolerance induction, and modulates the infant's microbiome, thus offering protection against autoimmune disorders.[37,38]

- *Childhood malignancies:* The safeguarding effects of breastfeeding against childhood cancers have been studied and reported to have lower risk of childhood leukemia,[39,40] lymphomas, and neuroblastoma as compared to non-breastfed children.[39] The lactoferrin, HMOs, stem cells, and HAMLET cells (human alpha-lactalbumin made lethal to tumor cells) are ascribed for this outcome.[40]

MATERNAL BENEFITS

Breastfeeding has incredible benefits on mother's health which can be discussed as short- and long-term advantages.

Short-term Benefits

Breastfeeding is associated with:
- Reduced risk of postpartum hemorrhage[41]
- Rapid uterine involution[42,43]
- Emotional bonding between mother and baby[41]
- Lower risk for postpartum psychiatric illnesses, namely baby blue and postpartum psychosis[41,43,44]
- Feeling a full sense of satisfaction of having achieved motherhood[41]
- Rapid resumption to pre-pregnancy weight[41,45]
- Longer birth spacing.[41]

Long-term Effects

Breastfeeding for longer duration is associated with lower risk of metabolic syndrome, overweight,[1,46] hypertension, and diabetes.[47-49] These effects can be explained by increased insulin sensitivity with practice of breastfeeding. Oxytocin released during breastfeeding prevents hypertension and Ghrelin along with protein peptide YY are gut hormones that regulate maternal appetite, and thus reduce the risk of these diseases.[50]

Mothers who breastfeed their babies are known to have greater protection against invasive breast cancer, ovarian cancers, and endometrial cancers. Breastfeeding for a year is known to reduce the risk of invasive breast cancers by 6%.[16,51] The probable reasons for this observation are sustained exfoliation of breast tissue during breastfeeding and the pronounced epithelial apoptosis at the end of lactation by eliminating the cells with deoxyribonucleic acid (DNA) damage and mutations.[52]

The occurrence of age-related health problems such as menopausal osteoporosis and fractures of long and spinal bones is also less with breastfeeding practice.[51]

TABLE 1: Benefits of breastfeeding to mother and baby and eco-economics.

Benefits to	Reduced risk of	Enhances
Newborn infant	• Neonatal sepsis • Hypothermia • Hypoglycemia • Necrotizing enterocolitis • Neonatal stress • Jaundice	• Analgesic property • Vaccination efficacy • Visual and hearing functions
Child	• Infections • Allergies • Metabolic disorders • Autoimmune disorders • Childhood malignancies	• Nutrition • Neurodevelopment • Dentition • Social security • Food security in emergency
Mother	• Postpartum hemorrhage • Postpartum psychosis • Metabolic syndromes • Gynecological malignancies • Osteoporosis • Fractures of long and spinal bones	• Emotional bonding • Sense of satisfaction • Faster resumption of pre-pregnancy weight • Birth spacing
Environmental		Planet-friendly
Economy		Cost-effective strategy

Economical Benefits

Breastfeeding has huge economic impact on the nation. It has been estimated that around 300 billion dollars of economic loss occurs globally every year due to lower intelligence associated with non-breastfeeding. In India, it has been estimated that 7,000 crores could be saved annually with improved breastfeeding practices.[16,51]

Environmental Benefits

Breastfeeding is planet-friendly; studies have shown that optimal breastfeeding is associated with reduced risk of greenhouse effects, deforestation, global warming, and ecological imbalances.[52-54] The summary of the benefits of breastfeeding is outlined in **Table 1**. For detailed information on the benefits of breastfeeding, one can refer to different studies in **Table 2**.

KEY MESSAGES

- Breastfeeding is the standard method of infant feeding for the optimal growth, development, and health of children.
- Its benefits last throughout the duration of life.
- It lays good foundation for long quality of life.
- It has dose-dependent response.
- Breastfeeding provides food security, especially in low-middle-income countries.
- It is the lifeline during natural calamities.

TABLE 2: The list of studies showing the benefits of breastfeeding.

Study	Population	Outcome	Variables	Studies (n)	Age range of outcome	Pooled effect (95% CI)	Remarks
Gupta et al. 2017[55]	0–23 months	Mortality due to infectious diseases	Exclusive versus predominant breastfeeding	3	<6 months	OR 0.59 (0.41–0.85)	Low and middle income countries (LMICs) involved
Altobelli et al. 2020[4]	Preterm	NEC	Human milk (breastfeeding + donor milk) versus formula feeds	6 RCTs		RR 0.62 (0.42–0.93)	
Altobelli et al. 2020[4]	Preterm	NEC	Human milk (breastfeeding + donor milk) versus formula feeds	3 observational studies		RR 0.74 (0.63–0.91)	
Hauck et al. 2011[7]	Term	SIDS	Breastfeeding of any amount for any duration	18 case control studies		SOR 0.55 (0.44–0.69)	Effect is stronger when breastfeeding is exclusive
Bowatte et al. 2015[15]	Term	Otitis media	Exclusive versus non exclusive breastfeeding			OR 0.57 (0.44–0.75)	
Bowatte et al. 2015[15]	Term	Otitis media	More versus less			OR 0.67 (0.59–0.76)	
Bowatte et al. 2015[15]	Term	Otitis media	Ever versus never breastfeeding			OR 0.67 (0.56–0.80)	
Horta et al. 2013[16]	Term	Admission for respiratory infections	More versus less breastfeeding	17	<2 years	RR 0.43 (0.33–0.55)	

Contd...

Contd...

Study	Population	Outcome	Variables	Studies (n)	Age range of outcome	Pooled effect (95% CI)	Remarks
Horta et al. 2013[16]	Term	Admission to hospital for diarrhoea	More versus less breastfeeding	9	<5 years	RR 0.28 (0.16–0.50)	Three RCTs showed protection against diarrhea
Lodge et al. 2015[20]	Term, preterm	Asthma or wheezing	More versus less breastfeeding	29	5–18 years	OR 0.91 (0.85–0.98)	Small and inconclusive protective effect
Horta BL 2015[16]	Term and preterm	Intelligence Quotient	Never versus ever More versus less Breastfeeding	17	>1 year	Mean difference 3.44 (2.30–4.58)	Mean difference was 2.62 (1.25-3.98) after adjusting for maternal IQ
Horta et al. 2015[24]	Term, preterm	Overweight or obesity	Never versus ever, Longer versus shorter (Breast feeding, bottle-feeding, formula feeding)	113	Childhood, adolescence, adulthood	OR 0.74 (0.70–0.78)	Quality of evidence is high for protection
Horta et al. 2015[19]	Term, preterm	Type 2 DM	Never versus ever, Longer versus shorter (Breastfeeding, bottle-feeding, formula feeding)	11	Childhood, adolescence, adulthood	OR 0.65 (0.49–0.86)	Restricted evidence on protection
Barclay et al. 2009[32]	Term, preterm	Pediatric Inflammatory bowel disease	Any exposure to breast milk (Breastfeeding, breast milk feeding)	7	<16 years of age (early onset of disease	OR 0.69 (0.51–0.94)	The quality of existing data is poor

Contd...

Contd...

Study	Population	Outcome	Variables	Studies (n)	Age range of outcome	Pooled effect (95% CI)	Remarks
Henriksson C et al.[34]	Term and low birth weight	Celiac disease	More versus less (Breastfeeding versus formula feeding)	4	Up to 8.4 years	(OR 0.665; 95% CI 0.481 to 0.891)	
Yan Zeng et al. 2020[28]	Term, preterm (VLBW)	ADHD	Never versus ever (Breastfeeding for 1, 3, 6 and 12 months)	10		OR 0.70 (0.52–0.93)	Dose dependent response seen in further analysis
Amitay et al. 2015[40]	Population based studies	Childhood leukemia	No/shorter versus any/ longer duration of breastfeeding	18		OR 0.81 (0.73–0.89)	All the studies had to be case control
Peres et al. 2015[13]	Term, low birth weight	Malocclusion	Never versus ever, longer versus shorter Pacifier use was also studied	41	Till adulthood	OR 0.32 (0.25–0.40)	
Tham et al. 2015[14]	Term, preterm	Dental caries	Breastfeeding >12 months versus ≤12 months	4	<6 years	OR 2.69 (1.28–5.64)	Most studies are conducted in high income countries and do not control for introduction of sugar drinks

(ADHD: attention-deficit/hyperactivity disorder; CI: confidence interval; DM: diabetes mellitus; IQ: intelligence quotient; LMICs: low- and middle-income countries; NEC: necrotizing enterocolitis; OR: odds ratio; RCTs: randomized controlled trials; RR: risk ratio; SIDS: sudden infant death syndrome; SOR: strand OR; VLBW: very low birth weight)

REFERENCES

1. Victora CG, Bahl R, Barros AJ, França GV, Horton S, Krasevec J, et al. Breastfeeding in the 21st century: epidemiology, mechanisms, and lifelong effect. Lancet. 2016;387(10017):475-90.
2. Uwaezuoke SN. Kangaroo mother care in resource-limited settings: implementation, health benefits, and cost-effectiveness. Res Reports Neonatol. 2017;7:11-8.
3. Ip S, Chung M, Raman G, Chew P, Magula N, DeVine D, et al. Breastfeeding and maternal and infant health outcomes in developed countries. Rockville, MD, USA: Agency for Healthcare Research and Quality; 2007.
4. Altobelli E, Angeletti PM, Verrotti A, Petrocelli R. The Impact of Human Milk on Necrotizing Enterocolitis: A Systematic Review and Meta-Analysis. Nutrients. 2020;12(5):1322.
5. Uruakpa FO, Ismond MA, Akobundu EN. Colostrum and its benefits: a review. Nutr Res. 2002;22(6):755-67.
6. Kenaley KM, Greenspan J, Aghai ZH. Exclusive breastfeeding and dehydration fever in newborns during the first days of life. J Matern Fetal Neonatal Med. 2020;33(4):593-7.
7. Hauck FR, Thompson JM, Tanabe KO, Moon RY, Vennemann MM. Breastfeeding and reduced risk of sudden infant death syndrome: a meta-analysis. Pediatrics. 2011;128(1):103-10.
8. Vennemann MM, Bajanowski T, Brinkmann B, Jorch G, Yücesan K, Sauerland C, et al. Does Breastfeeding Reduce the Risk of Sudden Infant Death Syndrome? Pediatrics. 2009;123(3):e406-10.
9. Carbajal R, Veerapen S, Couderc S, Jugie M, Ville Y. Analgesic effect of breastfeeding in term neonates: randomised controlled trial. BMJ. 2003;326(7379):13.
10. Dòrea JG. Breastfeeding is an essential complement to vaccination. Acta Paediatr. 2009;98(8):1244-50.
11. Carlson SE, Werkman SH, Rhodes PG, Tolley EA. Visual-acuity development in healthy preterm infants: Effect of marine-oil supplementation. Am J Clin Nutr. 1993;58:35-42.
12. Syahrir L, Fadlyana E, Effendi S. Comparison of language and visual-motor developments between exclusively and non-exclusively breastfed infants through cognitive adaptive test/clinical linguistic and auditory milestone scale. Paediatr Indones. 2009;49(6):337-41.
13. Peres KG, Barros AJ, Peres MA, Victora CG. Effects of breastfeeding and sucking habits on malocclusion in a birth cohort study. Revista de Saude Publica. 2007;41:343-50.
14. Tham R, Bowatte G, Dharmage SC, Tan DJ, Lau MX, Dai X, et al. Breastfeeding and the risk of dental caries: a systematic review and meta-analysis. Acta Paediatr. 2015;104: 62-84.
15. Bowatte G, Tham R, Allen KJ, Tan DJ, Lau M, Dai X, et al. Breastfeeding and childhood acute otitis media: a systematic review and meta-analysis. Acta Paediatr. 2015;104:85-95.
16. Horta BL, Victora CG; World Health Organization. (2013). Short-term effects of breastfeeding: a systematic review on the benefits of breastfeeding on diarrhoea and pneumonia mortality. [online] Available from https://www.who.int/publications/i/item/9789241506120 [Last accessed November, 2023].
17. Li C, Liu Y, Jiang Y, Xu N, Lei J. Immunomodulatory constituents of human breast milk and immunity from bronchiolitis. Ital J Pediatr. 2017;43(1):8.
18. Mårild S, Hansson S, Jodal U, Oden A, Svedberg K. Protective effect of breastfeeding against urinary tract infection. Acta Paediatr. 2004;93(2):164-7.
19. Howie PW. Protective effect of breastfeeding against infection in the first and second six months of life in Integrating Population Outcomes, Biological Mechanisms, and Research Methods in the Study of Human Milk and Lactation. Boston, MA: Springer; 2002. pp. 141-7.
20. Lodge CJ, Tan DJ, Lau MX, Dai X, Tham R, Lowe AJ, et al. Breastfeeding and asthma and allergies: a systematic review and meta-analysis. Acta Paediatr. 2015;104:38-53.
21. Bloch AM, Mimouni D, Mimouni M, Gdalevich M. Does breastfeeding protect against allergic rhinitis during childhood?

A meta-analysis of prospective studies. Acta Paediatr. 2002;91(3):275-9.
22. Wendy H. Oddy Breastfeeding, Childhood Asthma, and Allergic Disease. Ann Nutr Metab. 2017;70(2):26-36.
23. Bar S, Milanaik R, Adesman A. Long-term neurodevelopmental benefits of breastfeeding. Curr Opin Pediatr. 2016;28(4): 559-66.
24. Horta BL, Loret de Mola C, Victora CG. Breastfeeding and intelligence: a systematic review and meta-analysis. Acta Paediatr. 2015;104:14-9.
25. McCrory C, Murray A. The effect of breastfeeding on neurodevelopment in infancy. Matern Child Health J. 2013;17(9): 1680-8.
26. Kanazawa S. Breastfeeding is positively associated with child intelligence even net of parental IQ. Dev Psychol. 2015;51(12):1683.
27. Ghozy S, Tran L, Naveed S, Quynh TTH, Helmy Zayan A, Waqas A, et al. Association of breastfeeding status with risk of autism spectrum disorder: a systematic review, dose-response analysis and meta-analysis. Asian J Psychiatr. 2020;48:101916.
28. Zeng Y, Tang Y, Tang J, Shi J, Zhang L, Zhu T, et al. Association between the different duration of breastfeeding and attention deficit/hyperactivity disorder in children: a systematic review and meta-analysis. Nutr Neurosci. 2018;27:1-3.
29. Binns C, Lee M, Low WY. The long-term public health benefits of breastfeeding. Asia Pac J Public Health. 2016;28(1):7-14.
30. Davis MK. Breastfeeding and chronic disease in childhood and adolescence. Pediatr Clin North Am. 2001;48(1):125-41.
31. Kelishadi R, Farajian S. The protective effects of breastfeeding on chronic non-communicable diseases in adulthood: a review of evidence. Adv Biomed Res. 2014;3:3.
32. Barclay AR, Russell RK, Wilson ML, Gilmour WH, Satsangi J, Wilson DC. Systematic review: the role of breastfeeding in the development of pediatric inflammatory bowel disease. J Pediatr. 2009;155(3):421-6.
33. Klement E, Cohen RV, Boxman J, Joseph A, Reif S. Breastfeeding and risk of inflammatory bowel disease: a systematic review with meta-analysis. Am J Clin Nutr. 2004;80:1342-52.
34. Henriksson C, Boström AM, Wiklund IE. What effect does breastfeeding have on coeliac disease? A systematic review update. Evid Based Med. 2013;18(3):98-103.
35. Conradi S, Malzahn U, Paul F, Quill S, Harms L, Then Bergh F, et al. Breastfeeding is associated with lower risk for multiple sclerosis. Mult Scler. 2013;19(5):553-8.
36. Pisacane A, Buffolano W, Grillo G, Gaudiosi C. Infant feeding and Schönlein–Henoch purpura. Acta Paediatr. 1992;81(8):630.
37. Silano M, Agostoni C, Sanz Y, Guandalini S. Infant feeding and risk of developing celiac disease: a systematic review. BMJ Open. 2016;6:e009163.
38. Vieira Borba V, Sharif K, Shoenfeld Y. Breastfeeding and autoimmunity: Programing health from the beginning. Am J Reprod Immunol. 2018;79(1).
39. Martin RM, Gunnell D, Owen CG, Smith GD. Breastfeeding and childhood cancer: a systematic review with meta-analysis. Int J Cancer. 2005;117(6):1020-31.
40. Amitay EL, Keinan-Boker L. Breastfeeding and childhood leukemia incidence: a meta-analysis and systematic review. JAMA Pediatr. 2015;169(6):e151025.
41. Schwarz EB, Nothnagle M. The maternal health benefits of breastfeeding. Am Fam Physician. 2015;91(9):602-4.
42. Chua S. Influence of breastfeeding and nipple stimulation on postpartum uterine activity. Brit J Obstet Gynaecol. 1994;101:804-5.
43. Li J, Kendall GE, Henderson S, Downie J, Landsborough L, Oddy WH. Maternal psychosocial well-being in pregnancy and breastfeeding duration. Acta Paediatr. 2008;97(2):221-5.
44. Pope CJ, Mazmanian D. Breastfeeding and postpartum depression: an overview and methodological recommendations for future research. Depress Res Treat. 2016:4765310.
45. Baker JL, Gamborg M, Heitmann BL, Lissner L, Sørensen TI, Rasmussen KM. Breastfeeding

reduces postpartum weight retention. Am J Clin Nutr. 2008;88(6):1543-51.
46. Horta BL, Loret de Mola C, Victora CG. Long-term consequences of breastfeeding on cholesterol, obesity, systolic blood pressure, and type 2 diabetes: a systematic review and meta-analysis. Acta Paediatr. 2015;104:30-7.
47. Park S, Choi NK. Breastfeeding and maternal hypertension. Am J Hypertens. 2018;31(5):615-21.
48. Choi SR, Kim YM, Cho MS, Kim SH, Shim YS. Association between duration of breastfeeding and metabolic syndrome: The Korean National Health and Nutrition Examination Surveys. J Womens Health (Larchmt). 2017;26(4):361-7.
49. Chowdhury R, Sinha B, Sankar MJ, Taneja S, Bhandari N, Rollins N, et al. Breastfeeding and Maternal Health Outcomes: A Systematic Review and Meta-analysis. Acta Paediatr. 2015;104:96-113.
50. Shangshin Park, Nam-Kyong Choi. Breastfeeding and maternal hypertension. Am J Hypertens. 2018;31(5):615-21.
51. Rollins NC, Bhandari N, Hajeebhoy N, Horton S, Lutter CK, Martines JC, et al. Why Invest, and What It Will Take to Improve Breastfeeding Practices? Lancet. 2016;387(10017):491-504.
52. Walters DD, Phan LT, Mathisen R. The Cost of Not Breastfeeding: Global Results From a New Tool. Health Policy Plan. 2019;34(6):407-17.
53. Brahm P, Valdes V. Benefits of Breastfeeding and Risks Associated With Not Breastfeeding. Rev Chil Pediatr. 2017;88(1):15-21.
54. McLain AC, Frongillo EA, Hess SY, Piwoz EG. Comparison of Methods Used to Estimate the Global Burden of Disease Related to Undernutrition and Suboptimal Breastfeeding. Adv Nutr. 2019;10(3):380-90.
55. Gupta S. Natarajan S, Chandra Kumar et al. Complementary feeding at 4 vs. 6 months of age for preterm infants born at less than 34 weeks of gestation: a randomised, open-label, multicentre trial. The Lancet Global Health. 2017;5(5):e501-11.

CHAPTER 7

Harms from Delayed Initiation of Breastfeeding

Latha GS, Durgappa H, Megha Pai

"Early initiation of breastfeeding is critical for the survival of infants"

INTRODUCTION

Early initiation of breastfeeding has positive impacts on the health of the baby and mother. The World Health Organization (WHO) has recommended early initiation of breastfeeding preferably within 1 hour of delivery.[1] The mother and baby are "a biologically inseparable unit", especially in hours immediately after delivery. Immediate uninterrupted skin-to-skin contact between mother and baby increases the duration of exclusive breastfeeding practices and this has a dose-dependent response.[2,3] Despite the various strategies across the world to promote breastfeeding practices, the desired goal is not accomplished.

MAGNITUDE OF THE PROBLEM

The prevalence of delayed initiation of breastfeeding varies from 5-86% across the globe.[4,5] In India, according to National Family Health Survey 5 (NFHS-5), only 42% of newborn infants have been initiated breastfeeding within 1 hour of delivery.[6]

The factors influencing delayed initiation of breastfeeding include home deliveries, difficult deliveries, cesarean section, maternal separation, a sick baby, and lack of support and assistance. The delayed initiation of breastfeeding has negative impacts on the health of the baby and the mother.[7-11]

Impacts on the Baby

Delayed initiation of breastfeeding has negative impacts on the survival of infants. Studies have shown that early initiation of breastfeeding preferably within 1 hour of delivery is associated with a 22% reduced risk of neonatal mortality. Delay in the initiation of breastfeeding by 1 hour (2-23 hours) increases the risk of neonatal mortality by 33% and further delay by 24 hours doubles the risk of neonatal mortality (60%). Hence, it is important to ensure an early start of breastfeeding following delivery.[11-16]

The delayed initiation of breastfeeding is also associated with an increased risk of administration of prelacteal feeds (PLF), which has deleterious effects on the newborn baby.

Prelacteal feed is any solid or liquid administered before the initiation of breastfeeding. The common PLF include

> **BOX 1:** Impacts of delayed initiation of breastfeeding on baby and mother.
>
> *Impacts on the baby:*
> - Deprivation of colostrum
> - Altered microbiota in the gut
> - Hypothermia
> - Hypoglycemia
> - Neonatal sepsis
> - Prelacteal feeds
> - Diarrhea
> - Botulinum toxicity
> - Latching difficulties
>
> *Impacts on the mother:*
> - Loss of infant–mother bonding
> - Loss of immediate benefits of breastfeeding
> - Psychological stress
> - Breastfeeding difficulties

milk other than breast milk, infant milk substitutes, sugar water, honey, etc.[17] The factors influencing PLF administration include lack of awareness, absence of antenatal counseling, home deliveries, social and religious customs, myths on colostrum, etc.[18]

A recent survey has reported that globally, 51% of newborns are fed with PLF. The PLF affect the timely initiation of breastfeeding and exclusive breastfeeding practices. Other studies have also revealed that suboptimal breastfeeding and PLF contribute to 45% of neonatal mortality, 30% of diarrheal deaths, and 18% of respiratory deaths around the globe. PLF also reduces the immunological benefits that are gained from colostrum and increases the susceptibility to infections.[19]

Impacts on the Mother

Prelacteal feeds interfere with the bonding between the baby and the mother and the mother will also lose all the short-term benefits of breastfeeding.[20] The impacts of delayed initiation of breastfeeding on baby and mother are mentioned in **Box 1**.

WAYS TO OVERCOME[21,22]

- Antenatal counseling on the benefits of breastfeeding
- Immediate uninterrupted skin-to-skin contact between mother and baby
- Offer timely skilled practical assistance and support to the mother
- Mother–baby-friendly environment
- Adopting Baby-Friendly Hospital Initiative (BFHI) in centers where maternal and child services are provided
- In the case of cesarean deliveries, breast crawl can be practiced.

KEY MESSAGES

- Early initiation of breastfeeding has positive impacts on the health of the baby and the mother.
- Immediate uninterrupted skin-to-skin contact between mother and baby is associated with an increase in the duration of exclusive breastfeeding practices and it has a dose-dependent response.
- Half of the primiparous women face difficulties in achieving a successful technique of breastfeeding after delivery.
- Offering timely skilled practical assistance and support is of great importance.
- All the health professionals involved in the care of mother and baby should join the hands in promotion, protection, and support of breastfeeding.
- Adopting and implementing BFHI in the centers for mother and baby care
- The mother–baby-friendly environment is important for the early start of breastfeeding.
- Collective societal responsibility is critical in the promotion of breastfeeding practices.

REFERENCES

1. World Health Organization. Guideline: protecting, promoting, and supporting breastfeeding in facilities providing maternity and newborn services. Geneva: World Health Organization; 2017.
2. Moore ER, Bergman N, Anderson GC, Medley N. Early skin-to-skin contact for mothers and their healthy newborn infants. Cochrane Database Syst Rev. 2016;11(11):CD003519.
3. Stevens J, Schmied V, Burns E, Dahlen H. Immediate or early skin-to-skin contact after a Caesarean section: a review of the literature. Matern Child Nutr. 2014;10(4):456-73.
4. United Nations International Children's Emergency Fund (UNICEF). (2015). The State of the World's Children 2015: Reimagine the future: Innovation for every child. [online] Available from https//www.uncef.org/media/84891/file/SCWC-2015 [Last accessed November, 2023].
5. Raihana S, Alam A, Chad N, Huda TM, Dibley MJ. Delayed Initiation of Breastfeeding and Role of Mode and Place of Childbirth: Evidence from Health Surveys in 58 Low- and Middle-Income Countries (2012-2017). Int J Environ Res Public Health. 2021;18(11):5976.
6. Bhatia N, Rathi K, Arora C, Choedon T, Rajurkar P, Thakur R, et al. (2022). Analysis of Key Nutrition Indicators Based on National Family Health Survey, NFHS 4 (2015-16) and NFHS 5 (2019-2021). [online] Available from https://osf.io/r9ybf/ [Last accessed November, 2023].
7. Rao MR, Fathima N. A critical analysis of factors for delayed initiation of breastfeeding in a district-level hospital. Int J Reprod Contracept Obstet Gynecol. 2018;7(12):4840-4.
8. Bruno Tongun J, Sebit MB, Mukunya D, Ndeezi G, Nankabirwa V, Tylleskar T, et al. Factors associated with delayed initiation of breastfeeding: a cross-sectional study in South Sudan. Int Breastfeed J. 2018;13(1):1-7.
9. Berde AS, Yalcin SS. Determinants of early initiation of breastfeeding in Nigeria: a population-based study using the 2013 demographic and health survey data. BMC Pregnancy Childbirth. 2016;16(1):1-9.
10. Takahashi K, Ganchimeg T, Ota E, Vogel JP, Souza JP, Laopaiboon M, et al. Prevalence of early initiation of breastfeeding and determinants of delayed initiation of breastfeeding: secondary analysis of the WHO Global Survey. Sci Rep. 2017;7:44868.
11. Smith ER, Hurt L, Chowdhury R, Sinha B, Fawzi W, Edmond KM; NEOVITA Study Group. Delayed breastfeeding initiation and infant survival: a systematic review and meta-analysis. PloS One. 2017;12(7):e0180722.
12. Khan J, Vesel L, Bahl R, Martines JC. Timing of breastfeeding initiation and exclusivity of breastfeeding during the first month of life: effects on neonatal mortality and morbidity—a systematic review and meta-analysis. Matern Child Health J. 2015;19(3):468-79.
13. NEOVITA Study Group. Timing of initiation, patterns of breastfeeding, and infant survival: prospective analysis of pooled data from three randomized trials. Lancet Glob Health. 2016;4(4):e266-75.
14. Mugadza G, Zvinavashe M, Gumbo FZ, Pedersen BS. Early breastfeeding initiation and incidence of neonatal sepsis in Chipinge District Zimbabwe. Int J Contemp Pediatr. 2018;5(1):1-5.
15. Li Z, Mannava P, Murray JC, Sobel HL, Jatobatu A, Calibo A, et al. Association between early essential newborn care and breastfeeding outcomes in eight countries in Asia and the Pacific: a cross-sectional observational study. BMJ Glob Health. 2020;5(8):e002581.
16. Edmond KM, Kirkwood BR, Amenga-Etego S, Owusu-Agyei S, Hurt LS. Effect of early infant feeding practices on infection-specific neonatal mortality: an investigation of the causal links with observational data from rural Ghana. Am J Clin Nutr. 2007;86(4):1126-31.
17. Eloni V, Virginia P, Neda S. Prelacteal feeding practices and their determinants in India: a systematic review. Indian J Nutr Dietetics. 2018;55(2):232-8.

18. Tekaly G, Kassa M, Belete T, Tasew H, Mariye T, Teshale T. Prelacteal feeding practice and associated factors among mothers having children less than two years of age in Aksum town, Tigray, Ethiopia, 2017: a cross-sectional study. BMC Pediatr. 2018;18(1):310.
19. Temesgen H, Negesse A, Woyraw W, Getaneh T, Yigizaw M. Prelacteal feeding and associated factors in Ethiopia: systematic review and meta-analysis. Int Breastfeed J. 2018;13(1):1-2.
20. Matthiesen AS, Ransjö-Arvidson AB, Nissen E, Uvnäs-Moberg K. Postpartum maternal oxytocin release by newborns: effects of infant hand massage and sucking. Birth. 2001;28(1):13-9.
21. Victora CG, Bahl R, Barros AJ, França GV, Horton S, Krasevec J, et al. Breastfeeding in the 21st century: epidemiology, mechanisms, and lifelong effect. Lancet. 2016;387(10017):475-90.
22. Gupta AR, Thakur NE. Infant and young feeding practices in India: current status and progress towards SDG targets. Proc Indian Nat Sci Acad. 2018;84(4):853-65.

CHAPTER 8

Maternal Nutrition and Quality of Breast Milk

Padmashri S Kudachi

"The mother has to have enough food in order to produce enough milk in order to breastfeed, but she has to know that she should breastfeed. That's an education issue".
—Catherine Bertini

INTRODUCTION

In the process of evolution of human beings from Homo sapiens, the quality of food we consume today has changed tremendously under the influence of western diet and more processed food. It is very critical for the mothers to choose and eat wisely as it affects the growth and development of the fetus in the womb and breastfed babies in the postpartum phase as well. Very few studies have observed the direct link between the maternal diet and composition of the breast milk with varied conclusions. The present chapter will discuss the association of maternal diet and breast milk composition in terms of macronutrients and micronutrients.

Mother's milk is the best nutrition for the newborn; hence, nutrition of the mother is of prime importance. The composition of human milk is influenced by numerous factors apart from diet, including mother's lifestyle, gender of the infant, genetics, environment, etc.[1]

The breast milk consists of 60–75 kcal /100 mL of energy, carbohydrate (lactose 6.9–7.2%), protein (0.8–0.9%), and fat (3–5%). It also contains minerals and nitrogen compounds.[2]

MACRONUTRIENTS

Dietary Fat and Quality of Breast Milk

Maternal diet rich in fat, carbohydrate, and protein increases milk fat concentration.[3] It is observed that consumption of macronutrients in the maternal diet does not affect the breast milk macronutrient content; however, fatty acid levels are linked to immediate food intake.[4,5] Diet rich in edible oils and fish oils during pregnancy is known to increase these essential fatty acids.[6] High consumption freshwater fish in women showed more than recommended levels of omega-3 fatty acids in the breast milk, which makes us reanalyze the present recommendations of the infant formulae food and optimize the maternal intake.[7,8]

Both the monounsaturated fatty acids (MUFA) and polyunsaturated fatty acids (PUFA) in breast milk are correlated with intake in the mother.[9-11] Supplementation of docosahexaenoic acid (DHA) in mother increases the breast milk fatty acid levels proportionately[12] and the PUFAs significantly increase in mature milk.[13-17] Administration of arachidonic acid (AA) in combination with eicosapentaenoic acid (EPA) and DHA is known to increase these fatty acids in the breast milk compared to administration of AA alone.[18]

It is shown that obese mothers secrete more saturated fatty acids and less of PUFA in the breast milk compared to normal weighing mothers, which affects weight gain of newborns in the initial few months, which may also influence the health of the child later.[19] The fetal nervous system is very sensitive to the maternal dietary supply of essential fatty acids and long-chain fatty acids,[20,21] such as omega-3 and omega-6 fatty acids, known to benefit the growth of the newborn and its brain development.[22] Low-level fatty acids in the maternal diet will adversely affect the fetal brain; hence, quality of mother's diet is important.[23] This finding is supported by many studies which demonstrated better psychomotor skills at the age of 30 months and intelligence of children in long term, when mothers were given DHA supplement.[24,25] Breast milk fatty acid is also dependent on the protein intake of mother as both metabolism of lipid and protein are linked. Low intake of protein is known to cause decreased supply of DHA from mother to fetus, causing adverse effects on the brain development.[26]

Energy Content

Maternal nutrition also influences the energy levels along with fat composition in breast milk.[27] High dairy food consumption increases the breast milk lipid content[28] and high lipid leads to more energy output.[29,30] Few studies have shown that low energy consumption in the mother affects the milk production, while majority research has suggested no change in milk production despite low provision of calories in the mother's diet.[3] The decreased energy intake in the obese mothers did not change the growth of their babies,[31] indicating that the diet restriction (energy) leads to weight loss among mothers, which neither changes the production of milk nor affects the growth of infants.[32,33]

In contrast to the findings mentioned earlier, there are studies that report the essential fatty acids such as omega-3 and omega-6 levels did not match with breast milk levels in spite of the positive correlation of the lipid composition with mother's nutrition.[22] Few other studies have demonstrated no correlations with maternal intake of fatty acids and breast milk,[34] nor with vegetarian and nonvegetarian food, referring to fat and micronutrients.[35] A study which reported no difference in the milk lipids compared to undernourished and the well-nourished mothers states that the long-term diet and body stores of the mother influence the lipids in the breast milk rather than the intestinal absorption of lipids.[36] It is also observed in few studies that prenatal administration of omega-3 fatty acids failed to demonstrate the favorable effect on neurodevelopment and cognitive outcome in the newborn.[37,38]

Dietary Protein and Quality of Breast Milk

Majority of the studies have shown that there is no relation with protein intake (animal protein and vegetarian diet) and breast milk content.[39-41] However, a study in the past has reported that milk samples of mothers who consumed more proteins in the diet showed significantly high levels of proteins.[42] It was also shown that the quality of breast milk may be associated with body composition of the mother rather than the diet.[43]

MICRONUTRIENTS/MINERALS

The maternal micronutrient intake is below the recommended values in >50% of cases.[44] It has been studied that some of the micronutrients in breast milk are influenced by mother's diet such as vitamins A, B_2, D, and E and niacin; although all micronutrients in breast milk may not reflect the maternal intake.[45] Vitamin E levels, especially in transitional milk, are reported to be more in mothers with high vitamin E intake and their serum levels.[46]

Group 1 nutrients (B vitamins) are known to be associated with maternal dietary intake[47] and vitamin B_6 levels are reported to vary with dietary intake during gestational period and postpartum phase,[48] while breast milk concentration of group 2 nutrients (folate, iron, zinc, copper, and calcium) are independent of maternal food intake.[3] Another study has reported that iodine in breast milk varies with maternal intake levels.[49] Iodine intake needs to be normal, although excess of iodine can also produce adverse effects in fetus, which is rare compared to iodine deficiency.[50]

Vitamin B_{12} deficiency in infants leads to serious neurological symptoms which can be prevented by vitamin supplementation in infants.[51] Breastfed infants rarely suffer from vitamin C deficiency irrespective of maternal diet or supplementation of vitamin to infants.[52] Vitamin D levels in the infant depends on the vitamin status of the mother and supplementation of vitamin D in mother is known to prevent deficiency in the baby.[53] In contrast to these reports, it is shown that most of the trace elements have not shown any association with maternal nutrition; however, manganese seems to be influenced by maternal intake.[54-56]

Although the quality of milk is not much affected by maternal diet,[57] there is growing evidence which suggests that infants do not escape the effect of nutrient deficiency in mother during pregnancy and lactation, especially referring to the critical nutrients such as DHA, choline, folate, iodine, and vitamin D.[58-61] Choline is known to have important role in memory.[62] Some of the essential and nonessential trace minerals found in breast milk could be the result of mother's diet and environment or could have been consumed as smoke.[63]

In short, the studies have shown inconsistent association between maternal diet and breast milk nutrients. Among all the nutrients, fatty acids in human milk seem to be sensitive to maternal diet and in turn influence the infant brain development.[64] In Indian scenario too, it is reported that breast milk composition remains relatively constant irrespective of mother's nutrition, which is similar to other previous study reports.[65] The colostrum milk also does not vary much between well-nourished and poorly nourished mothers; however, fat and protein content may reflect mother's nutritional status.[66] Maternal diet may have more effect on milk composition in later postpartum phase rather than initial period of lactation.[67] Mothers with optimal nutrition can make healthy babies;[68] hence, taking care of mother's nutrition will positively favor the infant's overall growth.[69] It is advisable to maintain good nutrition of mothers, especially in developing countries such as India.

Recent findings suggest exclusive breastfeeding for 6 months might also be associated with micronutrient deficiencies in infants, which has led to prescribing nutrient supplementation during infancy. However, this discussion needs to be supported by more research before concluding the insufficiency of exclusive breastfeeding.

The review analysis reinforce the finding that vitamins (B and D) and DHA concentrations are affected by maternal nutrition.[70] The dietary guidelines suggested especially for Indian community are to be considered for mothers and growing infants, which ensure regaining birth weight and optimal growth of a child at various phases to attain complete genetic potential.[71]

KEY MESSAGES

- The studies have shown inconsistent association between maternal diet and breast milk nutrients.
- Among all the nutrients, fatty acids in human milk seem to be sensitive to maternal diet and in turn influence the infant brain development.
- The fetal nervous system is very sensitive to the maternal dietary supply of essential fatty acids.
- The critical nutrients such as DHA, choline, folate, iodine, and vitamin D need to be optimally supplied in mother.
- Mothers with optimal nutrition can give birth to healthy babies.

REFERENCES

1. Bravi F, Wiens F, Decarli A, Dal Pont A, Agostoni C, Ferraroni M. Impact of maternal nutrition on breast-milk composition: a systematic review. Am J Clin Nutr. 2016; 104(3):646-62.
2. Jenness R. The composition of human milk. Semin Perinatol. 1979;3(3):225-39.
3. Samuel TM, Zhou Q, Giuffrida F, Munblit D, Verhasselt V, Thakkar SK. Nutritional and Non-nutritional Composition of Human Milk Is Modulated by Maternal, Infant, and Methodological Factors. Front Nutr. 2020;7:576133.
4. Aumeistere L, Ciproviča I, Zavadska D, Andersons J, Volkovs V, Ceļmalniece K. Impact of Maternal Diet on Human Milk Composition Among Lactating Women in Latvia. Medicina (Kaunas). 2019;55(5):173.
5. Segura SA, Ansótegui JA, Díaz-Gómez NM. The importance of maternal nutrition during breastfeeding: do breastfeeding mothers need nutritional supplements? Anales de Pediatría. 2016;84(6):347-e1.
6. Zhang J, Wang Y, Meng L, Wang C, Zhao W, Chen J, et al. Maternal and neonatal plasma n-3 and n-6 fatty acids of pregnant women and neonates in three regions in China with contrasting dietary patterns. Asia Pac J Clin Nutr. 2009;18(3):377-88.
7. Muskiet FA, van Goor SA, Kuipers RS, Velzing-Aarts FV, Smit EN, Bouwstra H, et al. Long-chain polyunsaturated fatty acids in maternal and infant nutrition. Prostaglandins Leukot Essent Fatty Acids. 2006;75(3):135-44.
8. Kuipers RS, Fokkema MR, Smit EN, van der Meulen J, Boersma ER, Muskiet FA. High contents of both docosahexaenoic and arachidonic acids in milk of women consuming fish from lake Kitangiri (Tanzania): targets for infant formulae close to our ancient diet? Prostaglandins Leukot Essent Fatty Acids. 2005;72(4):279-88.
9. Antonakou A, Skenderi KP, Chiou A, Anastasiou CA, Bakoula C, Matalas AL. Breast milk fat concentration and fatty acid pattern during the first six months in exclusively breastfeeding Greek women. Eur J Nutr. 2013;52:963-73.
10. Lee PS, Wickramasinghe VP, Lamabadusuriya SP, Duncan AW, Wainscott G, Weeraman JD, et al. Breast milk DHA levels in Sri Lankan mothers vary significantly in three locations that have different access to dietary fish. Ceylon Med J. 2013;58:51-5.
11. Nishimura RY, Barbieri P, Castro GS, Jordão AA Jr, Perdoná Gda S, Sartorelli DS. Dietary polyunsaturated fatty acid intake during late pregnancy affects fatty acid composition of mature breast milk. Nutrition. 2014;30(6): 685-9.
12. Sherry CL, Oliver JS, Marriage BJ. Docosahexaenoic acid supplementation in lactating women increases breast milk and plasma docosahexaenoic acid

concentrations and alters infant omega 6:3 fatty acid ratio. Prostaglandins Leukot Essent Fatty Acids. 2015;95:63-9.
13. Scopesi F, Ciangherotti S, Lantieri PB, Risso D, Bertini I, Campone F, et al. Maternal dietary PUFAs intake and human milk content relationships during the first month of lactation. Clin Nutr. 2001;20:393-7.
14. Calvo-Lerma J, Selma-Royo M, Hervas D, Yang B, Intonen L, González S, et al. Breast Milk Lipidome Is Associated With Maternal Diet and Infants' Growth. Front Nutr. 2022;9:854786.
15. Olang B, Hajifaraji M, Ali MA, Hellstrand S, Palesh M, Azadnyia E, et al. Docosahexaenoic Acid in Breast Milk Reflects Maternal Fish Intake in Iranian Mothers. Food Nutr Sci. 2012;3(4).
16. Jagodic M, Potočnik D, Tratnik JS, Mazej D, Pavlin M, Trdin A, et al. Selected elements and fatty acid composition in human milk as indicators of seafood dietary habits. Environ Res. 2020;180:108820.
17. Carlson SE. Docosahexaenoic acid supplementation in pregnancy and lactation. Am J Clin Nutr. 2009;89(2):678S-84S.
18. Smit EN, Koopmann M, Boersma ER, Muskiet FA. Effect of supplementation of arachidonic acid (AA) or a combination of AA plus docosahexaenoic acid on breastmilk fatty acid composition. Prostaglandins Leukot Essent Fatty Acids. 2000;62(6):335-40.
19. Mäkelä J, Linderborg K, Niinikoski H. Breast milk fatty acid composition differs between overweight and normal weight women: the STEPS Study. Eur J Nutr. 2013;52(2):727-35.
20. van Goor SA, Dijck-Brouwer DA, Fokkema MR, van der Iest TH, Muskiet FA. Maternal and fetal brain contents of docosahexaenoic acid (DHA) and arachidonic acid (AA) at various essential fatty acid (EFA), DHA, and AA dietary intakes during pregnancy in mice. Prostaglandins Leukot Essent Fatty Acids. 2008;78(3):159-69.
21. McCann JC, Ames BN. Is docosahexaenoic acid, an n-3 long-chain polyunsaturated fatty acid, required for development of normal brain function? An overview of evidence from cognitive and behavioral tests in humans and animals. Am J Clin Nutr. 2005;82:281-95.
22. Rocquelin G, Tapsoba S, Dop MC, Mbemba F, Traissac P, Martin-Prével Y. Lipid content and essential fatty acid (EFA) composition of mature Congolese breast milk are influenced by mothers' nutritional status: impact on infants' EFA supply. Eur J Clin Nutr. 1998;52(3):164-71.
23. Dijck-Brouwer DA, Hadders-Algra M, Bouwstra H, Decsi T, Boehm G, Martini IA, et al. Lower fetal status of docosahexaenoic acid, arachidonic acid and essential fatty acids is associated with less favorable neonatal neurological condition. Prostaglandins Leukot Essent Fatty Acids. 2005;72(1):21-8.
24. Jensen CL, Voigt RG, Llorente AM, Peters SU, Prager TC, Zou YL, et al. Effects of early maternal docosahexaenoic acid intake on neuropsychological status and visual acuity at five years of age of breast-fed term infants. J Pediatr. 2010;157(6):900-5.
25. Helland IB, Smith L, Saarem K, Saugstad OD, Drevon CA. Maternal supplementation with very-long-chain n-3 fatty acids during pregnancy and lactation augments children's IQ at 4 years of age. Pediatrics. 2003;111:e39-44.
26. Burdge GC, Dunn RL, Wootton SA, Jackson AA. Effect of reduced dietary protein intake on hepatic and plasma essential fatty acid concentrations in the adult female rat: effect of pregnancy and consequences for accumulation of arachidonic and docosahexaenoic acids in fetal liver and brain. Br J Nutr. 2002;88(4):379-87.
27. Bzikowska A, Czerwonogrodzka-Senczyna A, Weker H, Wesołowska A. Correlation between human milk composition and maternal nutritional status. Rocz Panstw Zakl Hig. 2018;69(4):363-7.
28. Park Y, McGuire MK, Behr R, McGuire MA, Evans MA, Shultz TD. High-fat dairy product consumption increases delta 9c, 11t-18:2 (rumenic acid) and total lipid concentrations of human milk. Lipids. 1999;34(6):543-9.
29. Innis SM. Human milk: maternal dietary lipids and infant development. Proc Nutr Soc. 2007;66(3):397-404.

30. Mohammad MA, Sunehag AL, Haymond MW. Effect of dietary macronutrient composition under moderate hypocaloric intake on maternal adaptation during lactation Am J Clin Nutr. 2009;89:1821-7.
31. Lovelady CA, Garner KE, Moreno KL, Williams JP. The Effect of Weight Loss in Overweight, Lactating Women on the Growth of Their Infants. New Engl J Med. 2000;342(7):449-53.
32. Vashi R, Hooley R, Butler R, Geisel J, Philpotts L. Breast imaging of the pregnant and lactating patient: physiologic changes and common benign entities. AJR Am J Roentgenol. 2013;200(2):329-36.
33. Huynh DTT, Tran NT, Nguyen LT, Berde Y, Low YL. Impact of maternal nutritional supplementation in conjunction with a breastfeeding support program on breastfeeding performance, birth, and growth outcomes in a Vietnamese population. J Matern Fetal Neonatal Med. 2018;31:1586-94.
34. Mellies MJ, Ishikawa TT, Gartside P, Burton K, MacGee J, Allen K, et al. Effects of varying maternal dietary cholesterol and phytosterol in lactating women and their infants. Am J Clin Nutr. 1978;31:1347-54.
35. Finley DA, Lonnerdal B, Dewey KG, Grivetti LE. Inorganic constituents of breast milk from vegetarian and nonvegetarian women: relationships with each other and with organic constituents. J Nutr. 1985;115:772-81.
36. Del Prado M, Villalpando S, Elizondo A, Rodríguez M, Demmelmair H, Koletzko B. Contribution of dietary and newly formed arachidonic acid to human milk lipids in women eating a low-fat diet. Am J Clin Nutr. 2001;74(2):242-7.
37. Hadders-Algra M. Prenatal long-chain polyunsaturated fatty acid status: the importance of a balanced intake of docosahexaenoic acid and arachidonic acid. J Perinat Med. 2008;36(2):101-9.
38. Crawford MA, Golfetto I, Ghebremeskel K, Min Y, Moodley T, Poston L, et al. The potential role for arachidonic and docosahexaenoic acids in protection against some central nervous system injuries in preterm infants. Lipids. 2003;38(4):303-15.
39. Boniglia C, Carratu B, Chiarotti F, Giammarioli S, Sanzini E. Influence of maternal protein intake on nitrogen fractions of human milk. Int J Vitam Nutr Res. 2003;73:447-52.
40. Ding M, Li W, Zhang Y, Wang X, Zhao A, Zhao X. Amino acid composition of lactating mother's milk and confinement diet in rural North China. Asia Pac J Clin Nutr. 2010;19(3):344-9.
41. Quinn EA, Largado F, Power M, Kuzawa CW. Predictors of breast milk macronutrient composition in Filipino mothers. Am J Hum Biol. 2012;24:533-40.
42. Forsum E, Lönnerdal B. Effect of protein intake on protein and nitrogen composition of breast milk. Am J Clin Nutr. 1980;33(8)1809-13.
43. Bzikowska-Jura A, Czerwonogrodzka-Senczyna A, Olędzka G, Szostak-Węgierek D, Weker H, Wesołowska A. Maternal Nutrition and Body Composition During Breastfeeding: Association with Human Milk Composition. Nutrients. 2018;10(10):1379.
44. Gibson RS, Rahmannia S, Diana A, Leong C, Haszard JJ, Hampel D, et al. Association of maternal diet, micronutrient status, and milk volume with milk micronutrient concentrations in Indonesian mothers at 2 and 5 months postpartum. Am J Clin Nutr. 2020;112(4):1039-50.
45. Daniels L, Gibson RS, Diana A, Haszard JJ, Rahmannia S, Luftimas DE, et al. Micronutrient intakes of lactating mothers and their association with breast milk concentrations and micronutrient adequacy of exclusively breastfed Indonesian infants. Am J Clin Nutr. 2019;110(2):391-400.
46. Ortega RM, López-Sobaler AM, Andrés P, Martínez RM, Quintas ME, Requejo AM. Maternal vitamin E status during the third trimester of pregnancy in Spanish women: Influence on breast milk vitamin E concentration. Nutr Res. 1999;19(1):25-36.
47. Allen LH. B Vitamins in Breast Milk: Relative Importance of Maternal Status and Intake, and Effects on Infant Status and Function. Adv Nutrition. 2012;3(3):362-9.
48. Roepke JLB, Kirksey A. Vitamin B6 nutriture during pregnancy and lactation I. Vitamin

B6 intake, levels of the vitamin in biological fluids, and condition of the infant at birth. Am J Clin Nutr. 1979;32(11):2249-56.
49. Azizi F, Smyth P. Breastfeeding and maternal and infant iodine nutrition. Clin Endocrinol (Oxf). 2009;70(5):803-9.
50. Pearce EN. Effects of iodine deficiency in pregnancy. J Trace Elem Med Biol. 2012;26:2-3.
51. Graham SM, Arvela OM, Wise GA. Long-term neurologic consequences of nutritional vitamin B12 deficiency in infants. J Pediatr. 1992;121(5-part-P1):710-4.
52. Salmenperä L. Vitamin C nutrition during prolonged lactation: optimal in infants while marginal in some mothers. Am J Clin Nutr. 1984;40(5):1050-6.
53. Dawodu A, Tsang RC. Maternal Vitamin D Status: Effect on Milk Vitamin D Content and Vitamin D Status of Breastfeeding Infants. Adv Nutr. 2012;3(3):353-61.
54. Vuori E, Mäkinen SM, Kara R, Kuitunen P. The effects of the dietary intakes of copper, iron, manganese, and zinc on the trace element content of human milk. Am J Clin Nutr. 1980;33(2):227-31.
55. Aumeistere L, Ciproviča I, Zavadska D, Bavrins K, Borisova A. Zinc Content in Breast Milk and Its Association with Maternal Diet. Nutrients. 2018;10(10):1438.
56. Bianchi MLP, Cruz A, Zanetti MA, Dore JG. Dietary intake of selenium and its concentration in breast milk. Biol Trace Elem Res. 1999;70(3):273-7.
57. Valentine CJ, Wagner CL. Nutritional management of the breastfeeding dyad. Pediatr Clin North Am. 2013;60:261-74.
58. Zeisel SH. Is maternal diet supplementation beneficial? Optimal development of infant depends on mother's diet. Am J Clin Nutr. 2009;89(2):685S-7S.
59. Zeisel SH. Choline: critical role during fetal development and dietary requirements in adults. Annu Rev Nutr. 2006;26:229-50.
60. Hermoso M, Vollhardt C, Bergmann K, Koletzko B. Critical Micronutrients in Pregnancy, Lactation, and Infancy: Considerations on Vitamin D, Folic Acid, and Iron, and Priorities for Future Research. Ann Nutr Metab. 2011;59(1):5-9.
61. Emmett PM, Rogers IS. Properties of human milk and their relationship with maternal nutrition. Early Hum Dev. 1997:49 (Suppl):S7-28.
62. Meck WH, Smith RA, Williams CL. Pre- and postnatal choline supplementation produces long-term facilitation of spatial memory. Dev Psychobiol. 1988;21:339-53.
63. Leotsinidis M, Alexopoulos A, Kostopoulou-Farri E. Toxic and essential trace elements in human milk from Greek lactating women: association with dietary habits and other factors. Chemosphere. 2005;61:238-47.
64. Innis SM. Impact of maternal diet on human milk composition and neurological development of infants. Am J Clin Nutr. 2014;99(3):734S-41S.
65. Kothari N, Nakul KP, Jayashree M. Effect of maternal nutritional status on the human milk composition. J Pediatr Assoc India. 2018;7(2):94.
66. Garg M, Thirupuram S, Saha K. Colostrum Composition, Maternal Diet, and Nutrition in North India. J Trop Pediatr. 1988;34(2): 79-87.
67. Nommsen LA, Lovelady CA, Heinig MJ, Lönnerdal B, Dewey KG. Determinants of energy, protein, lipid, and lactose concentrations in human milk during the first 12 months of lactation: the DARLING Study. Am J Clin Nutr. 1991;53(2):457-65.
68. Hanafy MM, Morsey MRA, Seddick Y, Habib YA, el-Lozy M. Maternal Nutrition and Lactation Performance. J Trop Pediatr Environ Child Health. 1972;18(3):187-91.
69. Picciano MF, McGuire MK. Use of dietary supplements by pregnant and lactating women in North America. Am J Clin Nutr. 2009;89(2):663S-7S.
70. Chapman DJ, Nommsen-Rivers L. Impact of Maternal Nutritional Status on Human Milk Quality and Infant Outcomes: An Update on Key Nutrients. Adv Nutr. 2012;3(3):351-2.
71. Manual A. Dietary guidelines for Indians. Nat Inst Nutr. 2011;2:89-117.

CHAPTER 9

Micronutrients in Infants and Children

Sumitha Nayak, Sangappa M Dhaded, Satishkumar D, Durgappa H

"Micronutrient deficiency is a hidden hunger in infants and children"

■ INTRODUCTION

Children under 5 years are a vulnerable group as they are liable to develop malnutrition and diseases with higher morbidity and mortality. According to the data of the World Health Organization (WHO) in 2020, almost 149 million children under the age of 5 years were estimated to be stunted, 45 million were estimated as wasted, and 38.9 million were overweight and obese.[1] Undernutrition is responsible for almost 45% of deaths in the under-5 age group.[1] Micronutrients, together with the macronutrients, are extremely critical for optimal growth and development. These are substances like vitamins or minerals, required by the body in extremely small amounts, yet are vital for maintaining good health.[2] While deficiencies of these micronutrients may be severe and life-threatening, they can also result in subtle clinical changes that interfere with attaining optimal growth and development goals. Low- and middle-income countries (LMIC) suffer from a disproportionate burden. Hence, it is important to prevent as well as identify and address these deficiencies at an early stage.

■ WHAT ARE MICRONUTRIENTS?

Micronutrient is a generalized, broad term that refers to essential dietary ingredients such as vitamins and minerals, which are essentially obtained from the diet. These are required in extremely small quantities to maintain the normal cellular and molecular functions of the body.[3]

Some of the micronutrients required by the body include[4] iron, iodine, folate, vitamin A, vitamin D, zinc, selenium, etc.

Review of the available data shows that in India, there are 6,000 deaths per day in the category of under-5 age group, of which at least 50% are due to micronutrient deficiencies (MND).[5]

The United Nations has declared the decade from 2016 to 2025 as the United Nations Decade of Action on Nutrition.[1] This aims at setting a target to address all forms of malnutrition, as well as to meet the sustainable development goals (SDG) 2 and 3 of the WHO, which focus on better nutritional intake and elimination of micronutrient deficiency.

CAUSE AND IMPACT OF MICRONUTRIENT DEFICIENCY

Micronutrient deficiency has been found to be extremely high in the vulnerable population of <5 years of age and among pregnant women. These deficiencies usually do not occur alone, but multiple MND are known to coexist.[3]

The reasons for larger number of cases of micronutrient deficiency in the LMIC are multifold, such as poor consumption of the foods which are rich in micronutrients, lack of dietary diversity, and frequent infections, inflammation, and chronic illness that result in poor absorption of nutrients.[6]

The impact of MND is seen in the society and individuals, resulting in:
- Poorer health
- Lower educational achievements
- Lower earning potentials due to reduced work capacity[3]
- There is an increased risk of morbidity and mortality, along with higher rates of perinatal complications.
- This could result in an intergenerational cycle of deficiency, wherein the deficits get perpetuated, thus limiting the achievement of maximal potential.[3] Some of the effects of MND may be visible, while the subtle effects like mental clarity, lowered energy levels may not be obviously noted.[2] However, as we understand that these MND are preventable, it gives us an opportunity to provide interventions that offer best return on investment, in terms of eliminating the cause and the scope of the MND.[3]
- Interventions in the first 1,000 days with a coordinated commitment to scale up the nutrition can indeed go a long way in breaking this intergenerational cycle of MND.[3]

Iron

Iron is an extremely important mineral. It is essential for a wide variety of body components. It is needed for the adequacy of hemoglobin and for the optimal functioning of myoglobin, enzymes, and cytochromes.[3] In the human body, iron is transported along with an iron-binding globulin and transferrin. Synthesis of heme occurs in the cytosol and mitochondria of the erythrocytes. A series of reactions produces a ring structure called coproporphyrinogen III, which is then converted to protoporphyrin IX, into which iron is incorporated to produce heme.[7,8]

Iron deficiency is the most common micronutrient globally and affects over 30% of the world's population.[3] Around 40% of children under five years of age and 30% of pregnant women suffer from iron deficiency anemia.[9]

Iron deficiency anemia disrupts the endocrine functions and immune systems, making children more vulnerable to diseases. In pregnancy, there is increase in iron needs for mental growth and development of the fetus. Maternal anemia results in 20% of deaths, besides other complications such as low birth weight, premature delivery, and other perinatal complications. Those infants born to iron-deficient mothers have more likelihood of themselves being iron deficient and developing cognitive and physical impairments.[3]

Studies have shown that iron supplementation given between 0 and 6 months in those infants who are born with lower iron stores gives better motor development, as compared to later supplementation.[10] The meta-analysis of studies also showed that there was a relationship between cognitive outcomes and iron status, pointing toward the existence of the iron-related neural changes.[10]

Effects of Iron Deficiency[4,10,11]

The effects of iron deficiency include:
- Iron deficiency anemia
- Socioemotional behavior issues
- Irreversible effects on psychomotor skills and cognition and attention deficits
- Lower effort tolerance
- Pica
- Altered immunity
- Cerebral venous thrombosis.[4]

The most important reason for iron deficiency in children is due to improper nutrition. Diet which is inadequate in iron-containing foods, prolonged breastfeeding, prematurity and low birth weight, low socioeconomic status, maternal iron deficiency, poverty, and recurrent infections are some predisposing factors to iron deficiency in children.[3,4,11]

Daily requirements of iron vary with age, which are as follows:[4]
- From 6 to 60 months of age: 1–2 mg/kg/day
- Below 6 months: 2–3 mg/kg/day
- In case infant weighs < 1,500 g at birth, start iron supplementation from 2 weeks of age and in case the infant weighs over 1,500 g at birth, start supplementation from 6 to 8 weeks of age.

Iodine

Iodine is an essential micronutrient for adequate development in the early years. According to the WHO data, there is a 37% prevalence of iodine deficiency in school-aged children.[4]

The primary function of iodine is the synthesis of thyroid hormone, essential for the regulation of human growth and brain development.[3,11] Maternal requirement for iodine increases by over 50% during pregnancy to meet the needs of the growing fetus. If not adequately supplemented in pregnancy, there can be irreversible brain damage, neurological complications, and mental retardation, together referred to as iodine deficiency disorder (IDD).[3,4,11]

Global data shows around 2 billion population has inadequate iodine status and almost 30% of the school children are iodine deficient.[3] Iodine is essential in the production of thyroxine (T4) and triiodothyronine (T3). TSH (thyroid-stimulating hormone), produced by the anterior pituitary, increases the iodine uptake by the thyroid gland and stimulates the production and release of T3 and T4.[12] In the absence of adequate levels of iodine, the thyroid gland enlarges in size in an attempt to trap more iodine and goiter results.

Functions of Iodine

Iodine plays a role in the immune response. It is beneficial for mammary dysplasia and fibrocystic bone disease.[12] Iodine deficiency can manifest as goiter, hypo- or hyperthyroidism and the most severe presentation of cretinism.[4,11,12] According to recent data available, IDD leads to higher neonatal mortality, miscarriages, hearing impairment, congenital anomalies with permanent neuromotor damage, and diminished intellectual capacity and growth.[13]

The WHO considers iodine deficiency as the leading cause of preventable brain damage in the fetus and infant and psychomotor retardation in young adults.[11,13]

Salt is used as a traditional vehicle for delivering iodine to the population at a very affordable cost of production, despite which only 68% of households use iodized table salt.[3]

The daily requirements of iodine vary with age, which are as follows:[12]
- 0–6 months: 110 µg/day
- 7–12 months: 130 µg/day
- 1–8 years: 90 µg/day.

Folate

Folate is an umbrella term which describes a family of complex compounds that structurally resemble folic acid.[11] Folate occurs naturally in food, while folic acid is a synthetic form. It is more bioavailable and is converted following a series of reductions to tetrahydrofolate, which is involved in deoxyribonucleic acid (DNA) synthesis, repair, and stability.[3]

Functions of Folate

Folate has the capacity to alter DNA metabolism by altering the DNA methylation and is considered to be concerned with DNA mutations. Folate-dependent reactions convert homocysteine to methionine.[14] Folate deficiency is associated with impaired cell division and megaloblastic or macrocytic anemia.[14] It is also associated with the development of neural tube defects during pregnancy, low birth weight, preterm delivery, and fetal growth retardation.[11,14]

Folate deficiency is known to present with ulcers on the oral mucosa and tongue, gastrointestinal symptoms, and elevated blood homocysteine concentration.[14] Women of reproductive age, pregnant women, and young children are considered at high risk for folate deficiency.[3] However, no credible estimates of global folate deficiency are available.[3] Folate is susceptible to heat and prolonged storage and dissolves in water.[11]

Daily requirement of folate varies with age. Although a wide range of food contains folate, the level of adequate intake (AI) indicates levels which ensure nutritional adequacy.[14]

Recommended daily allowance for folate includes:[14]
- 0–6 months: 65 µg/day
- 7–12 months: 80 µg/day
- 1–3 years: 150 µg/day
- 3–8 years: 200 µg/day.

Folate has been postulated to play a role in prevention of several diseases such as autism spectrum disease and immunomodulate cancers and protection against stroke, dementia, cognitive disorders, and Alzheimer's disease.[13]

Vitamin A

Vitamin A is a fat-soluble vitamin that is also present in an inactive form in nature as provitamin A. Vitamin A deficiency is a public health problem in over 50% of the countries, especially in Africa and South-East Asia. According to the WHO data, every year an estimated quarter-to-half a million children with vitamin A deficiency develop blindness and half of them die within 1 year of losing their sight.[15]

Functions of Vitamin A

Provitamin A carotenoids are converted to retinal and retinoic acid, which are used by the body.[3,11] Retinol-binding protein, which utilizes zinc for its production, is involved in mobilizing the vitamin A stores from the liver and transport to other tissues of the body.[11]

Vitamin A deficiency is the single most important preventable cause of blindness in children. Early signs of deficiency include changes in the eyes such as development of Bitot spots, xerophthalmia, night blindness, and corneal ulceration.[11] Vitamin A plays an important role in the maintenance of immune status and protect against diseases of the gastrointestinal and respiratory tract and viral infections such as measles.[11,16]

Vitamin A is extremely valuable for the structural and functional integrity of mucosal cells (which act as innate barriers), regulation of number and function of natural killer (NK) cells, oxidative burst activity of the macrophages, downregulation of interferon gamma (IFN-γ) production, regulation of production of interleukin 2 (IL-2), and tumor necrosis factor alpha, and required for normal functioning of β cells. Vitamin A also has a role in differentiation of T helper 1 and T helper 2 cells.[16]

In case of vitamin A deficiency, children are more prone to develop severe infections of the respiratory, intestinal, and urinary tracts, which may also result in fatal diseases.[11]

Daily requirements of vitamin A vary with age, which are as follows:[17]
- 0–6 months: 400 µg/day
- 7–12 months: 500 µg/day
- 1–3 years: 300 µg/day
- 4–8 years: 400 µg/day.

Vitamin D

Vitamin D deficiency (VDD) is known to occur across all countries of the world and can be associated with growth failure and rickets in children.[18,19] Despite exposure to sunlight, VDD is prevalent among 50–90% of Indian children.[19] While nearly 90% of vitamin D requirements are met by the action of the ultraviolet B radiations on the skin, 10% of the requirements need to be met by the diet.

Vitamin D is metabolized in the liver to form 25-OHD (calcifediol), which is further metabolized in the kidney to form $1,25(OH)_2$ vitamin D (calcitriol), which is unstable but active.[19] The vitamin D-binding protein binds both these forms and circulates for endocrine and systemic functions.

Functions of Vitamin D

Calcitriol is known to stimulate antimicrobial peptides in epithelial cells of the respiratory tract, gastrointestinal tract, and renal epithelial barrier.[16]

Vitamin D deficiency may result in increased severity, morbidity, and mortality from infections and increased risks of autoimmune diseases.[16,20]

Recommended daily requirements of Vitamin D are as follows:[18,20]
- 0–1 year of age is 400 IU/day.

Risk factors for VDD in children[20] include children on anticonvulsant therapy, chronic diseases with malabsorption, dark skin pigmentation, insufficient sunlight exposure, exclusive breastfeeding without vitamin D supplementation, and low-maternal vitamin D levels.

Zinc

Undernutrition is a major challenge in children all over the globe. This affects their growth and development. According to Centers for Disease Control and Prevention (CDC) data, 17.3% of the global population is at risk of zinc deficiency and this could reach up top 30% in some parts of the world.[21] Across the world, approximately 165 million children are stunted, while 52 million children are wasted.[22] Most of these children have zinc deficiency beside other MND. Low school performance, lower work capacity that impacts the economic productivity as adults, and higher morbidity and mortality are some of the associated problems.[22]

Zinc is one of the most ubiquitous trace elements that is useful for a variety of human functions. It could be critical in human growth and development. Deficiency occurs due to inadequate intake, poor quality diet, increased excretion, increased demand, or a combination of these factors.[23,24]

Functions of Zinc

Zinc helps to maintain the integrity of the skin and mucosal membranes.[16] It also participates in various functions such as cell division and growth, electrolyte absorption, neurotransmission, immune response, enzymatic catalysis, functional modification of membrane proteins, and gene-regulatory proteins and hormonal receptors. All these roles help in DNA and ribonucleic acid (RNA) synthesis, protein metabolism, and overall growth and development of the body.[21]

Zinc plays a major role in maintaining the immune functions and put by enhancing the NK cell cytotoxic and phagocyte activity; it has a role in INF-Interferon production, modulating cytokine release and acts as a anti-inflammatory agent.[16] Zinc also plays a role in antibody production, especially immunoglobulin G (IgG) and maintains immune tolerance.[16] Zinc supplements have been helpful in blunting severe cases of malaria in children.[11] Zinc is a constituent of metalloenzymes that are essential for biological processes. Both vitamin A and zinc play a fundamental role in regeneration of intestinal mucosa.

The daily recommended allowance of zinc is:
- 0-6 months: 2 mg/day
- 7-12 months: 3 mg/day
- 1-3 years: 3 mg/day
- 4-8 years: 5 mg/day.

Dietary deficiency of zinc occurs because phytates and fibers in the diet that inhibits the absorption of zinc.[11] A recent Cochrane review of 80 trials that included children from 6 months to 12 years of age has shown that zinc supplementation is associated with better linear growth and decreased mortality related to infections and to other causes.[3] The number of preterm births was also known to decrease with zinc supplementation which was given during pregnancy.[3]

Selenium

Selenium has emerged as an exciting micronutrient as it has the capability of maintaining good health. Reports show that selenium deficiency is not widely studied, despite it being prevalent in over half a billion people worldwide.[25] Plant foods contain varying levels of selenium, which are reflective of the soil levels of selenium.[26] Some meats and sea food can also provide selenium.

Selenium is important for the production of selenoproteins which are crucial for the antioxidants that prevent cellular damage from free radicals.[11,16] It is involved in the immune functions by affecting the leukocyte and NK cell function, proliferation of T cells, improving T helper cell counts, and increasing IFN-γ and antibody levels.[11]

Hence, low levels of selenium result in increased viral virulence, decreased response to vaccination, and increased likelihood of respiratory tract infection in the first 6 weeks of life.[11] Skeletal muscle is the most common site of storage of selenium, accounting for 28-46% of the selenium pool.[27]

The daily recommended dietary allowance of selenium is:
- 0-6 months: 15 µg/day
- 7-12 months: 20 µg/day
- 1-3 years: 20 µg/day
- 4-8 years: 30 µg/day.

Certain specific diseases are associated with selenium deficiency, which include:[26,27]
- Keshan disease: Cardiomyopathy that occurs in children with selenium deficiency
- Kashin-Beck disease: It results in osteoarthropathy affecting joints of ankles, knees, elbows, hands, and fingers of children and adolescents.

TABLE 1: Overview of the importance of micronutrients and their daily requirements.

Micronutrients	Role	Mechanism of action	RDA
Iron	• Growth and development • Hemoglobin synthesis	• Heme formation • Oxygen transfer • Electron transfer	From 6 to 60 months age: 1–2 mg/kg/day Below 6 months: 23 mg/kg/day
Iodine	• Regulation of BMR • Neurodevelopment • Reproduction	Thyroid hormone synthesis	6 months: 110 µg 7–12 months: 130 µg 1–8 years: 90 µg
Folic acid	Amino acid and nucleotide synthesis	One carbon group transfer	0–6 months: 65 µg 7–12 months: 80 µg 1–4 years: 150 µg 4–8 years: 200 µg
Vitamin A	• Epithelialization • Gene regulation • Dark vision	• Gene expression • Growth factor	0–6 months: 400 µg 7–12 months: 500 µg 1–3 years: 300 µg 4–8 years: 400 µg
Vitamin D	• Bone mineralization • Calcium homeostasis	Gene expression	0–1 year: 400 IU
Zinc	• Cofactor for enzymes • Immune function • Growth and tissue repair	Regulation of gene expression factors	0–6 months: 2 mg 7–12 months: 3 mg 1–3 years: 3 mg 4–8 years: 4 mg
Selenium	• Antioxidant • Prevention of cell damage	Constituent of glutathione peroxidase	50–200 µg

(BMR: basal metabolic rate; RDA: recommended dietary allowance)

- Myxedematous endemic cretinism: This is associated with mental retardation. This occurs in infants born to mothers who are deficient in selenium and iodine. Elevated blood levels of selenium above 1,000 ng/mL have been shown to cause *selenosis*. This is associated with gastrointestinal upset, hair loss, white blotchy nails, garlic breath odor, fatigue, irritability, and mild nerve damage.[26] For a detailed overview of the importance of micronutrients, refer to **Table 1**.

KEY MESSAGES

- Micronutrients are invaluable substances that maintain the normal cellular and molecular functions of the body.
- Some micronutrients such as iron and iodine are essential for normal neurodevelopment.
- The recommended daily allowance of each micronutrient varies with age.
- These micronutrients are essential to maintain the normal immune functions of the body.
- Reduced levels of micronutrients are associated with deficiency diseases.
- Higher rates of infection and some immune deficiency disorders may occur when there is micronutrient deficiency in the body.

REFERENCES

1. World Health Organization. (2021). Malnutrition. [online] Available from:

https://www.who.int/news-room/fact-sheets/detail/malnutrition [Last accessed November, 2023].
2. World Health Organization. Micronutrients. [online]. Available from: https://www.who.int/health-topics/micronutrients#tab=tab_1 [Last accessed November, 2023].
3. Bailey RL, West Jr KP, Black RE. The epidemiology of global micronutrient deficiencies. Ann Nutr Metab. 2015;66 (Suppl 2):22-33.
4. Bharadva K, Mishra S, Tiwari S, Yadav B, Deshmukh U, Elizabeth KE, et al. Prevention of micronutrient deficiencies in young children: consensus statement from infant and young child feeding chapter of Indian Academy of Pediatrics. Indian Pediatr. 2019;56:577-86.
5. Verma R, Chawla S, Dhankar M. Importance of micronutrient supplementation program in childhood to reduce child mortality: The Haryana experience. Int J Prev Med. 2016;7:87.
6. Tam E, Keats EC, Rind F, Das JK, Bhutta AZA. Micronutrient supplementation and fortification interventions on health and development outcomes among children under five in low and middle income countries: a systematic review. Nutrients. 2020;12:289.
7. Harvard University. (2002). Hemoglobin synthesis. [online] Available from: https://sickle.bwh.harvard.edu/hbsynthesis.html [Last accessed November, 2023].
8. Farid Y, Bowman NS, Lecat P. Biochemistry, Hemoglobin synthesis. In: StatPearls [Internet]. Treasure Island (FL): StatPearls Publishing; 2023.
9. Centers for Disease Control and Prevention. (2022). Micronutrient facts. [online] Available from: https://www.cdc.gov/nutrition/micronutrient-malnutrition/micronutrients/index.html [Last accessed November, 2023].
10. McCann S, Amado MP, Moore SE. The role of iron in development: a systematic review. Nutrients. 2020;12(7):2001.
11. Ekweagwu E, Agwu AE, Madukwe E. The role of micronutrients in child health: a review of the literature. Afr J Biotechnol. 2008;7(21):3804-10.
12. National Institutes of Health. Office of Dietary Supplements. (2023). Iodine. [online] Available from: https://ods.od.nih.gov/factsheets/Iodine-HealthProfessional/ [Last accessed November, 2023].
13. Morales-Suárez-Varela M, Peraita-Costa I, Llopis-Morales A, Llopis-Gonzalez A. Assessment of Dietary Iodine Intake in School Age Children: The Cross-Sectional ANIVA Study. Nutrients. 2018;10(12):1884.
14. National Institutes of Health. Office of Dietary Supplements. (2022). Folate. [online] Available from: https://ods.od.nih.gov/factsheets/Folate-HealthProfessional/ [Last accessed November, 2023].
15. World Health Organization. (2023). Nutrition landscape information system. Vitamin A deficiency. [online] Available from: https://www.who.int/data/nutrition/nlis/info/vitamin-a-deficiency [Last accessed November, 2023].
16. Gombart AF, Pierre A, Maggini S. A review of micronutrients and the immune system working in harmony to reduce risk of infection. Nutrients. 2020;12:236.
17. National Institutes of Health. Office of Dietary Supplements. (2022). Vitamin A and Carotenoids. [online] Available from: https://ods.od.nih.gov/factsheets/VitaminA-HealthProfessional/ [Last accessed November, 2023].
18. Gupta P, Dabas A, Seth A, Bhatia VL, Khadgawat R, Kumar P, et al. Indian Academy of Pediatrics revised (2021) guidelines on prevention and treatment of vitamin D deficiency and rickets. Indian Pediatr. 2022;59(2):142-58.
19. Surve S, Chauhan S, Amdekar Y, Joshi B. Vitamin D deficiency in children: an update on its prevalence, therapeutics, and knowledge gaps. Indian J Nutr. 2017;4(3).
20. Casey CF, Slawson DC, Neal LR. Vitamin D supplementation in infants, children, and adolescents. Am Fam Physician. 2010;81(6):745-8.
21. Centers for Disease Control and Prevention. (2022). Nutrition. [online]

Available from: https://www.cdc.gov/nutrition/micronutrient-malnutrition/micronutrients/index.html [Last accessed November, 2023].
22. Liu E, Pimpin L, Shulkin M, Kranz S, Duggan CP, Mozaffarian D, et al. Effect of zinc supplementation on growth outcomes in children under 5 years of age. Nutrients. 2018;10(3):377.
23. Abdollahi M, Ajami M, Abdollahi Z, Kalantari N, Houshiarrad A, Fozouni F, et al. Zinc supplementation is an effective and feasible strategy to prevent retardation in 6 to 24 month children: a pragmatic, double blind randomised trial. Helyon. 2019;5(11):e02581.
24. National Institutes of Health. Office of Dietary Supplements. (2022). Zinc. [online] Available from: https://ods.od.nih.gov/factsheets/Zinc-HealthProfessional/ [Last accessed November, 2023].
25. Gashu D, Stoecker BJ, Bougma K, Adish A, Haki GD, Marquis GS. Stunting, selenium deficiency, and anemia are associated with poor cognitive performance in preschool children from rural Ethiopia. Nutr J. 2015;15:38.
26. Centers for Disease Control and Prevention. (2023). Trace elements: Selenium. [online] Available from: https://www.cdc.gov/nutritionreport/pdf/nr_ch4b.pdf [Last accessed November, 2023].
27. National Institutes of Health. Office of Dietary Supplements. (2021). Selenium. [online] Available from: https://ods.od.nih.gov/factsheets/Selenium-HealthProfessional/ [Last accessed November, 2023].

SECTION 2
Methods of Infant and Young Child Feeding

10. **Mother–Baby-Friendly Environment**
    Ramesh R Pol, Shivanand I, Ganashree B, Durgappa H

11. **Kangaroo Mother Care**
    Abhishek S Aradhya, Kanya Mukhopadhyay

12. **Breastfeeding Technique**
    Suman Rao PN, Durgappa H

13. **Feeding in Preterm and Low Birthweight Infants**
    Manisha Bhandankar, Tanmaya Metgud, Durgappa H

14. **Breastfeeding and Working Mother**
    Shrikanth Kulkarni, Anu Sachdeva

15. **Breastfeeding and Maternal Medications**
    Sandeep R, Madhu B Jagalasar

16. **Complementary Feeding**
    KV Raghunath, Vishwanath B, Durgappa H

17. **Functional Gastrointestinal Disorders in Infants and Toddlers**
    B Shantharam Baliga, Jayashree K, Durgappa H

CHAPTER 10

Mother–Baby-Friendly Environment

Ramesh R Pol, Shivanand I, Ganashree B, Durgappa H

"There is a world of difference between insisting on someone's doing something and establishing an atmosphere in which that person can grow into wanting to do it."
—**Fred Rogers**

INTRODUCTION

Feeding the infant is the most important bonding factor in the journey of motherhood. It is a learned skill which requires patience and practice and is one of the important determinants of child health, development, nutrition, and survival. Breastfeeding is emotionally satisfying and relaxing to the mother because of release of oxytocin, which reduces stress levels in the mother and increase the bonding behavior to her baby. However for some mothers, breastfeeding can become demanding, physically exhausting, and uncomfortable at times. Most of the primigravida mothers experience doubts about their ability to care for a newborn. Successful breastfeeding requires education, support, and good atmosphere that values and understands breastfeeding.

Mother needs to be happy and relaxed while feeding her baby and make breastfeeding a joyful experience. Such atmosphere can be created by adequate sleep and nutrition of mother, physical activity, and being surrounded by supportive people.

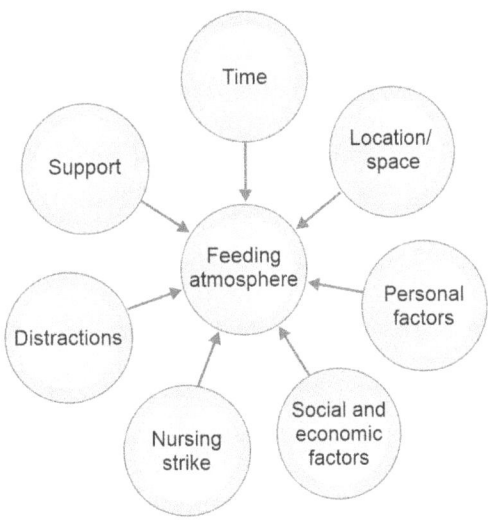

Fig.1: Factors influencing feeding atmosphere.

Critical factors that are important are maternal employment, maternal role satisfaction, maternal nutrition, family stability, paternal attitude toward maternal employment, and the quality of time spent with the children[1] **(Fig. 1)**.

Nursing mothers who play a vital role in household chores may find it challenging to devote adequate time for their newborn as well as for themselves. Moreover, a working mother must balance her personal and professional life while taking care of her newborn, which adds on to the stress. Many women express guilt of having not been able to take care of the baby sufficiently. The flexible working hours with limited hours for work with adequate breaks for feeding would favor the nursing environment. Adequate space for both mother and child with proper ventilation and lighting is ideal. Overcrowding should be avoided. Mothers feel that home is the best place to have good nursing/feeding atmosphere. Privacy for feeding is necessary and provides comfort, especially at workplaces and public places (e.g., restaurants, feeding lounges at fuel stations, railway stations, bus stations, etc.).

The overall support to mother should be started from antenatal period with positive reinforcement during antenatal visit in the form of counseling of the mother, father, and other family members by healthcare professionals regarding exclusive breastfeeding and importance of breast milk.[2] The distractions in the form of prelacteal feeds and advertisements of formula feed have to be discouraged. Education material which is noncommercial and without advertising breast milk substitutes, bottles, or nipples should be shared with mother.

Personal and socioeconomic factors such as uncomfortable feeling while feeding in public places surrounded by strangers and feeling of not having sufficient milk synthesis can hinder breastfeeding practice. Other factors such as physical pain, discomfort, and health problems of mother are associated with poor feeding.[3] Marital issues and multiple births (twins/triplets) also affect the feeding atmosphere, especially in nuclear family. Most of the Indian mothers hesitate to breastfeed their babies at public places.[3] Babies of working mothers at times are not breastfed because of unavailability of mother and other issues associated with work stress.

A nursing strike is when a baby refuses to breastfeed after nursing well for few weeks or months. The common causes are illness, pain or discomfort, strange taste or odor, distractions, stuffy nose, recently changed nursing pattern, and sore gums during teething.

FACTORS CREATING IDEAL FEEDING ATMOSPHERE

Ideal feeding atmosphere is created by the following factors:

At Hospital

Establish a written Baby-Friendly Hospital Initiative (BFHI) hospital policy. Educate the mother and family about the importance of breast milk and breastfeeding. Display appropriate educational materials such as pictures, magazines, posters, and large photos of breastfeeding mothers from variety of ethnic and cultural backgrounds at-hospital reception area, in wards, etc. The educational material containing newborn growth patterns, feeding, and sleep patterns of breastfed babies would impact the mother. It is also advised to educate the mother about management of growth spurts, recognition of hunger and satiety cues, latch-on and positioning, management of sore nipples, mastitis, blocked ducts, engorgement, reflux, normal stooling and voiding patterns, maintaining lactation when separated from the infant (e.g., during illness, prematurity, and return to work), postpartum depression, maternal medication use, and maternal illness during breastfeeding.[4,5]

Peer counseling is useful in postnatal care (PNC) wards and when baby is admitted in neonatal intensive care unit (NICU). Mother feels more comfortable by exchanging her feeding information with peers from similar ethnic and cultural backgrounds.

At Home

At home, a separate room needs to be earmarked for mother and baby during the antenatal period itself, where the mother feels comfortable and relaxed. Further, that room can be decorated with relevant mother and baby pictures; playing of relaxing music and peaceful atmosphere can help the mother relax completely. Support of family members is of immense help in the form of accompanying the mother for newborn baby care and taking care of other children in the family.

At Workplace

Women work in both formal (offices, hospitals, educational institutes, and factories) and informal sectors (farms, streets, markets, and construction sites). Hence, mother-friendly workplace and separate, identified breastfeeding locations make a huge difference in the baby care. Private facilities or space with creches, comfortable chairs, and mini refrigerator for storage of expressed breast milk will be favorable in newborn care.

The support of employers is important to encourage breastfeeding employees by providing guidance on the facilities necessary to ensure that this is possible through various incentives such as flexible hours, time off, and facilities for breastfeeding or expressing and storing breast milk.[6]

At Public Place

The priority of the mother is to breast feed when the baby is hungry, irrespective of the place and surrounding. The scarf or nursing cover can be used while feeding in public areas to maintain privacy, while care is to be taken to not create too hot temperature and supervise for comfortable breathing of the baby.

■ KEY MESSAGES

- Breastfeeding is a physiological norm.
- "Mother–baby friendly environment" is critical to establish successful breastfeeding practice in health care centers, workplaces, and public places.
- Collective societal responsibility is essential in promotion of breastfeeding.

■ REFERENCES

1. Employment and away from home activities while breastfeeding. In: Lawrence RA, Lawrence RM (Eds). Breastfeeding: A Guide for the Medical Profession, 8th edition. Philadelphia: Elsevier; 2016. pp. 650-66.
2. World Health Organization. Protecting, promoting, and supporting breastfeeding in facilities providing maternity and newborn services. Geneva: World Health Organization; 2017.
3. Kong SKF, Lee DTF. Factors influencing decision to breastfeed. J Adv Nurs. 2004;46(4): 369-79.
4. The Breastfeeding-Friendly Medical Office. In: Schanler RJ (Ed). Breastfeeding Handbook for Physicians, 2nd edition. Washington DC: American Academy of Pediatrics; 2014. pp. 229-30.
5. Protocol 14: Breastfeeding Friendly Physician's Office, Part 1: Optimizing Care for Infants and Children. In: Lawrence RA, Lawrence RM (Eds). Breastfeeding: A Guide for the Medical Profession, 8th edition. Philadelphia: Elsevier; 2016. pp. 897-900.
6. World Health Organization. (2015). National breastfeeding policy and action plan 2015-2020. [online] Available from: https://extranet.who.int/nutrition/gina/en/node/23607# [Last accessed November, 2023].

CHAPTER 11

Kangaroo Mother Care

Abhishek S Aradhya, Kanya Mukhopadhyay

"Mothers and babies form an inseparable biological and social unit; the health and nutrition of one group cannot be divorced from the health and nutrition of the other".
—**World Health Organization**

INTRODUCTION

Kangaroo mother care (KMC) is the most cost-effective strategy for the care of premature and low birth weight (LBW) babies, especially in low-middle-income countries with resource-limited settings. Immediate uninterrupted skin-to-skin contact between mother and baby has profound positive effect on neonatal outcome. KMC has been known to reduce mortality by 40%, among hospitalized patients with birth weight <2 kg, started when they are clinically stable. Recent studies have demonstrated that immediate KMC between mother and baby is associated with further 25% reduction in the neonatal mortality. Therefore, it is critical to establish mother and newborn intensive care unit (ICU) to support KMC practices.[1]

In India, premature and LBW babies account for 28% of total deliveries. One in every seven babies born globally is a LBW (<2,500 g) baby.[2] LBW babies are either born too early (preterm) or have intrauterine growth retardation (IUGR). LBW babies have inherent challenges with temperature regulation, infections, feeding difficulties, growth delay, neurodevelopmental delay, and thereby higher risk of morbidity and mortality. These babies require special care in the hospital with anticipation of morbidities as mentioned earlier in the form of intensive care, warmth (warmer/incubator), etc., adding a cost burden for the caregivers. KMC offers an effective solution to most of it. Dr Edgar Rey and Dr Hector Martinez first conceptualized KMC in neonates at Bogota (Columbia) way back in 1978 as an alternative to providing warmth instead of an incubator in resource-limited settings. KMC involves providing early, prolonged, and continuous skin-to-skin contact for LBW babies by either mother or other caregiver for optimum growth and development. Almost four decades from its conception, KMC is now a standard of care for LBW not only for giving warmth but also to provide nutrition, neurosensory stimulation, and prevention of nosocomial infections irrespective of the settings.

COMPONENTS OF KANGAROO MOTHER CARE

Kangaroo mother care involves the following three major components:[3]
1. Kangaroo position
2. Kangaroo feeding policy
3. Kangaroo early discharge and follow-up.

Kangaroo Position

The baby is placed vertically in between the mother's breasts, chest-to-chest. The baby's head is slightly extended and turned to one side. Avoid either hyperextension or forward flexion of the head. Hips are abducted, flexed in a "frog position" and arms should be flexed. The baby's abdomen should not be compressed and should be at the mother's epigastrium with enough room for abdominal breathing **(Fig. 1)**. Mother's breathing will also stimulate the baby. With this position, the baby's eyes can see mother, smell breast milk, feed on milk, listen to the mother's voice, and warmth is obtained through the skin. Thus, KMC provides early stimulation for all the sense organs of the baby. The mother can either sit on a semi-reclining chair or sleep on a bed with adjustable bed rest. Avoid supine posture as it can cause reflux and vomiting.

Avoid interruptions of skin-to-skin contact unless it is necessary, such as changing diapers/mother needing expression of milk, etc. Each session of KMC should be given for not less than 1 hour to avoid the stress of frequent positioning of the baby. With the binder/cloth tied to the mother's chest to secure the baby, the mother can walk, stand, or engage in educational/recreational activities. This mobility can also help longer duration of KMC and make mother's extended stay less boring.

Kangaroo Feeding

The baby can be directly breastfed depending on the baby's gestation or clinical condition while in kangaroo position. Otherwise, gavage feeds can be given during the session.

Kangaroo Early Discharge and Follow-Up

Early discharge is one of the key components of KMC as warmth is taken care for the LBW baby by KMC and if there is adequate weight gain in hospital. Follow-up is required to ensure adequate growth and to continue support to the mother for KMC and breastfeeding.

BENEFITS OF KANGAROO MOTHER CARE

During KMC, skin-to-skin contact from the mother maintains thermal control of the baby and also provides a source of nutrition by stimulating lactation and early multi-sensory stimulation. Apart from better thermal stability, babies on KMC have shown to have better cardiorespiratory stability, modulation of pain responses, increased duration of quiet sleep, improved cerebral blood flow, etc.[4] A total of 21 studies including 3,042 neonates from the recent Cochrane meta-analysis[5] has shown the following benefits (evidence from Cochrane meta-analysis is summarized in **Box 1**):

- In hospital: Less risk of hypothermia, nosocomial sepsis, and mortality; better exclusive breastfeeding at discharge
- *At latest follow-up:* Better growth and continued effects of better survival, exclusive breastfeeding (even up to 1–3 months), and less sepsis

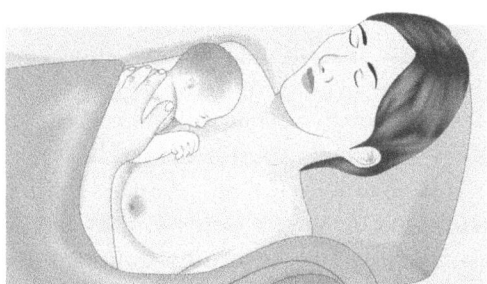

Fig. 1: Kangaroo mother care (including Indian mother).

BOX 1: Benefits of KMC.

Physiological benefits:
- Maintaining thermoneutral temperature (natural incubator)
- Improves exclusive breastfeeding
- Cardiorespiratory stability (HR, RR, and SpO_2)
- Growth and development (improves weight, length, and head circumference)
- Stress and pain relief during minor procedures
- Improved early cognitive performance, learning, and behavior
- Cost-effective, natural, acceptable, feasible, and safe
- Infant survival

Psychological benefits:
- Emotional bonding between mother and baby
- Confidence of the mother
- Competency in the mother and family members
- Parental sensitivity to infant cues
- Positive attitude in mothers toward KMC
- Prevents postpartum psychosis

Clinical benefits:
- Reduced risk of:
  – Hypothermia
  – Hypoglycemia
  – Sepsis
  – NEC
  – Apnea
  – Hospital readmissions
  – Hospital stay and early discharge from the hospital

(HR: heart rate; KMC: kangaroo mother care; NEC: necrotizing enterocolitis; RR: respiratory rate; SpO_2: peripheral oxygen saturation)

Long-term effects of KMC are mediated through multiple factors such as increased physiological stability, decreased infections, reduction of stress and pain, and better exclusive breastfeeding rates. At 1 year of age, a systematic review[6] of 13 studies reported better self-regulation of babies who received KMC compared to controls, while possibly due to heterogeneity of studies, no effect could be demonstrated on cognitive or motor development, socioemotional skills, and temperament. However at 20 years, follow-up from an randomized controlled trial (RCT) cohort[7] (62% from the original RCT cohort) showed children with KMC compared to traditional care had reduced school absenteeism, externalization, aggressiveness, and socio-deviant conduct of young adults. These results indicate that probably KMC mothers were more protective and nurturing. Another outcome reported by this cohort was that KMC children had a larger volume of the left caudate nucleus and linear regression was related to KMC duration, fragility index at birth, and fine motor skills at 20 years.[8] Thus possibly, KMC would have helped these vulnerable neonates to have better compensation or plasticity in the periventricular region to have larger volumes.

ELIGIBILITY FOR KANGAROO MOTHER CARE

Neonate

All stable LBW babies are eligible for KMC. The definition of "stable LBW babies" is not precise and is independent of gestation and weight. Most units initiate KMC once babies are hemodynamically stable, off respiratory support, and with no significant morbidities such as jaundice, umbilical lines, etc. for continuous KMC. Conventionally, KMC is started after stabilization usually after 3 days. Two RCTs including one Indian study has shown KMC can be initiated early (within 3 days) and was associated with better exclusive breast milk feeding postdischarge.[9,10]

Another concern in resource-limited settings is up to two thirds of LBW babies would have died before becoming stable for KMC. With this challenge of survival, the impact of mortality benefit of KMC is estimated to decrease from 40% to just 13% in actual practice in these settings.[11] Hence, short sessions of KMC can be considered for babies with minimal oxygen/continuous positive airway pressure (CPAP) or intravenous (IV) fluids with close monitoring. Limited evidence shows the feasibility of KMC even on ventilation (CPAP/mechanical ventilation) but needs close monitoring with adequate nurses.[9,12,13]

Mother

All mothers can provide KMC. Mothers need to be motivated, free from a serious illness, and maintain good hygiene (wash hands, clean clothes, and daily bath/sponge).

Foster Kangaroo Mother Care

Traditionally, KMC is provided by mothers; however, fathers and other close family members can also be provided with an opportunity to provide continuous skin-to-skin contact with an aim to involve them as part of care of the preterm. Involvement of father becomes essential especially when mother is ill or not available in an outborn unit in the initial days or mother needs a break for food or rest. In an RCT,[14] kangaroo father care (KFC) compared to KMC had similar physiological stability and stress levels of infants as measured by salivary cortisol levels; thus, KFC is feasible and must be encouraged. Likewise, grandmothers or aunts can also provide continuous skin-to-skin contact whenever mother is unavailable.

KANGAROO MOTHER CARE PROCEDURES

Counseling

Follow general principles while counseling—B, ALPAC (build rapport, ask and listen, praise, advice and confirmation from parents). Once a LBW neonate becomes eligible, mother preferably both parents are counseled about KMC. They need to be explained on the positioning, benefits, and dressing requirements. Benefits in addition to growth outcomes such as physiological stability, survival outcomes, and better breastfeeding rates are also stressed. It is also preferable to get them peer counseling with another mother providing KMC to boost the mother's confidence. If any mother is expected to deliver a preterm baby, counseling can start antenatally.

Dress Requirements

Mother needs to wear front open dresses as per local culture. Customized apparels if available can be used to ease ambulation such as Mamma pod (developed by IIT Delhi and AIIMS), KEM kangaroo bag, CAREPLUS wrap (Laerdal), etc. Baby is dressed in a cap, gloves, socks, and a front open shirt with a diaper.

Human Resource for Kangaroo Mother Care

There is no need for an additional staff for providing KMC. It is essential for the same nurse caring for the baby to be aware of eligibility for KMC, able to motivate mothers, and continue monitoring while on KMC.

Positioning and Monitoring

The baby is kept upright between mother's breasts with skin-to-contact in a comfortable position as described earlier. Culturally acceptable privacy standards must be provided for the mother. The baby needs frequent monitoring for temperature (axillary measurement), breathing, and also the neck of the baby need not be too flexed nor too extended. It is preferable to have continuous pulse oximetry monitoring for babies with apnea/respiratory support.

Duration in a Day

Continuous KMC involves providing continuous skin-to-skin contact without breaking except for change of nappy. Intermittent KMC involves practice of skin-to-skin contact alternated with a warmer/incubator. Each session of KMC should be at least for 1 hour. Total daily duration should be minimum 4–6 hours.

Discontinue

Kangaroo mother care can be discontinued once the baby attains term gestation or 2.5 kg weight. Weaning from KMC can also be considered if the baby wriggles (uncomfortable) or becomes fussy and cries on skin-to-skin contact.

KANGAROO MOTHER CARE IN THE COMMUNITY

In hospital, KMC is now standard of care irrespective of settings and has shown to reduce hypothermia, sepsis, and mortality. Most of these babies are discharged early from the hospital to the community. Although there is considerable need and interest in this intervention in the community, there is only limited evidence on its impact in the community. A single RCT in this regard has shown better survival by 28 days (29%) and 6 months of age (24%) in term small for gestational age (SGA) and in late preterm. This community-initiated KMC was delivered to parents through healthcare workers by home visits.[14,15] Although survival was better, the same cohort had no difference in neurodevelopment outcomes by 12 months of age and further long-term data is awaited.[16]

KANGAROO MOTHER CARE IN INDIA—GOVERNMENT POLICIES

Kangaroo mother care is proved well beyond doubt as a low-cost intervention to improve survival. Despite that, global uptake of KMC for eligible babies is <5%.[17] In 2014, as part of India Newborn Action Plan (INAP), KMC was included as a specific intervention to reduce morbidity and mortality. One of the priority actions was to establish special newborn care units (SNCUs) with attached KMC wards (with 8 beds per unit) and KMC coverage target was set to 50% by 2020 and 90% by 2030.[18,19] In 2017 as part of National Health Policy, integrated approach to newborn care through family participatory care (FPC) was piloted at facilities which involved KMC as one of the components.

Out of 712 SNCUs in India in 2017, around 265 had a KMC unit. However, only 15% of these units had recommended 8 beds. Available data indicates in six states that KMC coverage is above 20% in eligible babies, while in remaining states, it ranges between 0 and 20%.[20] There are three main challenges of KMC in the public sector, which are as follows:

1. Motivation of healthcare workers to practice and advocate KMC
2. Another key issue in the public sector is designated spaces for practice of KMC. Apart from funding gaps in existing facilities, there is challenge of identification of space for creation of KMC ward.
3. There is an urgent need to have a KMC indicator as part of Hospital Management Information System (HMIS) of SNCU to capture the actual coverage.

Apart from government initiatives, five major institutes from the country (PGIMER, AIIMS, KEM, IOG (Chennai), and KGMU) are part of KMC India initiative. The objective of this network is to disseminate knowledge and skills to healthcare professionals, guide parents, and to assist in research and generate evidence about feasibility of KMC in the community and healthcare facilities.

CHALLENGES IN EFFECTIVE UTILIZATION OF KANGAROO MOTHER CARE

There are several barriers and enablers for effective utilization of KMC and can be at the level of mothers, nurses, and also at the health system level.[21-24] KMC practices can be audited in the unit to assess performance.

RESEARCH DIRECTIONS

- What is the optimum duration of KMC needed to achieve an impact on neonatal mortality and other critical outcomes?
- What is the optimal follow-up frequency for mothers providing KMC after discharge from the facility?
- Safety of KMC for babies on respiratory support/early initiation of KMC
- Can KMC be effectively initiated and sustained in the community setting?
- What is the best model for implementation of KMC in various settings?

KEY MESSAGES

- KMC has now moved from being an alternative to nonavailability of warming devices to standard-of-care irrespective of the settings.
- KMC not only improves thermal control but also has benefits in terms of improving lactation, greater physiological stability, less nosocomial infections, and thereby better survival.
- The effect of KMC is long lasting, even up to 20 years from the intervention. While the benefits of KMC are proven well beyond doubt in stable LBW, there is also increasing literature to support its use with careful monitoring even in recovering neonates on respiratory support (O_2/CPAP).
- Research needs to focus on effective implementation of KMC at various levels by handling barriers and facilitation of enablers through quality improvement strategies to save lives.

REFERENCES

1. WHO Immediate KMC Study Group. Immediate "kangaroo mother care" and survival of infants with low birth weight. New Engl J Med. 2021;384(21):2028-38.
2. Blencowe H, Krasevec J, de Onis M, Black RE, An X, Stevens GA, et al. National, regional, and worldwide estimates of low birthweight in 2015, with trends from 2000: a systematic analysis. Lancet Glob Health. 2019;7(7):e849-60.
3. World Health Organization. Kangaroo mother care: a practical guide. Department of Reproductive Health and Research, Geneva: World Health Organization; 2003.
4. Nyqvist KH, Anderson GC, Bergman N, Cattaneo A, Charpak N, Davanzo R, et al. Towards universal Kangaroo Mother Care: recommendations and report from the First European conference and Seventh International Workshop on Kangaroo Mother Care. Acta Paediatr. 2010;99(6):820-6.
5. Conde-Agudelo A, Díaz-Rossello JL. Kangaroo mother care to reduce morbidity and mortality in low birth weight infants. Cochrane Database Syst Rev. 2016;8:CD002771.
6. Akbari E, Binnoon-Erez N, Rodrigues M, Ricci A, Schneider J, Madigan S, et al. Kangaroo mother care and infant biopsychosocial outcomes in the first year: A meta-analysis. Early Hum Dev. 2018;122:22-31.
7. Charpak N, Ruiz-Peláez JG, Figueroa de CZ, Charpak Y. A randomized, controlled trial of kangaroo mother care: results of follow-up at 1 year of corrected age. Pediatrics. 2001;108(5):1072-9.
8. Charpak N, Tessier R, Ruiz JG, Hernandez JT, Uriza F, Villegas J, et al. Twenty-year Follow-up of Kangaroo Mother Care Versus Traditional Care. Pediatrics. 2017;139(1):e20162063.

9. Jayaraman D, Mukhopadhyay K, Bhalla AK, Dhaliwal LK. Randomized Controlled Trial on Effect of Intermittent Early Versus Late Kangaroo Mother Care on Human Milk Feeding in low-birth-weight Neonates. J Hum Lact. 2017;33(3):533-9.
10. Nagai S, Andrianarimanana D, Rabesandratana N, Yonemoto N, Nakayama T, Mori R. Earlier versus later continuous Kangaroo Mother Care (KMC) for stable low-birth-weight infants: a randomized controlled trial. Acta Paediatr. 2010;99(6):827-35.
11. World Health Organization (WHO). Maternal, Newborn, Child and Adolescent Health Department Study Protocol. A multi-country randomized clinical trial to evaluate the impact of continuous KMC initiated immediately after birth compared to KMC initiated after stabilization in newborns with birth weight 1.0 to <1.8kg on their survival in low-resource settings. Geneva: World Health Organization; 2018. pp. 1-60.
12. Bisanalli S, Nesargi S, Govindu RM, Rao SP. Kangaroo Mother Care in Hospitalized Low Birth-Weight Infants on Respiratory Support: A Feasibility and Safety Study. Adv Neonatal Care. 2019;19(6):E21-5.
13. Gale G, Franck L, Lund C. Skin-to-skin (kangaroo) holding of the intubated premature infant. Neonatal Netw. 1993;12(6):49-57.
14. Srinath BK, Shah J, Kumar P, Shah PS. Kangaroo care by fathers and mothers: comparison of physiological and stress responses in preterm infants. J Perinatol. 2016;36(5):401-4.
15. Mazumder S, Taneja S, Dube B, Bhatia K, Ghosh R, Shekhar M, et al. Effect of community-initiated kangaroo mother care on survival of infants with low birthweight: a randomised controlled trial. Lancet. 2019;394(10210):1724-36.
16. Taneja S, Sinha B, Upadhyay RP, Mazumder S, Sommerfelt H, Martines J, et al. Community initiated kangaroo mother care and early child development in low birth weight infants in India: a randomized controlled trial. BMC Pediatr. 2020;20(1):1-2.
17. Bhutta ZA, Das JK, Bahl R, Lawn JE, Salam RA, Paul VK, et al. Lancet Newborn Interventions Review Group, Lancet Every Newborn Study Group. Can available interventions end preventable deaths in mothers, newborn babies, and stillbirths, and at what cost. Lancet. 2014;384(9940):347-70.
18. India Ministry of Health and Family Welfare (MOHFW) (2014a). India Newborn Action Plan. [online] Available from: https://nhm.gov.in/index4.php?lang=1&level=0&linkid=153&lid=174 [Last accessed November, 2023].
19. India Ministry of Health and Family Welfare (MOHFW). National Health Mission (2014b). Kangaroo Mother Care and Optimal Feeding of Low Birth Weight Infants: Operational Guidelines. [online] Available from: https://nhm.gov.in/images/pdf/programmes/child-health/guidelines/Operational_Guidelines-KMC_&_Optimal_feeding_of_Low_Birth_Weight_Infants.pdf [Last accessed November, 2023].
20. USAID Maternal and Child Survival Program. (2019). Kangaroo Mother Care in India. [online] Available from: https://www.mcsprogram.org/wp-content/uploads/dlm_uploads/2019/01/India-KAP-Summary-Sheet.pdf [Last accessed November, 2023].
21. Seidman G, Unnikrishnan S, Kenny E, Myslinski S, Cairns-Smith S, Mulligan B, et al. Barriers and enablers of kangaroo mother care practice: a systematic review. PLoS One. 2015;10(5):e0125643.
22. Vesel L, Bergh A-M, Kerber KJ, Valsangkar B, Mazia G, Moxon SG, et al. Kangaroo mother care: a multi-country analysis of health system bottlenecks and potential solutions. BMC Pregnancy Childbirth. 2015;15 (Suppl 2):S5.
23. Chan G, Bergelson I, Smith ER, Skotnes T, Wall S. Barriers and enablers of kangaroo mother care implementation from a health systems perspective: a systematic review. Health Policy Plan. 2017;32(10):1466-75.
24. Cattaneo A, Amani A, Charpak N, De Leon-Mendoza S, Moxon S, Nimbalkar S, et al. Report on an international workshop on Kangaroo mother care: lessons learned and a vision for the future. BMC Pregnancy Childbirth. 2018;18:170.

CHAPTER 12

Breastfeeding Technique

Suman Rao PN, Durgappa H

"Breastfeeding—A confidence trick"
—**World Health Organization**

■ INTRODUCTION

Breastfeeding is a physiological norm for optimal health of infants and young children. The World Health Organization (WHO) has recommended exclusive breastfeeding for 6 months, continued breastfeeding up to 2 years or beyond, and appropriate, adequate, safe complementary feeding at 6 months.[1]

■ MAGNITUDE OF THE PROBLEM

Recent data has shown that only 37% of infants are exclusively breastfed below 6 months of age and 20% of infants are never breastfed across the globe.[2] In India, only 63% of infants are exclusively breastfed below 6 months of age.[3]

Though most mothers have determination to breastfeed their babies, they often find difficulties at initiation and maintenance of breastfeeding. Recent evidence shows that half of the primiparous women find difficulty at initiation of breastfeeding in the postpartum period. Hence, it is important to ensure "mother–baby-friendly environment" and "timely skilled practical assistance and support" which will facilitate the breastfeeding practices.[4]

■ TECHNIQUE OF BREASTFEEDING

The mothers can attain any comfortable position to breastfeed their baby according to their convenience and comfort. The correct method of breastfeeding includes proper position of the mother and baby and support to breast. The proper *positioning and latching* on to breast is the most fundamental step in the establishment of effective breastfeeding practices.[5]

- *Position of the mother:* Mother can sit comfortably on armless chair with back straight and foot resting on the footrest with cushion pillow to support the baby.
- *Position of the baby:* Hold the baby as close to abdomen as possible, in aligned position with whole body supported, without causing the twisting of the head. Keep the hand of the baby by the side of the mother so that it does not come in the way of feeding. Baby's face should be facing the breast and nose should be in front of the nipple.
- *Breast support:* Support the breast with other hand while feeding the baby. Then initiate the rooting reflex with the help of nipple. The moment baby opens the

mouth you bring the baby to the breast instead of bending yourself toward the baby and make sure that signs of good attachment are achieved.[5]

Signs of good attachment[5,6] (Figs. 1A to D)

- Baby's mouth should be wide open
- Lower lip is turned outward
- Chin touching the breast
- Only upper portion of the areola is visible.

In most circumstances, good attachment can be achieved. However in certain situations, mothers may find difficulty in getting good attachment. The common causes for not latching on include delayed initiation of breastfeeding, prelacteal feeds administration, difficult deliveries, nipple confusion, bottle-feeding, pacifiers use, flat or retracted nipple, lack of technical assistance and support, lack of confidence, negative attitude of the mother toward lactation and baby's factors such as tongue tie, cleft lip, and palate, neuromotor incoordination disorders, nursing strike, oral thrush, spasm of jaw muscles, and maternal separation.[7] It is also important to predict the problems of breastfeeding in the mother which can be assessed by "Latch score".

Latch Score

Latch score is a useful tool to predict the duration of breastfeeding and identify the problems of breastfeeding both in mother and baby so that appropriate interventions can be initiated before discharge. Latch score

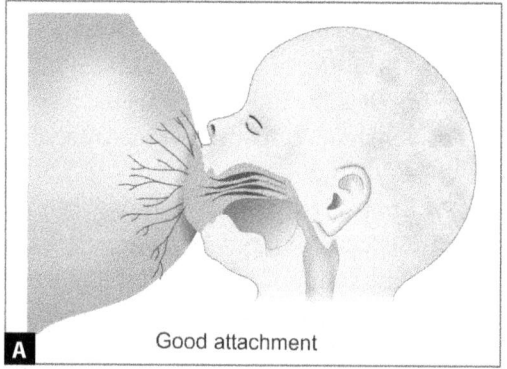 Good attachment

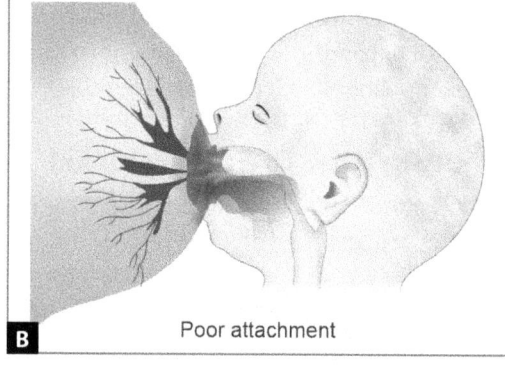 Poor attachment

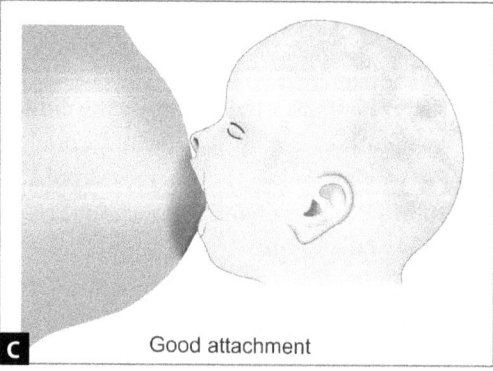 Good attachment

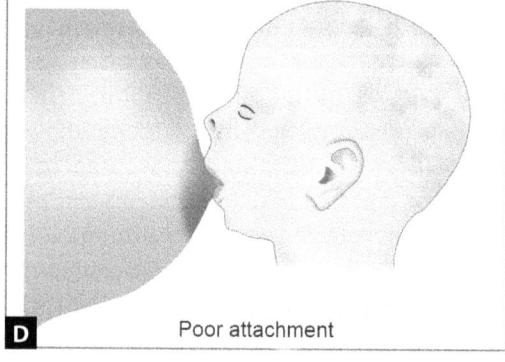 Poor attachment

Figs. 1A to D: Good attachment and poor attachment.

is assessed between 8 and 48 hours of delivery. If the score is >8, this infers there is high chance of exclusive breastfeeding for next 6 months of age and if score is <8, this infers mother is having difficulty in feeding the baby and needs intervention at this point of time.[8] For details, refer to **Table 1**.

HOW LONG TO FEED THE BABY?

Once good latching is achieved, continue to breastfeed the baby for 10–15 minutes so that baby gets both foremilk and hindmilk, then switch over to other side of the breast and continue to feed the baby for 10–15 minutes. The total duration of breastfeeding should be 20–30 minutes. It is also important to burp the baby for 10–15 minutes or till swallowed air is expelled out. Practice baby-led feeding. Then assess for adequacy of breast milk secretion in the baby and mother and mother should also learn to identify and respond to the early signs of hunger cues in the baby.

Signs of Hunger Cues

The early feeding cues include sucking movements and sucking sounds, hand-to-mouth movements, rapid eye movements, soft cooing or sighing sounds, lip smacking, and baby becoming restless. In case of premature babies, it is important to ensure feeding every 2 hourly as in the initial days of delivery, these babies may not exhibit the signs of hunger cues and it is also important to note that "cry is the late sign of hunger" and hence, one should not be waiting till baby cries.[9] *Make sure that mother is getting adequate milk secretion and there is adequate milk transfer to baby.*

- *Assessment of adequacy of breast milk secretion:* One can indirectly assess the adequacy of breast milk secretion in both baby and mother.[7]
- *Assessment in the baby:* If the baby is passing urine more than six times, stool frequency is more than three times in 24

TABLE 1: Latch score.

	2	1	0
L Latch	• Grasps breast • Tongue down • Lips flanged • Rhythmic sucking	• Repeated attempts for sustained latch or suck • Hold nipple in mouth • Stimulate to suck	• Too sleepy or reluctant • No latch achieved
A Audible swallowing	Spontaneous, intermittent, and frequent	A few with stimulation	None
T Type of nipple	Everts after stimulation	Flat	Inverted
C Comfort	• Soft • Nontender	• Filling • Reddened/small • Blisters, bruises • Mild/moderate discomfort	Engorged, cracked bleeding, large blisters or bruises, severe discomfort
H Hold	No assist from staff, mother able to position/hold infant	• Minimal assist (i.e., elevate head of bed, place pillows for support) • Teach one side, mother does other • Staffs holds and then mother takes over	Full assist (staff holds infant at breast)

hours and is gaining weight 20–30 g per day—indicates baby is getting adequate milk intake.
- *Assessment in the mother:* One can also assess adequacy of breast milk secretion in the mother. Mother experiences fullness in the breast before feeding the baby. After feeding, breasts become soft and flabby and mother feels thirsty. The mother experiences slight pain during letdown reflex when gush of milk flows and she can also witness the dribbling of milk from other side of the breast and mother can also appreciate deep, slow, and rhythmic swallowing clicking sounds while feeding the baby.[5]

There are various positions/methods of breastfeeding which mother can adapt to feed her baby depending on her comfort. The different methods adapted by the mother include[5] **(Figs. 2 and 3)**:
- *Cradle:* Most commonly practiced method among the mothers
- *Cross cradle:* Second most commonly practiced method
- *Football:* It is a good method to feed the babies, especially in twin deliveries.

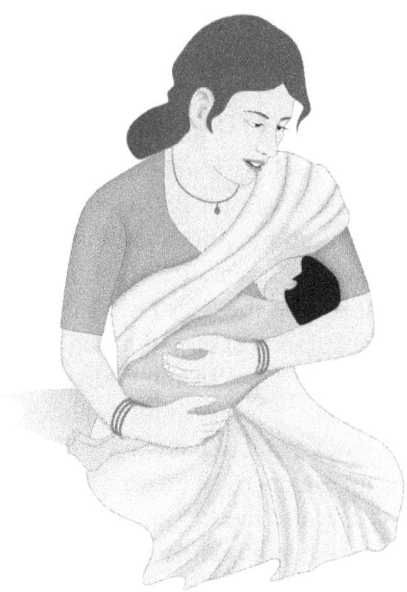

Fig. 2: Breastfeeding in cradle position.

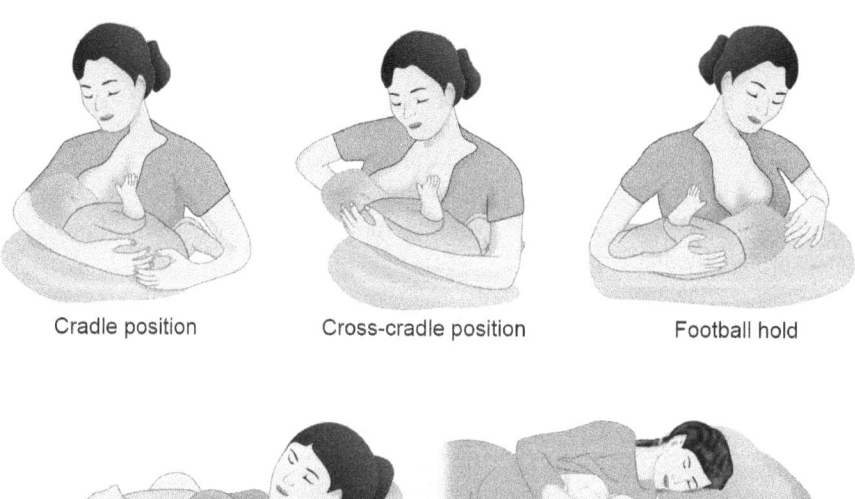

Fig. 3: Breastfeeding in side lying down position.

- *Leaning back:* This method is practiced when mother has undergone cesarean section (C-section) and is having large breast and oversupply of milk.
- *Side lying:* Whenever mother is exhausted and needs rest, she can feed the baby in side lying down position.

It is not uncommon to encounter feeding difficulties in the mothers in the postpartum period. The common situations include excessive crying, not latching well on to the breast, mother is restless, anxious, undergone C-Section, and too small infant to feed.

SOLUTIONS

Family-centered counseling is important. Educate the mother on physiological process of breastfeeding. Not all babies feed at the same time; babies need little time to learn to feed at the breast.[10,11]

Remedies

Comfortable environment is essential to feed the baby. The following steps are to be followed in difficult situations:
- Mothers need to be calm and cool.
- Comfort the baby by cuddling and gentle rocking.
- Attempt to feed when baby is quiet or sleepy in isolated slight dark room.
- If still finding difficulty, do not hesitate to seek the help of healthcare professionals.

Role of HealthCare Professionals

- Build confidence in the mother
- Observe the feeding technique and identify the steps to be corrected
- Praise the mother for good things that she does and do not point out the mistakes of the mother
- Optimize the technique of breastfeeding, i.e., positioning and latching
- In difficult situations, try with supplementary suckling technique (SST)
- Enable mother to express breast milk and feed the baby
- Educate the mother and family members on harmful effects of infant milk substitute

To ensure optimal infant feeding practices, it is always good to have "Breastfeeding Observation Aid Tool" to keep checks on the correct technique of breastfeeding.[12]

BREASTFEED OBSERVATION AID

Mother's name _____   Date_____

Baby's name _____   Baby's age_____

Signs that breastfeeding is going well: *Signs of possible difficulty:*

General:

Mother:
Mother looks healthy
Mother relaxed and comfortable
Signs of bonding between mother and baby

Mother:
Mother looks ill or depressed
Mother looks tense and uncomfortable
No mother/baby eye contact

Baby:
Baby looks healthy
Baby calm and relaxed
Baby reached or roots for breast if hungry

Baby:
Baby looks sleepy or ill
Baby is restless or crying
Baby does not reach or root

Breasts:
Breasts look healthy
No pain or discomfort
Breast well supported with fingers away from nipple
Nipple protractile

Breast look red, swollen, or sore
Breast or nipple painful
Breasts held with fingers and areola

Nipple flat, not retractile

Baby's position:
Baby's head and body in line
Baby held close to mother's body
Baby's whole body supported
Baby approaches breast, nose to nipple

Baby's neck and head twisted to feed
Baby not held close
Baby supported by head and neck only
Baby approaches breast, lower lip/chin to nipple

Baby's attachment:
More areola seen above the baby's top lip
Baby's mouth wide open
Lower lip turned outward
Baby's chin touches the breast

More areola seen below bottom lip
Baby's mouth not wide open
Lips pointing forward or turned in
Baby's chin not touching the breast

Suckling:
Slow, deep sucks with pauses
Cheeks round when suckling
Baby releases breast when finished
Mother notices signs of oxytocin reflex

Rapid shallow sucks
Cheeks pulled in when suckling
Mother takes baby off the breast
No signs of oxytocin reflex noticed

KEY MESSAGES

- Antenatal counseling on benefits of breastfeeding is important.
- Mother–baby-friendly environment facilitates for early initiation of breastfeeding.
- Early skin-to-skin contact between mother and baby enhances the rates of exclusive breastfeeding practices.
- Proper positioning and latching on to the breast is the fundamental step in the establishment of successful breastfeeding.
- Timely technical assistance and support is critical.
- Practice baby-led feeding and learn to identify hunger cues.
- Building the confidence in the mother is most important.

REFERENCES

1. World Health Organization. Guideline: protecting, promoting, and supporting breastfeeding in facilities providing maternity and newborn services. Geneva: World Health Organization; 2017.
2. Victora CG, Bahl R, Barros AJ, França GV, Horton S, Krasevec J, et al. Breastfeeding in the 21st century: epidemiology, mechanisms, and lifelong effect. Lancet. 2016;387(10017):475-90.
3. Bhatia N, Rathi K, Arora C, Choedon T, Rajurkar P, Thakur R, et al. (2022). Analysis of Key Nutrition Indicators Based on National Family Health Survey, NFHS 4 (2015-16) and NFHS 5 (2019-2021). [online] Available from: https://osf.io/r9ybf/ [Last accessed November, 2023].
4. World Health Organization. (2020). Protecting, promoting, and supporting breastfeeding in facilities providing maternity and newborn services: the revised Baby-Friendly Hospital Initiative: 2018 implementation guidance: frequently asked questions. [online] Available from: https://www.who.int/publications/i/item/9789240001459 [Last accessed November, 2023].
5. World Health Organization (WHO). Essential newborn care and breastfeeding: training modules. Copenhagen: WHO Regional Office for Europe; 2002.
6. Zakarija-Grković I, Šegvić O, Božinović T, Ćuže A, Lozančić T, Vučković A, et al. Hospital practices and breastfeeding rates before and after the UNICEF/WHO 20-hour course for maternity staff. J Hum Lact. 2012;28(3):389-99.
7. Neifert MR. Breastmilk transfer: positioning, latch-on, and screening for problems in milk transfer. Clin Obstet Gynecol. 2004;47(3):656-75.
8. Sowjanya SV, Venugopalan L. LATCH score as a predictor of exclusive breastfeeding at 6 weeks postpartum: a prospective cohort study. Breastfeed Med. 2018;13(6):444-9.
9. Tiwari S, Bharadva K, Yadav B, Malik S, Gangal P, Banapurmath CR, et al. Infant and young child feeding guidelines, 2016. Indian Pediatr. 2016;53(8):703-13.
10. Widström AM, Brimdyr K, Svensson K, Cadwell K, Nissen E. Skin-to-skin contact the first hour after birth, underlying implications and clinical practice. Acta Paediatr. 2019;108(7):1192-204.
11. Aryeetey R, Dykes F. Global implications of the new WHO and UNICEF implementation guidance on the revised Baby-Friendly Hospital Initiative. Matern Child Nutr. 2018;14(3):e12637.
12. Puapornpong P, Raungrongmorakot K, Suksamarnwong M, Ketsuwan S, Wongin S. The validity and reliability of the breastfeed observation aid in the exclusive breastfeeding predictions at six weeks postpartum. J Med Assoc Thai. 2018;101(7):919-24.

CHAPTER 13

Feeding in Preterm and Low Birthweight Infants

Manisha Bhandankar, Tanmaya Metgud, Durgappa H

"Being at the breast reminds the baby of being in the womb: there's that familiar heartbeat and soothing voice, as well as the warmth and comfort. And that makes the transition to the outside world a little easier"

—Jack Newman

◼ INTRODUCTION

Low birthweight (LBW) is an important risk factor contributing to high perinatal mortality and long-term morbidity. LBW neonates weigh <2,500 g and are further classified as "Very low birth weight" if they weigh <1,500 g and "Extremely low birth weight" if weighing <1,000 g at birth. These neonates can be result of preterm birth (before completion of 37 weeks), small for gestational age (SGA) (<10th centile weight for gestation), or both.

Approximately 8 million newborns are delivered LBW in India every year contributing to 18% of total birth as per the National Family Health Survey (NFHS)-5 (Year 2019-21).[1] Previous chapters have already highlighted the importance, benefits, and role of exclusive breastfeeding in newborns. In this chapter, we will discuss current recommendations with regards to feeding LBW and Preterm infants. Most of these recommendations are from the Clinical Practice Guidelines prepared by the National Neonatology Forum in January, 2020.[2]

Feeding in small vulnerable newborn (SVN) babies; preterm, LBW, and small for gestation is particularly challenging due to various maternal factors, immature sucking and swallowing reflexes and coordination, baby's specific nutritional needs, and limitations with feed tolerance after birth. This chapter discusses the type of milk, timing, quantity, and modes of feeding among LBW infants.[3]

◼ GENERAL PRINCIPLES

All neonates are required to be breastfed immediately after birth to induce lactation, prevent hypoglycemia, and establish mother-and-baby bonding. LBW and preterm neonates are in particular at higher risk of hypoglycemia due to lower glycogen stores in the liver at birth. Clinically stable LBW neonates weighing >1,800 g and more than 34 weeks' gestation can be managed at mother's side immediately after birth provided, they are adequately fed and closely monitored for hypoglycemia and temperature maintenance. Among LBW neonates born by cesarean section, it is likely that mother may not be able to start breastfeeding immediately after birth. In such cases, available suitable options should be adopted.

Which milk?
Currently, we have three options for neonates:
1. MOM: Mother's Own Milk
2. DHM: Donor Human Milk
3. Formula Milk.

Low birthweight infants including those with very low birth weight (VLBW) and Extremely low birth weight (ELBW) should be fed MOM. Those, who cannot be fed mother's own milk should be fed DHM (recommendation relevant for settings where safe and affordable milk-banking facilities are available or can be set up). Those who cannot be fed MOM or DHM should be fed standard infant formula (recommendation relevant for resource-limited settings).

Very low birthweight infants who cannot be fed mother's own milk or donor human milk should be given preterm infant formula if they fail to gain weight, despite adequate feeding with standard infant formula. VLBW infants who fail to gain weight despite adequate breast milk feeding should be given human milk fortifiers, (HMF) preferably those that are human milk based.

How?
- *Direct breastfeeding:* Stable LBW infants weighing more than 1,800 g and >34 weeks' gestation
- *Katori/spoon feeding:* Stable LBW and VLBW infants with gestational age >32 weeks. These infants may require additional intravenous (IV) fluids due limited feed tolerance in the first few days.
- *Gavage feeding:* Clinically unstable LBW, VLBW, and ELBW infants may require additional IV fluids to meet their nutritional and fluid demands. Bolus intermittent feeds are well tolerated in most groups.

Gavage feeding in neonates: Neonates who are not mature enough to suck and swallow feed but are stable enough to receive feeds can be started on tube feeds [Neonates with gestational age <32 weeks, late preterm and term neonates with respiratory distress, on continuous positive airway pressure (CPAP) or ventilator].

Placement of tube: Feeding tube can be inserted through oral cavity [orogastric (OG) tube] or nasal cavity [nasogastric (NG) tube]. There is no clear benefit of one route over the other. However, most neonatal units prefer OG tube placement.

Benefits and disadvantages of one route over the other can be discussed.

Length of NG tube/OG tube insertion is calculated by distance from bridge of nose-to-ear lobe and then from ear lobe to midway between xiphisternum and umbilicus (NEMU method).[4] Correct tube placement is checked by first aspirating and then pushing in 2 mL air and listening by stethoscope. Tube feeding lowers sucking function and its motor development in premature neonates.

There is no significant difference in somatic growth and incidence of necrotizing enterocolitis (NEC) between NG or OG feeding methods has been reported.[5] Third hourly feeding is recommended for infants weighing >1,250 g. Those weighing <1,250 g, second hourly feeding can be given. Once the infant is stable and ready for oral feeding, paladai feeding should be introduced.
- *Paladai feeding:* Studies have reported that premature neonates with over 30 weeks of gestational age and physiological stability can be safely fed by paladai and show better weight gain than cup feeding. Cup/paladai feeding is useful for the neonates

who have good swallowing ability but do not have appropriate sucking. It is also recommended for those neonates who cannot be breastfed to stimulate sucking by providing the neonate experience of oral feeding.
- *Oral swabbing:* Application of MOM to oral mucosa in extremely preterm neonates who are on ventilator or clinically unstable have been reported recently.[6] The outcome of the study like prevention of ventilator-associated pneumonia needs elaboration.

When?
Clinically stable LBW infants weighing >1,800 g and are able to breastfeed should be put to the breast as soon as possible after birth. These infants and mothers may need extra support to initiate and establish breastfeeding. The infant may be fed every 2-3 hourly or based on hunger cues.

Stable VLBW infants can be started on gavage or katori feeding within 24 hours of birth. Currently, there is lot of variation in practices for feeding preterm infants between 28 and 32 weeks and birthweight between 1,000 g and 1,500 g. Nangia *et al.* have reported that early total enteral feeding in stable VLBW infants is feasible and safe with decrease in NEC, sepsis, and hospital stay.[7]

MINIMAL ENTERAL NUTRITION

Sucking and swallowing coordination is known to be established between 32 and 34 weeks in preterm infants. Practice of feeding small volume of enteral feeds in order to stimulate development of immature gut is known as "Trophic Feeding" or "Minimal Enteral Nutrition". Initiation of trophic feeding at 10-20 mL/kg in hemodynamically stable VLBW newborns on first day (Expressed breast milk MOM or DHM) and progression of feeds at 20-30 mL/kg every day to reach target feeding at 150-180 mL/kg has not shown increase in the incidence of NEC, feed intolerance (FI), and combined outcome of NEC and FI. Slow feed advancement with delayed establishment of full enteral nutrition has been reported to be associated with increased chances of invasive infection.[8]

Abnormal antenatal Doppler study is a major factor that influences decision regarding early initiation and slow progression of feeds in VLBW and ELBW infants. Early enteral feeding (as early as 24 hours) can be initiated in Reversal of End Diastolic Flow (REDF) if there are no abdominal symptoms and signs.[9] Among preterm SGA babies with <29 weeks of gestation who have AREDF (Absent/Reversal of End Diastolic Flow), extreme caution has to be exercised while advancing feeds during the first 10 days of life.

NON-NUTRITIVE SUCKING

The National Neonatology Forum India recommends non-nutritive sucking (NNS) should be encouraged in preterm VLBW infants admitted in neonatal unit. This can be done in <32 weeks baby by providing sterile pacifier to suck while tube feeding or encouraging baby to suck on empty breast (after expression of milk) before feeding the baby. The World Health Organization (WHO) has recommended NNS as intervention to reduce the time to transition from gavage to full oral feeding, the time to transition from initiation of oral feeding to full oral feeding, and length of hospital stay.

METHOD OF MILK EXPRESSION

Mothers whose preterm infants are admitted in the neonatal unit should be encouraged to use either breast pumps (manual or electric) or perform manual expression as early as possible after birth to stimulate lactation. They should be counseled to regularly to express milk even when the infant is not on complete enteral nutrition to ensure higher volume of expressed breast milk as and when required; they may use manual breast pumps to do sequential expression (i.e., expression from one breast followed by that from the other) in the second week after delivery.

Mother should be sitting comfortably after washing hands. She can place a warm clean towel on the breast and gently massage the breasts till milk starts flowing. Then making a C-shaped hold on the areola of the breast, she gently squeezes the breast tissue simultaneously holding a sterile cup in front of the nipple so that milk can drip in it. Skilled professional support should be provided to lactating mothers whose babies are admitted in neonatal units to establish and sustain breastfeeding.

Low-cost interventions such as breast massage, breast warming, and relaxation techniques should be used to enhance breast milk supply in mothers whose preterm infants are admitted in the neonatal unit.

■ HUMAN MILK SUPPLEMENTS

Multinutrient fortification of breast milk can be initiated in preterm LBW infants with birthweight <1,800 g and receiving enteral feeding of at least 50–80 mL/kg/day.

The VLBW infants should be given vitamin D supplements at a dose ranging from 400 IU to 1,000 IU/day until 6 months of age.

The VLBW infants who are fed MOM or DHM should be given calcium (120–140 mg/kg/day) and phosphorus (60–90 mg/kg/day) supplementation during the first months of life.

The VLBW infants fed MOM or DHM should be given 2–4 mg/kg/day iron supplementation starting at 2 weeks until 6 months of age.

Daily oral vitamin A supplementation and routine zinc supplementation for LBW infants who are fed MOM or DHM is not recommended at the present time, because there is not enough evidence of benefits to support such a recommendation.

How to express breast milk by hand?

- Encourage the mothers to express breast milk by herself.
- Thorough hand washing is important to prevent contamination of expressed milk.
- Let the mother be comfortable in sitting position and hold a wide-mouthed clean container near her breast.
- Massage the breast gently for few minutes. Allow her to lean forward so that gravity is facilitating.
- Put her thumb on her breast above nipple and areola and her first finger on the breast below the nipple and areola, opposite the thumb. She supports the breast with her other fingers. Note that the thumb and index finger are approximately 4 cm from areola across the nipple making a C.
- Press her thumb and first finger slightly inwards toward the chest wall. Use rhythmical backward (Pushing back into chestwall) then forward movements to massage the breast.
- Apply the steady pressure inward toward the chest wall, not toward the nipple.
- Press and release, press and release as shown in the **Figure 1**.
- This should not hurt, if it hurts, the technique is wrong. At first no milk may come, but after pressing few times milk starts to drip out. It may flow in streams if the oxytocin reflex is active.
- Press the areola in the same way from the sides, to make sure that the milk is expressed from all the segments of the breast. She must press on the lactiferous sinuses beneath the areola.

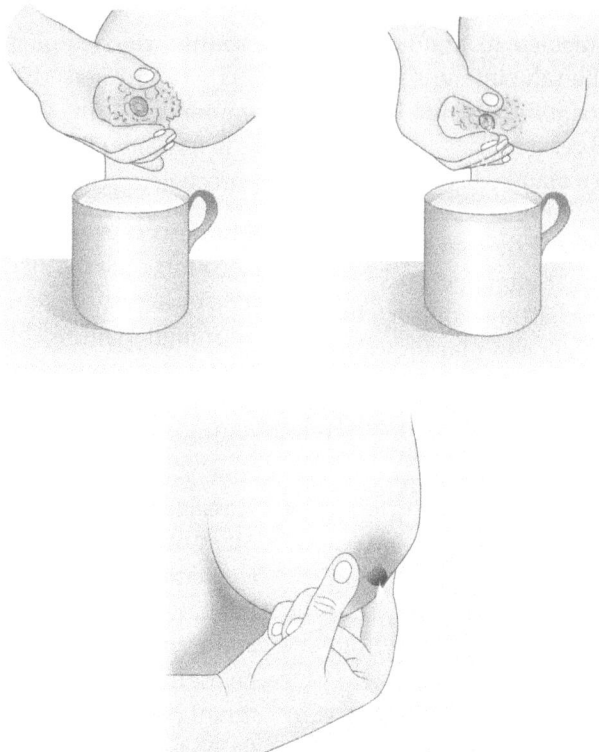

Fig. 1: Manual expression of milk.

- This technique is repeated as the hands rotate around the breast.
- Usually expression of milk from one breast takes around 3–5 minutes after which the milk flow slows, then express from other side and then repeat both sides.
- Avoid squeezing the nipple itself.

KEY MESSAGES

- Mother's Own Milk is the best.
- Minimal enteral nutrition is safe and beneficial with the earlier establishment of feeds, reduced length of stay, and reduced use of parenteral nutrition. Early and rapid enhancement is safe with close monitoring.
- For extremely preterm babies/ELBW, there is no good evidence to support delaying feeds excessively and MEN can be started once baby is hemodynamically stable.
- Stable VLBW babies tolerate early advancement to full feeds.
- In A/REDF, initiate and advance feeding with close monitoring. Optimal duration needed to establish full enteral feeds remains unclear. It should be based on baby's clinical response.

REFERENCES

1. International Institute for Population Sciences (IIPS) and ICF. (2021). National Family Health Survey (NFHS-5), 2019-21. [online] Available from: https://dhsprogram.com/pubs/pdf/FR375/FR375.pdf. [Last accessed November, 2023]. [Last accesses 2023].

2. Banait N, Basu S, Desai P, Dutta S, Shah S, Kumar P, et al. (2020). Clinical Practice Guidelines: Feeding of Low Birth Weight Neonates. [online] Available from: https://www.nnfi.org/assests/pdf/cpg-guidelines/Feeding%20of%20LBW-Key%20Recommendations.pdf. [Last accessed November, 2023]. [Last accesses 2023].
3. Hofmeyr GJ, Black RE, Rogozińska E, Heuer A, Walker N, Ashorn P, et al. Evidence-based antenatal interventions to reduce the incidence of small vulnerable newborns and their associated poor outcomes. Lancet. 2023 May;401(10389):1733-44.
4. Ziemer M, Carroll JS. Infant gavage reconsidered. Am J Nurs. 1978;78(9):1543-4.
5. Wang Y, Zhu W, Luo BR. Continuous feeding versus intermittent bolus feeding for premature infants with low birth weight: a meta-analysis of randomized controlled trials. Eur J Clin Nutr. 2019:1-9.
6. Maffei D, Brewer M, Codipilly C, Weinberger B, Schanler RJ. Early oral colostrum administration in preterm infants. J Perinatol. 2020;40(2):284-7.
7. Nangia S, Vadivel V, Thukral A, Saili A. Early total enteral feeding versus conventional enteral feeding in stable very-low-birth-weight infants: a randomised controlled trial. Neonatology. 2019;115(3):256-62.
8. Oddie SJ, Young L, McGuire W. Slow advancement of enteral feed volumes to prevent necrotising enterocolitis in very low birth weight infants. Cochrane Database Syst Rev. 2017;8(8):CD001241.
9. Aradhya AS, Mukhopadhyay K, Saini SS, Sundaram V, Dutta S, Kumar P. Feed intolerance in preterm neonates with antenatal reverse end diastolic flow (REDF) in umbilical artery: a retrospective cohort study. J Matern Fetal Neonatal Med. 2020;33(11):1846-52.

CHAPTER 14

Breastfeeding and Working Mother

Shrikanth Kulkarni, Anu Sachdeva

"While breastfeeding may not seem the right choice for every parent, it is the best choice for every baby."

—Amy Spangler

INTRODUCTION

The first 1,000 days of life (270 days of the intrauterine period and the first two years of age) are critical for nutritional intervention. Poor nutrition during this period increases the risk of infections, recurrent hospitalizations, malnutrition, and subsequent abnormal neurodevelopment, thus growing morbidity and mortality in children. Exclusive breastfeeding is to be given for 6 months, followed by its continuation with complementary feeds for a minimum of 2 years since maximum brain growth occurs during this period.

Suboptimal breastfeeding contributes to >8 million infant deaths, and countries lose >$300 billion annually because of low breastfeeding rates.[1] Globally, only 41% of infants are exclusively breastfed till 6 months of age, and breastfeeding rates decrease further with increasing infant age. The World Health Organization (WHO) has set a target of achieving at least a 50% exclusive breastfeeding rate by 2025. One of the recommended action plans is to empower women by giving them 6 months of paid maternity leave and having a policy that encourages them to breastfeed in the workplace and in public.[1] Global prevalence of breastfeeding at 12 months is highest in low-middle-income countries (LMICs) like sub-Saharan Africa, South Asia, and parts of Latin America (variable from 60% to 90%). In most high-income countries, the prevalence of breastfeeding at 12 months of age is <20%.[2]

According to the Indian National Family Health Survey-5 (2019-21), exclusive breastfeeding in children's feeding practices have improved except for the percentage of children younger than 3 years who were breastfed within an hour of birth, which remains unchanged from NFHS-4. The most significant improvement is in the rate of exclusively breastfed children under 6 months—from 55% in NFHS-4 to 64% in NFHS-5 **(Fig. 1)**. As the infant's age increases, the proportion of infants, who are not at all receiving breastfeeding, reduces. Returning to work too soon is a significant barrier to exclusive breastfeeding in the first 6 months and continuation of breastfeeding until the age of 2 years or longer.[3]

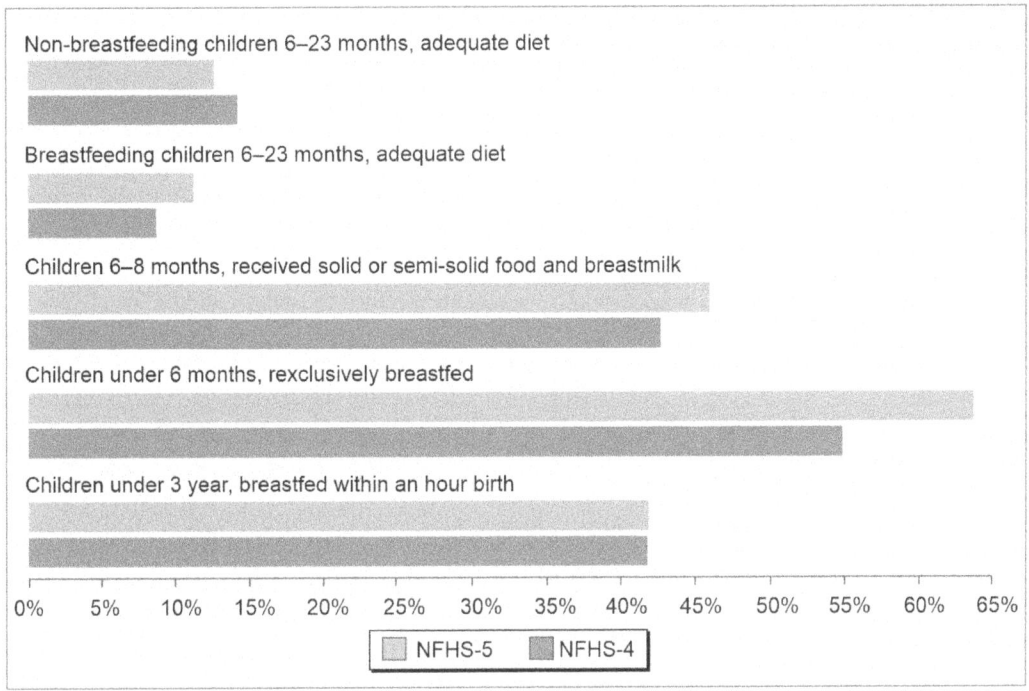

Fig. 1: Breastfeeding practices by age (NFHS-5). (NFHS-5: National Family Health Survey-5)

Most countries have maternity protection legislation, but only 53% (98/185) meet the International Labor Organization of minimum 14-week maternity leave, and only 23% meet or exceed their commendation of 18 weeks' leave.[4] An analysis of breastfeeding policies in the workplace in 182 countries showed that breastfeeding breaks with pay were guaranteed in 71%, unpaid breaks in 4%, and the rest, 25%, had no policy.[5] A study that evaluated breastfeeding practices among working women in South India demonstrated that only 11% of mothers exclusively breastfed for 6 months; significant barriers for low exclusive breastfeeding rates were shorter duration of maternity leave and non-availability of crèches.[6] Another study suggested that mothers working in informal sectors face multiple challenges to maintaining breastfeeding due to the lack of maternity benefits.[7] Data from Taiwan suggests that only 10.6% of mothers continue to breastfeed after returning to work, whereas the data from Indonesia is much better (62.5%).[8]

World Breastfeeding Week 2023 theme was "Enabling Breastfeeding: *Making a difference for working parents.*" The WHO and the United Nations International Children's Emergency Fund (UNICEF) advised all establishments (Government and private) to adopt family-friendly policies to improve breastfeeding rates among working women. Family-friendly policies include paid maternity leave for mothers and better breastfeeding practices at the workplace. Maternity leave helps mothers bond with their infants in early life and improves their exclusive breastfeeding rates. Mothers require time off from work to recover from birth and establish breastfeeding. When the breastfeeding mother returns to work, a continuation of breastfeeding will depend on

BOX 1: Barriers to breastfeeding in working mothers.
- Return to work too soon
- Feeling insecure or guilty about improper feeding to infant
- Unavailability of crèches/baby rooms
- No designated place for breastfeeding or expression of milk
- Prolonged separation from the infant
- Feeding time not coinciding with breaktime
- Lack of time for self
- Short break time
- Work stress
- Maintaining job performance
- Negative reactions of colleagues

having access to breastfeeding breaks; a safe, private, and hygienic space for expressing and storing breast milk; and affordable childcare at or near her workplace.[9] **Box 1** lists the potential barriers to breastfeeding in a working mother.

ADVANTAGES OF BETTER BREASTFEEDING PRACTICES AT THE WORKPLACE[2]

Better breastfeeding practices at the workplace lead to a longer duration of breastfeeding. A supportive work environment increases the exclusive breastfeeding rates and continuation of breastfeeding for 2 years **(Table 1)**.[10]

LAW RELATED TO IMPROVING BREASTFEEDING AMONG WORKING WOMEN IN INDIA

Maternal Benefit Act 2017[11]

This act was an amendment to the Maternity Benefit Act 1961 and is effective from April 2017. This act protects the women's employment during her maternity leave and provides her maternity benefit, full paid absence from work. This applies to all establishments of 10 or more employees. The following are the amendments to the act:

- To increase working women's maternity leave from 12 weeks to 26 weeks for the first two children. This can be availed 8 weeks before delivery and rest after childbirth. For mothers with two or more alive children benefit will be for 12 weeks.
- Maternity leave of 12 weeks for mothers adopting a child below 3 months of age and to the "commissioning mothers". The commissioning mother is a biological mother who uses her egg to develop an embryo planted in any other woman.
- *Creche facility:* Establishment with >50 employees to provide a creche for working mothers, and mothers will be allowed to make four visits to the child in the creche during working hours.
- Work from home may be permitted for mothers after 26 weeks' leave if possible.

Eligibility for Maternal Benefit Act 2017
Women must be working in the establishment for at least 80 days in the last 12 months to avail of the benefits.

Applicability of the Act
All establishments such as factories, mines, plantations, Government establishments, shops, or any other notified by the central government

Challenges/drawbacks of the Act
- Some of the companies/establishments may not hire women of childbearing age groups
- The financial burden on the employer because a temporary employee may have to be appointed in place of an absent employee or get work done by another existing employee.
- Women may lose more jobs.

TABLE 1: Effects of workplace interventions on Breastfeeding (BF) outcome measures.

	Exclusive breastfeeding till 6 months	Continued breastfeeding for 12–23 months	Any breastfeeding up to 6 months
The overall supportive work environment for BF	Four studies: RR 1.28 (0.98–1.69)	One study: RR 3.33 (1.43–10.0)	Four studies: RR 1.31 (1.1–1.56)
Maternal leave policy	Two studies: RR 1.52 (1.03–2.23)	No studies	One study: RR 0.99 (0.8–1.29)
Workplace support	Two studies: RR 1.08 (0.74–1.60)	No studies	One study: RR 1.25 (1.09–1.43)
Employment status	No studies	One study: RR 3.33 (1.43–10.0)	Two studies: RR 1.49 (1.12–1.98)

TABLE 2: Workplace breastfeeding policies across different countries.

	United States	United Kingdom	Indonesia	Taiwan	Pakistan
Maternity leave	Obligation for 6 months can be extended to 1 year	Obligation for 6 months can be extended to 1 year	Obligation for 3 months	Obligation for 6 months can be extended to 8 months	Obligation for 6 months, but the majority are returning to work in 9 weeks
Breastfeeding breaks	Obligation	Obligation	Suggested	Suggested	Suggested
Lactation facilities	Obligation	Obligation	Obligation	Suggested	NA
Childcare facilities	Obligation	Obligation	NA	NA	NA
Lactation consultation	Obligation	Obligation	NA	NA	NA

BREASTFEEDING POLICIES IN THE WORKPLACE ACROSS DIFFERENT COUNTRIES

High-income countries such as USA and UK have established lactation programs in the workplace, whereas many Asian countries still have not strictly implemented the same (Table 2).[8,12,13]

How to improve breastfeeding practices at the workplace?[14-16]

The following are a few measures to improve breastfeeding practices in the workplace.

- The concept of "Hirkanikaksh" may be considered at workplaces (Hirkanikaksh is a separate room at the workplace where mothers can breastfeed the baby and can also express milk and store it in a refrigerator during their working hours)
- To have a workplace lactation policy/program
- Work from home if possible
- Flexible work schedule with adequate break time
- Shift to office branches which are nearer to home if available

- If the working schedule is at night, try to shift to daytime work
- Availability of creches to care for the infant by a trusted individual
- Support from colleagues
- Increased breastfeeding at night and on weekends
- Good diet and family support
- Availability of healthcare professionals for consultation and counseling, including breastfeeding support groups.

GUIDANCE FOR BREASTFEEDING IN WORKING MOTHERS[14-16]

Advanced preparation will help the women to tackle the problem/s which can be encountered while returning to work.

Before delivery:
- Duration of maternity leave.
- Communicate the plan with the supervisor or employer.
- Discuss the option of a work schedule when returning to work.
- Identify whether the place is available for feeding or expression of breast milk.
- Discuss with other colleagues who were breastfeeding while returning to work.
- Inquiry about creches and child's caregivers.
- Discuss the plan with your spouse and family members.

After birth and during maternity leave:
- Early initiation of breastfeeding
- Avoidance of prelacteal feeds
- Exclusive breastfeeding till 6 months
- Avoidance of infant milk substitutes, artificial nipples, or bottles
- Make plans on how to continue breastfeeding during work.
- Try practicing the expression of milk a couple of weeks before joining work.
- Trial run of a workday schedule before maternity leave ends.
- To have a goal and motivation to continue breastfeeding even after joining the work

While returning to work:
- Make a timetable of work schedule and breastfeeding/expression of milk.
- Take the baby to the workplace if creche and a suitable environment for child care are available.
- Take out time from work and feed the baby.
- If creche is not available, breastfeed the baby just before leaving home and immediately after returning home, express the milk at the workplace and store it properly.
- To know how to store the expressed breast milk **(Table 3)**.
- Reduce stress at the workplace.
- A good diet with adequate rest
- Breastfeed frequently at night and on weekends.
- Consult support groups.
- Clarify all queries with healthcare professionals and consult if required.

Lactation room/Hirkanikaksh:
An ideal lactation room should meet the following criteria:[14]
- Easily accessible to women
- Clean, well-ventilated, and comfortable
- Ensure privacy.
- Availability of equipment for milk expression and storage
- Small table with a comfortable seat
- Water source and handwashing facility
- Manuals on Breastfeeding information
- Notice board to be placed outside the room (Don't disturb or don't enter the room without permission).

TABLE 3: Human milk storage guideline (CDC guidelines).[17]

Type of breast milk	Storage locations and temperatures		
	Room temperature (25°C)	Refrigerator (4°C)	Freezer (−18°C or colder)
Freshly expressed or pumped	4 hours	4 days	3 to 6 months
Thawed or previously frozen	1-2 hours	24 hours	Never refreeze after it is thawed
Leftover from feeding (baby didn't finish)	Use within 2 hours of feeding		

Lactation breaks:[14]
- At least 40 minutes of break in an 8-hour work schedule apart from lunch break
- Minimum of two to three breaks of 15-20 minutes for expression or direct breastfeeding.

Some atypical workplace settings or exceptional circumstances:
- *Healthcare and hospital:* Mothers may work as nurses, clerical staff, residents, faculty, technician, or housekeeping staff. Duty hours may be >8-hour shifts. In large hospitals, multiple lactation rooms may be required at places near emergency, OPD, operation theatre, etc. Special arrangements should be made for breastfeeding, and appropriate breaks should be provided.
- *Educational institutes:* Teaching and non-teaching staff, as well as students, could be mothers in educational institutes. Having a breastfeeding policy on campus is essential. Teachers and staff may cover one another during lactation breaks.
- *Shopping malls/wholesale traders/ restaurants:* Shopping malls should set up separate spaces for lactation for workers and the general public. This will benefit both businesses as well as families. A simple divider screen may be used for breastfeeding in smaller units to provide privacy. Restaurants should have flexible and shared spaces for feeding, such as an empty guest room, a small conference room, or an office area.

Sustaining the Workplace Lactation Programme[14]

- Recognize that the program is your contribution to society.
- Make a person in charge of the program.
- Continuously assess needs and try to fulfill them with existing opportunities and resources.
- The program should be implemented as per the local context and need.
- Justify continuous support with policies and mandates.
- Foster breastfeeding support groups.
- Build alliances between the local government and the social sector.

Coming back to the case scenario, the suggested plan for women regarding Breastfeeding after joining work:
- Women should get maternity leave of at least 6 months
- A timetable of work schedule and breastfeeding/expression of milk should be made
- Identify the lactation room in working place and check whether adequate facilities are available.

- Take the baby to the workplace if creche and a suitable environment for child care are available.
- Adequate lactation break/s should be ensured for a working woman.
- If crèche is not available, the mother can breastfeed the baby just before leaving home and immediately after coming home.
- In the above scenario, milk should be expressed and stored safely at the workplace.
- Mother should try practicing the expression of milk a couple of weeks before joining work.
- Mother should have a good diet with adequate rest and frequent breastfeeding at night time.

KEY MESSAGES

- Return to job is one of the most common reasons for switching over to top feeding.
- "Mother–baby-friendly workplace" is critical for the promotion of breastfeeding.
- Support from the family members, coworkers and employers is essential for improving breastfeeding practices at the workplace.

REFERENCES

1. World Health Organization. 10 facts on Breastfeeding [Internet]. [online] Available from: http://www.who.int/features/factfiles/breastfeeding/en/. [Last accessed November, 2023].
2. Victora CG, Bahl R, Barros AJD, França GVA, Horton S, Krasevec J, et al. breastfeeding in the 21st century: epidemiology, mechanisms, and lifelong effect. Lancet Lond Engl. 2016;387(10017):475-90.
3. International Institute for Population Sciences (IIPS) and ICF. 2021. National Family Health Survey (NFHS-5), 2019-21:India: Volume I. Mumbai: IIPS.
4. Addati L, Naomi C Katherine G. (2014). Maternity and paternity at work: Law and practice worldwide. [online] Available from: http://www.ilo.org/global/publications/ilo-bookstore/order-online/books/WCMS_242615/lang-en/index.htm. [Last accessed November, 2023].
5. Heymann J, Raub A, Earle A. Breastfeeding policy: a globally comparative analysis. Bull World Health Organ. 2013;91(6):398-406.
6. Ashoka A, Shwetha JH, Mahesh TK. A study of breastfeeding practices among working women in an urban area of Davangere, Karnataka, India. Int J Contemp Pediatr. 2016;3(2):645-8.
7. Horwood C, Surie A, Haskins L, Luthuli S, Hinton R, Chowdhury A, et al. Attitudes and perceptions about breastfeeding among female and male informal workers in India and South Africa. BMC Public Health. 2020;20(1):875.
8. Basrowi RW, Sastroasmoro S, Sulistomo AW, Bardosono S, Henderson A, Soemarko DS, et al. Challenges and Supports of Breastfeeding at Workplace in Indonesia. Pediatr Gastroenterol Hepatol Nutr. 2018;21(4):248-56.
9. World Breastfeeding Week 2019 Message. [online] Available from: https://www.who.int/news-room/commentaries/detail/world-breastfeeding-week-2019-message. [Last accessed November, 2023].
10. Rollins NC, Bhandari N, Hajeebhoy N, Horton S, Lutter CK, Martines JC, et al. Why invest, and what will it take to improve breastfeeding practices? Lancet Lond Engl. 2016;387(10017):491-504.
11. Ministry of Labour & Employment. Maternity Benefit Amendment Act, 2017. | [online]. Available from: https://labour.gov.in/whatsnew/maternity-benefit-amendment-act2017. [Last accessed November, 2023].
12. Murtagh L, Moulton AD. Working Mothers, Breastfeeding, and the Law. Am J Public Health. 2011;101(2):217-23.

13. Hirani SAA, Karmaliani R. Evidence-based workplace interventions to promote breastfeeding practices among Pakistani working mothers. Women Birth J Aust Coll Midwives. 2013;26(1):10-6.
14. Healthy beginnings for a better society breastfeeding in the workplace is possible: A toolkit [online]. Available from: http://www.ilo.org/manila/publications/WCMS_493121/lang-en/index.htm. [Last accessed November, 2023].
15. Tiwari S, Bharadva K, Yadav B, Malik S, Gangal P, Banapurmath CR, et al. Infant and Young Child Feeding Guidelines, 2016. Indian Pediatr. 2016;53(8):703-13.
16. Bettinelli ME. Breastfeeding policies and breastfeeding support programs in the mother's workplace. J Matern Fetal Neonatal Med. 2012;25Suppl 4:81-2.
17. Centers for Disease Control and Prevention. Breastfeeding Guidelines & Recommendations [online] Available from: https://www.cdc.gov/breastfeeding/recommendations/index.htm. [Last accessed November, 2023].

CHAPTER 15
Breastfeeding and Maternal Medications

Sandeep R, Madhu B Jagalasar

"Breastfeeding is not a choice; it is a responsibility"

INTRODUCTION

Breast milk nourishes the infant by providing the nutrients required for growth and development. It is the medium through which nutrients from the mother enters the baby after birth. Similarly, drugs consumed by the mother can also be secreted into breast milk. Although most drugs do not cause any harm, there is a risk to the growing infant.[1] Some drugs can have impact on lactation also. Hence, it is essential for healthcare workers to be aware of drugs which can be potentially harmful during lactation.

It is often challenging for healthcare workers to prescribe drugs during lactation as there is lack of evidence-based data on medication during lactation. This can result in hazardous decisions such as withholding medications to mother which could be necessary for her well-being. It can also lead to unnecessary formula feeding in babies.[2] In a developing nation like India, formula feeding can be harmful to the infant. There is an increased risk of mortality and infections such as diarrhea and otitis media.[3,4] Continuing breastfeeding is beneficial for both mother (long-term comorbidities such as cancer and diabetes and psychological benefits) and infant (improving immune system and improving developmental outcomes). Hence it is essential to understand the physiology of drug metabolism and its effects on infant, which can help in decision-making on prescribing drugs to the lactating mother.

BARRIERS TO BREASTFEEDING

A number of factors may contribute to ineffective establishment and maintaining effective breastfeeding. Few of them can be infant refusal, multiple births, returning to work, maternal health (physical/mental), localized issues, and concern about medication use. Healthcare workers may not be aware of the strategies to minimize infant exposure to drugs during breastfeeding or they may use the risk information of drugs during pregnancy to make decisions for breastfeeding which could not be the case.

Factors Affecting Transfer of Drugs from Maternal Plasma to Breast Milk

- *Mammary epithelial barrier:* Mammary epithelial cells in the alveolus form a semipermeable lipoid membrane separating plasma from breast milk.

During the first few days, the pores are open and after 1 week they close and do not allow larger molecules to enter. Molecular weights of less than about 200 Da pass readily through the pores into breast milk. Mastitis and maternal inflammation can affect this barrier.[5]
- pH of milk is typically slightly acidic (pH 7.1–7.2) relative to that of plasma; the ionized form of weak bases can concentrate in breast milk and weak acids are inhibited from passing into milk.[6]
- Highly protein-bound drugs are secreted into the milk in only low concentrations.[7]
- Lipid-soluble drugs tend to accumulate in milk fat, causing the total amount of drug in milk to increase, e.g., diazepam and phenytoin. The concentration of milk fat varies based on the time of feeding and day; hence, the concentration of such drugs also varies in the milk.[7]
- A few drugs get actively secreted into breast milk by transporters, e.g., Acyclovir, Methotrexate, and Iodide.[8]
- Passive diffusion is the most predominant way of transfer of drugs depended on the concentration of drug in maternal plasma.

The milk-to-(maternal) plasma (MP) drug concentration ratio (MP ratio) is commonly used as a parameter of a relative degree of drug excretion into milk, but not an absolute value of drug concentration in milk. This variable is calculated by using the following formula:

Milk to maternal plasma ratio
$$= C_{milk}/C_{plasma}$$

MP >1 indicates that medication accumulates in the breast milk. It does not indicate infant systemic exposure and value varies based on when the sampling was done to determine the value, as concentration varies in foremilk and hindmilk.[9] The detailed physiological changes in pregnancy and potential effects on pharmacokinetics are summarized in **Table 1**.

Neonatal Exposure

- Infant daily dose is calculated based on concentration in the milk and volume of milk ingested. It is important to know that the volume of milk in the first week is less and the concentration of drug also varies based on maternal plasma concentration and fat content in milk.

$$\text{Infant daily dose} = C_{milk}/V_{milk}/day$$

- Relative infant dose.

The infant daily dose should be compared to normal therapeutic doses, in order to assess whether a meaningful

TABLE 1: Physiological changes in pregnancy and potential effects on pharmacokinetics.[10]

Physiological change in pregnancy	Potential effect on pharmacokinetics of drugs
↓ Gastric emptying/small bowel motility	↑ Time to reach peak levels
↑ Gastric pH	↓ Absorption
↑ Vascularity and edema respiratory mucosa	↑ Absorption of inhaled drugs
↑ Minute ventilation	↓ Protein binding due to respiratory alkalosis
↑ Total body water, blood volume, and capillary hydrostatic pressure	↑ Volume of distribution of hydrophilic drugs
↑ Glomerular filtration rate	↑ Renal clearance
↓ Serum albumin	↑ Active fraction of drug
↑ CYP450 and ↑ UGT activity	↑ Metabolism

(UGT: UDP-glucuronosyltransferase)

pharmacological exposure is to be expected. For this purpose, the relative infant dose (RID) may be calculated as follows:

$$RID = \text{Infant dose (mg/kg/day)} / \text{Therapeutic dose (mg/kg/day)} \times 100\%$$

Relative infant dose of lower than 10% is often used as an arbitrary cutoff where breastfeeding is considered safe. This may not be applicable for drugs with wide therapeutic range and poor enteral absorption and in infants with glucose-6-phosphate dehydrogenase deficiency, in whom drug-induced hemolysis may occur at very low plasma concentrations of certain drugs.[11] The common drugs used during lactation are listed in **Table 2**.

TABLE 2: Commonly prescribed drugs.

Drugs	Rationale
Analgesics	• Acetaminophen is the safest analgesic • Nonsteroidal anti-inflammatory drugs such as aspirin should be used in low doses if given for long duration. High dose, long duration can cause Reye syndrome in infants during viral infections • Opioid analgesics should be used with caution, especially meperidine • Oral narcotics during breastfeeding can result in drowsiness and even death in infant[12]
Antibiotics	• Most antibiotics are safe during lactation • Tetracyclines can cause teeth discoloration and get deposited in bone. Most literature mentions it as contraindicated but can be used for short term • Chloramphenicol should be avoided as there is a risk of aplastic crisis even with low dose
Sedative/anxiolytics	• Diazepam and alprazolam can cause sedation and poor weight gain in infants. Withdrawal syndrome is also reported. Intermittent dose can be used with caution • Midazolam, lorazepam, and oxazepam have low levels in breast milk
Antihypertensives	• Propranolol and labetalol are considered safe. Other beta blockers such as atenolol and sotalol should be avoided[13]
Antidepressants	• Breastfeeding should be encouraged after discussing with the parents about the risk and benefit to mother–infant dyad • Paroxetine and sertraline are most likely suitable first-line agents • Fluoxetine, citalopram, and venlafaxine should be used with caution[14]
Antiepileptics	• Phenobarbitone can cause drowsiness and poor weight gain • Phenytoin and valproate are seen in low level in breast milk • Levetiracetam can be used safely; however, monitor for drowsiness and poor weight gain in infant • Carbamazepine should be used with caution and infant hepatic function; complete blood counts needs to be monitored, especially when multiple anticonvulsants are used
Anticancer drugs, Radioactive drugs	Breastfeeding is contraindicated
Alcohol, caffeine, tobacco	• Mother should not consume alcohol or should consume no more than one drink 2–3 hours before breast-feeding[15] • The ingestion of moderate amounts of caffeine should be safe • Because of the effects of second-hand smoke and the fact that nicotine is excreted in breast milk, smoking is contraindicated in breastfeeding women

DRUGS DURING PREGNANCY AFFECTING LACTATION

Galactagogues

Gastrointestinal motility drugs metoclopramide and domperidone are most commonly used off-label as galactagogues. Metoclopramide (centrally acting drug) and domperidone (peripheral dopamine antagonist) block dopamine D_2 receptors in the anterior pituitary and, in a limited number of clinical trials, they have had modest efficacy over placebo in initiating and maintaining lactation.[16] The best chance for efficacy is if the galactagogue is started within 3 weeks of delivery.[17] The safe duration of galactagogue therapy is controversial. The adverse effects of various herbs used as galactagogues are listed in **Table 3**.

LACTATION SUPPRESSION

The dopamine agonist bromocriptine was associated with maternal deaths from myocardial infarction and is no longer recommended. It has been replaced by a single 1-mg dose of long-acting cabergoline, ideally taken on the first postpartum day. The common adverse effects are nausea, headache, and dizziness. Cabergoline has

TABLE 3: Adverse effects of herbs used as galactagogues.

Herb	Adverse effects
Alfalfa Medicago sativa	Dose-related bleeding
Blessed thistle Cnicus benedictus	Gastric irritation and potential allergies, as it is part of the ragweed family
Dill Anethum graveolens	Alterations in sodium balance
Chaste tree Vital agnus-castus	Nausea, vomiting, irritation, pruritus, rash, headache, increased menstruation
Fennel Foeniculum vulgare	Allergic reactions, dermatitis (photo and contact)
Fenugreek seed Trigonella foenum-graecum	• Hypoglycemia, hypertension, diarrhea, and maple syrup body odor in mother • Allergy potential as part of the peanut family
Goats rue Galega officinalis	Hypoglycemia, hypotension, coughing, dose-related toxicity
Milk thistle (silymarin) Silybum marianum	Allergic reactions, diarrhea
Malunggay Moringa oleifera	Hypoglycemia, sedation
Raspberry leaf Rubus idaeus	Hypersensitivity reactions, changes in blood glucose
Damiana Turnera diffusa	Hepatotoxicity, confusion and hallucinations with high-dose *Turnera*
Shatavari Asparagus racemosus	Possible teratogenicity—avoid in pregnancy

been used, but bromocriptine should be avoided because of maternal deaths.

LactMed[14]

LactMed is a freely accessible, well-resourced, and peer-reviewed online database that can be downloaded as an app for mobile devices. It is updated to keep pace with new information, including published studies and drug approvals. It also incorporates information on complementary treatments.

The queries for the drugs used during pregnancy and lactation are listed in **Table 4**.

KEY MESSAGES

- Prescribe the drug at the lowest effective dose.
- Temporarily suspend breastfeeding (and express milk) for potentially toxic drugs, such as cytotoxic and radiopharmaceuticals.
- Feeding can be timed, based on half-life of the drug. Use drugs with shorter half-life.
- Feed infant/express the milk before taking the medicine. This is not applicable for drugs with longer half-life.
- Nursing mothers should not take dietary supplements unless composition and purity are known.

TABLE 4: Resources for pregnancy and lactation questions.

Reference	Comments
Drugs in pregnancy and lactation by Briggs et al.[18]	• Published approximately every 3 years • Provides information on medications in both pregnancy and lactation
LactMed https://www.ncbi.nim.nih.gov/books/NBK501922/?report=classic	• Free and available anywhere you have access to the internet (Recommend bookmarking this page on your desktop) • Compiled by experts and peer reviewed • Updated regularly • Provides information on medications in lactation only
Lexi-Drugs	• Updated regularly • Online and book form available • Requires a subscription • Has in-depth pregnancy information for many drugs in addition to standard information
Medications and Mother's Milk by Thomas W. Hale[19]	• Published every 2 years • Classifies medications based on risk with L1 being the safest and L5 being contraindicated • Provides information on medications in lactation only
Micromedex[20]	• Updated regularly • Requires a subscription • Contains TERIS and Shepard's Catalog of Teratogenic Agents • Provides US and Australian pregnancy drug risk classification along with additional detailed information when available • Provides the AAP and Thomson Lactation classification
TERIS	• Available online • Requires subscription • Also available with online subscription to Micromedex[20]

- Mothers undergoing general or regional anesthesia may resume breastfeeding as soon as they are awake and feel strong enough to do so.

REFERENCES

1. Ito S. Drug therapy for breast-feeding women. N Engl J Med. 2000;343:118-26.
2. Ito S, Lieu M, Chan W, Koren G. Continuing drug therapy while breastfeeding. Part 1. Common misconceptions of patients. Can Fam Physician. 1999;45:897-9.
3. Sankar MJ, Sinha B, Chowdhury R, Bhandari N, Taneja S, Martines J, et al. Optimal breastfeeding practices and infant and child mortality: a systematic review and meta-analysis. Acta Paediatr. 2015;104(467):3-13.
4. Duijts L, Jaddoe VW, Hofman A, Moll HA. Prolonged and Exclusive Breastfeeding Reduces the Risk of Infectious Diseases in Infancy. Pediatrics. 2010;126(1):e18-e25.
5. Hunt KM, Williams JE, Shafii B, Hunt MK, Behre R, Ting R, et al. Mastitis is associated with increased free fatty acids, somatic cell count, and interleukin-8 concentrations in human milk. Breastfeed Med. 2013;8:105-10.
6. Atkinson HC, Begg EJ. Prediction of drug distribution into human milk from physicochemical characteristics. Clin Pharmacokinet. 1990;18:151-67.
7. Anderson GD. Using pharmacokinetics to predict the effects of pregnancy and maternal-infant transfer of drugs during lactation. Expert Opin Drug Metab Toxicol. 2006;2:947-60.
8. Ito S, Alcorn J. Xenobiotic transporter expression and function in the human mammary gland. Adv Drug Deliv Rev. 2003;55:653-65.
9. Verstegen RHJ, Ito S. Drugs in lactation. J Obstet Gynaecol Res. 2019;45(3):522-31.
10. Anderson GD. Pregnancy-induced changes in pharmacokinetics: a mechanistic-based approach. Clin Pharmacokinet. 2005;44(10):989-1008.
11. Anderson PO. Drugs in Lactation. Pharm Res. 2018;35(3):45.
12. Lamvu G, Feranec J, Blanton E. Perioperative pain management: an update for obstetrician-gynecologists. Am J Obstet Gynecol. 2018;218(2):193-9.
13. Ito S. Drug therapy for breast-feeding women. N Engl J Med. 2000;343(2):118-26. [Erratum in: N Engl J Med 2000 Nov 2;343(18):1348].
14. Berle JO, Spigset O. Antidepressant use during breastfeeding. Curr Womens Health Rev. 2011;7(1):28-34.
15. Drugs and Lactation Database (LactMed) [Internet]. Bethesda (MD): National Library of Medicine (US); 2006-. Available from: https://www.ncbi.nlm.nih.gov/books/NBK501922/ [Last accessed November, 2023].
16. Donovan TJ, Buchanan K. Medications for increasing milk supply in mothers expressing breastmilk for their preterm hospitalized infants. Cochrane Database Syst Rev 2012:CD005544.
17. Ehrenkranz RA, Ackerman BA. Metoclopramide effect on faltering milk production by mothers of premature infants. Pediatrics 1986;78:614-20.
18. Briggs GG, Freeman RK, Yaffe SJ. Drugs in Pregnancy and Lactation, 9th edition. Baltimore, MD: Lippincott Williams & Wilkins; 2011.
19. Hale TW. Medication and Mother's Milk. 15th edition. Amarillo, TX: Hale Publishing; 2012.
20. Micromedex 2.0 [intranet database]. Greenwood Village, CO: Thomson Healthcare.

16. Complementary Feeding

KV Raghunath, Vishwanath B, Durgappa H

> *"Just because a child's parents are poor or uneducated is no reason to deprive the child of basic human rights to healthcare, education and proper nutrition"*
> —**Marian Wright Edelman**

INTRODUCTION

Complementary feeding is defined as the process starting when breast milk alone is no longer sufficient to meet the nutritional requirements of infants, and therefore other foods and liquids are needed, along with breast milk. The target age range for complementary feeding is generally taken to be 6–24 months of age, even though breastfeeding may continue beyond 2 years.[1]

Breastfeeding provides complete nutrition up to 6 months of age which alone is not sufficient to meet the demands of a growing child beyond 6 months. Hence, it is important to start appropriate, adequate, and safe complementary feeding at 6 months for the optimal growth and development of the child.[2] The period between 6 and 24 months of age is called "critical window period".[2,3] Any amount of undernutrition during this period is going to be permanent and irreversible, and it may contribute to late-onset chronic noncommunicable diseases such as diabetes, hypertension, and metabolic diseases later in the life. If it is a girl child, undernutrition may pass on to next generations which will have a negative impact on the health of an individual. Hence, it is crucial to ensure optimal nutrition during this period. The optimal nutrition has a positive impact on the health of children. The recent studies have shown that optimal complementary feeding could prevent 6% of under-5 deaths across the world. Therefore, timely start of complementary feeding is crucial for the good health of the children[4] (Fig. 1).

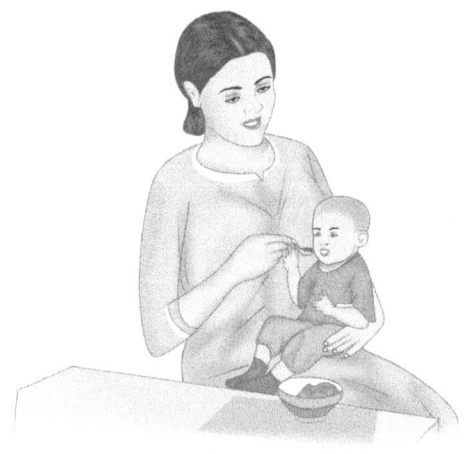

Fig. 1: Complementary feeding.

MAGNITUDE OF PROBLEM

Although most mothers and caretakers of children are aware of complementary feeding, the optimal complementary feeding is rarely being practiced. In India, according to recent reports, only 45.5% of infants between 6 and 8 months of age are started with complementary feeding. It is also astonishing to note that only 11% of children between 6 and 24 months of age receive adequate food across the country.[5]

PRINCIPLE OF SELECTION OF FOOD INGREDIENTS

Food ingredients selected for preparation of complementary feeding should be locally available, affordable, socially and culturally acceptable, safe, and easy to prepare.[2,3]

Diet Diversity

It is essential to include "diverse group of food ingredients" to ensure optimal nutrition to the child. Add fresh dark leafy vegetables which are a rich source of micronutrients. The nutritive value of food can also be enhanced by the process of fermentation or sprouting. In addition, cleaned seasonal fruits should be offered.[2]

The seven diverse groups of food ingredients include the following:
1. Pulses and grains, roots and tubers, legumes, and nuts (proteins)
2. Dark green leafy vegetables and leaves (vitamins and minerals)
3. Yellow, orange-colored fruits and vegetables (vitamin A)
4. Egg (protein)
5. Meat (protein); if family is vegetarian, increase the intake of milk and its products
6. Milk and milk products (calcium, proteins vitamins and fats)
7. Add a spoon of ghee/oil in the child's food (energy and palatability).

PREPARATION OF COMPLEMENTARY FOOD

Thorough hand wash and preparation of baby food under "good hygienic condition" is important to prevent contamination and infections. Always offer freshly prepared food to children and avoid storing prepared food for >2 hours. It is not necessary to add salt as these food ingredients have sufficient salt to meet the requirements of child. Avoid sugar and processed foods.[2]

The characteristics of good complementary feeding include the following:
- Rich in energy and adequate in good quality proteins, vitamins, and minerals.
- The consistency of complementary food should be soft, easily digestible, and just run off when the spoon is tilted.
- Low dietary bulk
- Minimal preparation is needed prior to feeding and easily digestible
- Free from antinutritional factors and low in indigestible fiber.

The World Health Organization has recommended complementary feeding guidelines, intended to optimize the feeding practices across the world. The 10 guiding principles[1] include the following:
1. Practice exclusive breastfeeding from birth to 6 months of age and introduce complementary foods at 6 months of age (180 days) while continuing to breastfeed.
2. Continue frequent, on-demand breastfeeding until 2 years of age or beyond.
3. Practice responsive feeding, applying the principles of psychosocial care.
4. Practice good hygiene and proper food handling.

TABLE 1: Energy requirements in children aged 6–23 months.

Age (months)	From breast milk (kcal/day)	To be supplemented in CF (kcal/day)	Total required (kcal/day)
6–8	415	200	615
9–11	386	300	686
12–23	344	550	894

(CF: complementary feed)

5. Start at 6 months of age with small amounts of food and increase the quantity as the child gets older, while maintaining frequent breastfeeding.
6. Gradually increase food consistency and variety as the infant grows older, adapting to the infant's requirements and abilities.
7. Increase the number of times that the child is fed complementary food as the child gets older.
8. Feed a variety of nutrient-rich foods to ensure that all nutrient needs are met.
9. Use fortified complementary foods or vitamin-mineral supplements for the infant, as needed.
10. Increase fluid intake during illness, including more frequent breastfeeding, and encourage the child to eat soft, favorite foods. After illness, give food more often than usual and encourage the child to eat more.

METHOD OF FEEDING

Practice responsive feeding, applying the principles of psychosocial care; the components of responsive feeding include the following:[1,3]
- Feed the baby under good hygienic conditions.
- Feed the child slowly and patiently.
- Encourage self-feeding and finger feeding.
- Stay with the baby throughout the duration of feed.
- Practice frequent feeding during and after illness.
- Praise the child when takes mouthful of food.
- Do not threaten the child to eat.
- Avoid monotonous food.
- Avoid distractions during feeding.

It is also important to ensure to fill the "energy gap" as mentioned in **Table 1**.[3]

There is always a dilemma among mothers and caretakers what to feed and how much to feed the baby. It is important to choose soft and easily digestible food items as mentioned in **Table 2**.[3]

It is also important to educate the mothers about rich sources of macronutrients and micronutrients as mentioned in Table 3.

EXAMPLES OF COMPLEMENTARY FOODS[6]

1. *Khichdi:*
   Rice—35 g
   Green gram dhal—10 g
   Leafy vegetables—2 tsp
   Fat—2 tsp
   Cumin (jeera)
   Method: Clean the rice and dhal and cook them in water with salt till the grains are soft and water is absorbed. Leafy vegetables can be added when the cereal/pulse is three fourth done. Cumin is fried in fat and added toward the end.
2. *Malted ragi porridge:*
   Malted ragi—30 g
   Roasted groundnut—15 g
   Jaggery—20 g

TABLE 2: Quantity, variety, and frequency of complementary feed.

Age (months)	Texture	Frequency	Quantity at each meal
6	Soft porridge, mashed vegetables	2 times per day + Frequent breastfeeds	2–3 tablespoon-full
7–8	Mashed food	3 times per day + Frequent breastfeeds	Increasing gradually to two third of 250-mL bowl
9–11	Finely chopped food or food that baby can pick up	3 meals + 1 snacks between meals + breastfeeds	Three fourth of 250-mL bowl
12–23	Family food, chopped or mashed if necessary	3 meals + 2 snacks between meals + breastfeeds	Full of 250-mL bowl or even more

TABLE 3: Good sources of nutrients.[3]

Protein-rich foods	Iron-rich foods	Vit C-rich foods	Vit A-rich foods	Iodine-rich foods
• Chicken	• Liver	• Guava	• Red pumpkin	• Spinach
• Fish	• Mutton	• Watermelon	• Carrot	• Lentils
• Mutton	• Eggs	• Orange	• Orange	• Kidney beans
• Eggs	• Prawn	• Cherry	• Jackfruit	• Figs
• Milk	• Pumpkin seeds	• Grapes	• Papaya	• Quinoa
• Seeds	• Sunflower seeds	• Black grapes	• Mangoes	• Almonds
• Sesame	• Peanut	• Sweet lime	• Dill leaves	• Green leafy vegetables
• Cashew nut	• Watercress seeds	• Strawberry	• Fenugreek leaves	• Soybeans
• Chickpeas	• Cowpeas	• Lemon	• Spinach	• Oats
• Peanut	• Turmeric	• Kiwi	• Colossian	• Potatoes
• Drumstick leaves	• Lotus stem	• Peach	• Chickpeas	
• Colossian	• Dry coconut	• Alma	• Millets	
• Spinach	• Spinach	• Capsicum	• Lentils	
• Cauliflower	• Radish leaves	• Green chili	• Red lentils	
• Pulses	• Dill leaves	• Green mango	• Chickpeas	
• Rice	• Pulses		• Soyabeans	

Method: Malted ragi, roasted groundnuts, and jaggery are powdered. Sufficient water is added and cooked.

3. *Wheat payasam:*

   Wheat—30 g

   Roasted Bengal gram flour—15 g

   Roasted and crushed groundnut—5 g

   Sugar—15 g

   Method: Roast whole wheat and powder. Add roasted Bengal gram flour, groundnut, and sugar. Cook with sufficient water.

4. *Kheer:*

   Vermicelli/Rice—30 g

   Milk—100 mL

   Water—as required

   Jaggery—20 g

   Method: Boil rice/vermicelli in water till half done. Add milk and bring to boil. Add jaggery and cook well.

Notes:
- All these recipes provide approximately 250 kcal. Add 5 g proteins, and amounts given are for two servings.
- Recipes Nos. 2 and 3 can be prepared and stored in airtight containers to be used whenever required.
- Nonvegetarian foods such as soft-boiled egg and minced meat may be introduced at the age of 6 months.

Maternal literacy and maternal feeding practices have a significant outcome on linear growth of the infant as shown by two studies from South East Asia.[7,8]

KEY MESSAGES

- Breastfeeding alone is not sufficient beyond 6 months of age to meet the growing needs of the child.
- The period between 6 and 24 months of age is "critical window" during which any amount of undernutrition will have permanent negative impacts on the health of the children.
- Therefore, it is crucial to start appropriate, adequate, and safe complementary feeding at 6 months of life.
- Thorough hand wash and preparation of infant food under good hygienic conditions are critical to preventing contamination and infections in the children.
- Always include "diverse group of food ingredients" to ensure optimal nutrition to child.
- Practice responsive feeding.
- Feed the baby slowly and patiently and do not threaten the child to eat.
- Encourage self and finger feeding.
- Encourage breastfeeding and complementary feeding during and after illnesses.
- Optimal complementary feeding is associated with 6% reduced risk of under-5 deaths.

REFERENCES

1. World Health Organization. Guiding principles for complementary feeding of the breastfed child. Geneva: World Health Organization; 2003. [online] Available from: https://www.who.int/publications/i/item/9275124604 [Last accessed November, 2023].
2. World Health Organization. Complementary feeding: report of the global consultation, and summary of guiding principles for complementary feeding of the breastfed child. [online] Available from: https://www.who.int/publications/i/item/924154614X [Last accessed November, 2023].
3. Tiwari S, Bharadva K, Yadav B, Malik S, Gangal P, Banapurmath CR, et al. Infant and young child feeding guidelines, 2016. Indian Pediatr. 2016;53(8):703-13.
4. Victora CG, Bahl R, Barros AJ, França GV, Horton S, Krasevec J, et al. Breastfeeding in the 21st century: epidemiology, mechanisms, and lifelong effect. Lancet. 2016;387(10017): 475-90.
5. Bhatia N, Rathi K, Arora C, Choedon T, Rajurkar P, Thakur R, et al. Analysis of Key Nutrition Indicators Based on National Family Health Survey, NFHS 4 (2015-16) and NFHS 5 (2019-2021). [online] Available from: https://osf.io/r9ybf [Last accessed November, 2023].
6. National Institute of Nutrition. (2011). Dietary guidelines for Indians: a Manual. 2nd edition. pp. 89-117. [online] Available from https://www.nin.res.in/downloads/DietaryGuidelinesforNINwebsite.pdf [Last accessed November, 2023].
7. Saleem AF, Mahmud S, Baig-Ansari N, Zaidi AK. Impact of maternal education about complementary feeding on their infants' nutritional outcomes in low-and middle-income households: a community-based randomized interventional study in Karachi, Pakistan. J Health Popul Nutr. 2014;32(4):623-33.
8. Kuriyan R, Kurpad AV. Complementary feeding patterns in India. Nutr Metab Cardiovasc Dis.2012;22(10):799-805.

CHAPTER 17

Functional Gastrointestinal Disorders in Infants and Toddlers

B Shantharam Baliga, Jayashree K, Durgappa H

"Mothers milk is soul food for babies. The babies of the world need a lot more soul food"
—Ina May Gaskin

INTRODUCTION

Functional gastrointestinal disorders (FGIDs) are the group of conditions occurring in infants and toddlers without structural or biochemical abnormalities.[1] After reviewing extensive literature, a committee of gastroenterologist in ROME formulated criteria for the diagnosis of FGIDs, called ROME criteria which define seven different FGIDs: Infantile colic, regurgitation, and functional constipation represent most common disorders, while infant dyschezia, Cyclic vomiting Syndrome (CVS), rumination and functional diarrhea account for <10% of conditions (*See* Box 1). Overall half of the healthy infants are affected with FGIDs across the world, and often multiple problems coexist.[2]

Pathophysiology of FGIDs is multifactorial, complex interplay of autonomic, psychosocial, dietary, microbial, and gastric sensorimotor disturbances.[3]

Though most FGIDs resolve spontaneously over time they often have behavioral and economic impact on the family. In majority of cases investigations are not necessary unless there are alarming signs and symptoms to suggest organic diseases in infants and toddlers. The pharmacotherapy is limited to infants having persistent constipation. There is evidence that specific strains of probiotic are found to be beneficial in infants with colic.[2]

Timely diagnosis and effective management are most important to alleviate the anxiety and stress among the parents and family members.

G1. GASTROESOPHAGEAL REFLUX

G1.Gastroesophageal reflux is involuntary retrograde passage of gastric content into esophagus and mouth with or without regurgitation or vomiting. It occurs in 50-60% of infants between 3 weeks and 12 months of age. Infants can have 4 or more than 4 episodes per day, otherwise these babies are healthy they are often called happy spitters[2] and usually it resolves in 95% of cases by the age of one year without any intervention.[5] It is important to differentiate from Gastroesophageal reflux disease (GERD) which is often associated with excessive crying, fussiness, irritability, arching, refusal

BOX 1: Revised ROME IV Criteria (2016)[1,4].

Functional gastrointestinal disorders in neonates and toddlers

G1. Infant regurgitation:
Diagnostic criteria for infant regurgitation must include both of the following in otherwise healthy infants with 3 weeks to 12 months of age:
- Regurgitation for 2 or more times per day for 3 or more weeks
- No retching, hematemesis, aspiration, apnea, failure to thrive, feeding or swallowing difficulties, or abnormal posturing

G2. Infant rumination syndrome
Diagnostic criteria for rumination syndrome must include all of the following for at least 2 months:
- Repetitive contractions of the abdominal muscles, diaphragm, and tongue
- Effortless regurgitation of gastric contents, which are either expelled from the mouth or re-chewed and re-swallowed
- Three or more of the following:
  1. Onset between 3 and 8 months
  2. Does not respond to management for gastroesophageal reflux disease and regurgitation
  3. Unaccompanied by signs of distress
  4. Does not occur during sleep and when the infant is interacting with individuals in the environment.

G3. Cyclic vomiting syndrome
Diagnostic criteria for cyclic vomiting syndrome must include all of the following:
- Two or more periods of unremitting paroxysmal vomiting with or without retching, lasting hours to days within a 6-month period
- Episodes are stereotypical in each patient
- Episodes are separated by weeks to months with return to baseline health between episodes of vomiting.

G4. Diagnostic criteria for Infantile Colic must include all of the following:
- Infant who is <5 months of age when the symptoms start and stop
- Recurrent and prolonged periods of infant crying fasting or irritability reported by caregivers that occur without obvious cause and cannot be prevented or resolved by caregivers
- No evidence of failure to thrive or fever or illness

"Fussing" refers to intermittent distressed vocalization and has been defined as "behavior that is not quite crying but not awake and content either." Infants often fluctuate between crying and fussing, so that the 2 symptoms are difficult to distinguish in practice

For Clinical Research purposes, a diagnosis of Infant colic must meet the preceding Diagnostic criteria and also include both of the following:
- Caregiver reports infant has cried or fussed for 3 or more hours per day during 3 or more days in 7 days in a telephone or face-to-face screening interview with a researcher or clinician
- Total 24-hour crying plus fussing in the selected group of infants is confirmed to be 3 hours or more when measured by at least one prospectively kept, 24-hour behavior diary

G5. Functional diarrhea
Diagnostic criteria for functional diarrhea must include all of the following:
- Daily painless, recurrent passage of 4 or more large, unformed stools
- Symptoms last more than 4 weeks
- Onset between 6 and 60 months of age
- No failure to thrive if caloric intake is adequate

G6. Infant dyschezia
Diagnostic criteria for infant dyschezia must include in an infant:
- At least 10 minutes of straining and crying before successful or unsuccessful passage of soft stools
- No other health problems

Contd...

Contd...

G7. Functional constipation
Diagnostic criteria for functional constipation must include all of the following:
One month of at least 2 of the following in infants up to 4 years of age:
- Two or fewer defecations per week
- History of excessive stool retention
- History of painful or hard bowel movements
- History of large-diameter stools
- Presence of a large fecal mass in the rectum in toilet-trained children, the following additional criteria may be used:
- At least 1 episode/week of incontinence after the acquisition of toileting skills
- History of large-diameter stools that may obstruct the toilet

to feed, abdominal pain, recurrent vomiting, sleep disturbances, recurrent pneumonia and failure to thrive[6] which has to be managed accordingly.

Management[7-10]

- Parental reassurance and education remain the cornerstone in the management of infants with regurgitation
- Gentle handling and burping after each feed are important.
- Prokinetic drugs such as domperidone may be tried in infants having frequent episodes of regurgitations.
- Modifications in the feeding positions and thickened infant feed at 6 months of age may help.
- Keeping the baby in prone position is discouraged as it is associated with sudden infant death syndrome.

G2. INFANT WITH RUMINATION SYNDROME

It involves habitual regurgitation of gastric content into mouth for the purpose of self-stimulation. A recent study showed the prevalence of 1.9%. It is self-stimulating behavior in the context of longstanding deprivation. Neglectful maternal behavior and lack of bonding between the mother and baby is found to be important reason for rumination.[1-3]

Treatment: Empathetic and responsive nurturing is important in alleviating the symptoms

G3. CYCLIC VOMITING SYNDROME

It is characterized by stereotyped episodes of vomiting lasting from hours to days and with interventions, returns to baseline health. Typically, the symptoms start at the same time of the day most commonly during late night or early morning hours. The duration symptoms found to be same in each patient over time of presentation. Once vomiting begins reaches its highest intensity during first hour and thereafter frequency tends to decrease. The episodes of cyclic vomiting syndrome (CVS) end as rapidly as they start and recovery occurs rapidly provided there is no fluid deficit or dyselectrolytemia. Frequently mothers are found to have migraine. Genetic and psychosocial factors are found to be playing a role in the CVS.[1-3]

G4. INFANTILE COLIC[11-19]

It is one of the common functional gastrointestinal disorders in infants often mounting distress among the parents and is even challenging for healthcare professional to differentiate it from serious underlying organic conditions in office practice. The term "colic" stems from the Greek "kolikos", the adjective of "kolon", which means intestine.

Magnitude: Globally, 20% of infants are reported to be having infantile colic between 3 weeks and 3 months of age.

Pathophysiology: The exact etiology is not known; however, the following mechanisms have been proposed to explain infantile colic:
- Gut dysbiosis means imbalance in the gut microbiota; recent evidences have found that infants with colic had slower colonization, lower diversity, and stability of microbiota in the gut.
- Chronic gut inflammation and increased permeability: This is indicated by elevated concentration of fecal calprotectin, a biomarker of intestinal neutrophilic infiltration.
- More recently, infants with colic had higher serum concentration of proinflammatory cytokines and chemokines, including IL-8 and CC-chemokine ligand 4 than infants without colic indicating low-grade gut inflammation.
- Gram-negative bacteria such as species of *Escherichia* and *Bacteroidetes* can induce gut inflammation through the presence of lipopolysaccharides (LPS) on their outer membrane and thus might pathogenically be linked to colic. Pathogen-associated LPS can activate production of pro-inflammatory cytokines and chemokines, provoking pro-inflammatory response.
- Behavioral factors: Such as parental over or under stimulation.
- Recently, a study from Egypt showed that *H. pylori* stool antigen was positive in 81.8% of infants having colic and 23.3% infants without colic. It was also found that *H. pylori* alters host immune response which in turn leads to non-commensal bacterial colonization and altered gut microflora.
- The other gastrointestinal theories proposed for infantile colic are: immaturity of enteric nervous system which leads to intestinal contraction and colic, increased motilin receptors which causes intestinal hyperperistalsis, and cow milk hypersensitivity. Some children, especially with family history of atopy, are sensitive to cow milk protein.

Clinical presentation: Paroxysmal inconsolable cry, fussiness, and irritability associated with flushing of face, fisting of hands, frowning and flexion of legs toward abdomen occurring in infants in the evening hours of the day. Wessel and colleagues described the presentations of infantile colic in 1954, as infant crying >3 hours a day, >3 days a week for >3 weeks (Rule of 3) otherwise, healthy child. Later on, due to difficult in keeping the record of cry for 3 hours the definition of infantile colic was modified by ROME 4 committee in 2016. The ROME IV criteria are "An infant who is <5 months of age when symptoms start and stop; recurrent and prolonged periods of infant crying, fussing or irritability reported by caregivers that occur without any obvious cause and cannot be prevented or resolved by caregivers; no evidence of infant failure to thrive, fever, or illness".

Management
- Parental counseling and education about benign nature of the condition remains cornerstone in the management.
- Dietary modifications in the mother: *Avoid milk and milk products and observe for 2 weeks if colic persists despite diet modification then continue to take regular diet.*
- Lactase enzyme supplementation may be beneficial in relieving colic in infants

- Probiotic supplementation with *Lactobacillus reuteri* at a dose of 10 CFUs once daily to breastfed infants less than 6 months of age resulted in significantly greater improvement in colic symptoms at the end of treatment (21 or 28 days) compared to controls.
- Pain relieving agents: not recommended below 6 months of age
- General measures include: burping after each feed, gentle rocking, attention diversion, taking the baby out, a car ride might help in comforting the baby.
- Outcome: as it is normal spectrum of cry will resolve by 3 months of age.

G5. FUNCTIONAL DIARRHEA[1,20]

It is important to be aware of normal stool pattern in infants to avoid unnecessary administration of drugs. Normally, the breastfed infants may pass stools up to 7 times per day which is golden yellow to greenish in color, small quantity, and non-foul smelling; otherwise, these babies are active, feeding well and growing normally.

Treatment

- Parental reassurance and education about physiological nature of stool pattern
- It is important to monitor growth parameters, which help in counseling the parents.

G6. DYSCHEZIA[1]

Infants strain for many minutes, scream, cry, and turn red or purple in the face with each effort to defecate. The symptoms may persist for 10-20 minutes and infants pass several stools per day. The symptoms begin in the first month of age and tend to disappear after 3-4 weeks. In one study, it was reported that at the age of 1 and 3 months, the dyschezia was prevalent in 3.9% and 0.9% of infants, respectively.

Treatment

- Effective counseling and reassurance to parents and care givers are most important.
- Avoid rectal stimulation as it may cause injury to rectum and become habitual.
- Laxatives are not necessary.

G7. FUNCTIONAL CONSTIPATION[20-30]

It is common problem in children with an estimated prevalence of 9% across the world. Functional constipation accounts for 95% of all cases of constipation and 5% of cases are due to underlying organic diseases.

Pathophysiology: Prolonged withholding behavior to evacuate the stool is the most important factor involved in the pathogenesis of functional constipation in children.

Rectum reabsorbs water content from the retained stool resulting in hardening of the stool which further leads to fecal impaction, stretching of rectal mucosa, decreased sensation, incontinence and difficulty in evacuation of stool, thus repeating the vicious cycle.

Clinical picture includes constipation pain during defecation bleeding due to fissures and abdominal pain.

Treatment

- Dis-impaction is the primary step in the management of functional constipation in children
- Polyethylene glycol is the recommended choice, given in the dose of 1-1.5 g/kg mixed in 6-8 OZ of water or juice over 3 hours is found to be efficient and safe in relieving functional constipation. If no significant response, then repeat the dose next day.

- Maintenance therapy to keep stool soft—0.2–0.8 g/kg/day for 2–3 months is effective in resolving the functional constipation.
- Parental reassurance and education and behavioral therapy are important.
- Regular sitting on toilet for 5–10 minutes at the same time every day with same meal.
- Encourage to take normal fiber-containing diet with plenty of oral fluids.
- Encourage exercise activities.

KEY MESSAGES

- Functional gastrointestinal disorders are conditions occurring in infants and toddlers without any structural or biochemical abnormalities.
- Timely diagnosis and effective management are important in avoiding unnecessary expensive investigations and therapeutic interventions
- Most FGIDs are benign in nature and resolve spontaneously over a period of time.
- Parental reassurance and education remains the cornerstone in the management of most FGIDs of infants and toddlers.

REFERENCES

1. Zeevenhooven J, Koppen IJ, Benninga MA. The new Rome IV criteria for functional gastrointestinal disorders in infants and toddlers. Pediatr Gastroenterol Hepatol Nutr. 2017;20(1):1-3.
2. Salvatore S, Vandenplas Y. Functional Gastrointestinal Disorders in Infants and Toddlers. In Pediatric Neurogastroenterology: Gastrointestinal Motility Disorders and Disorders of Gut Brain Interaction in Children. Cham: Springer International Publishing; 2023. pp. 465-75.
3. Boronat AC, Ferreira-Maia AP, Matijasevich A, Wang YP. Epidemiology of functional gastrointestinal disorders in children and adolescents: a systematic review. World Journal of Gastroenterology. 2017; 23(21):3915.
4. Koppen IJ, Nurko S, Saps M, Di Lorenzo C, Benninga MA. The pediatric Rome IV criteria: what's new?. Expert Rev Gastroenterol Hepatol. 2017;11(3):193-201.
5. Czinn SJ, Blanchard S. Gastroesophageal reflux disease in neonates and infants. Pediatr Drugs. 2013;15(1):19-27.
6. Hyman PE. Gastroesophageal reflux: one reason why baby won't eat. J Pediatr. 1994;125(6):S103-9.
7. Rosen R, Vandenplas Y, Singendonk M, Cabana M, Di Lorenzo C, Gottrand F, et al. Pediatric gastroesophageal reflux clinical practice guidelines: joint recommendations of the North American Society for Pediatric Gastroenterology, Hepatology, and Nutrition (NASPGHAN) and the European Society for Pediatric Gastroenterology, Hepatology, and Nutrition (ESPGHAN). Journal of pediatric gastroenterology and nutrition. 2018;66(3):516.
8. Poddar U. Gastroesophageal reflux disease (GERD) in children. Paediatrics and international child health. 2019;39(1):7-12.
9. Sherman PM, Hassall E, Fagundes-Neto U, Gold BD, Kato S, Koletzko S et al. A global, evidence-based consensus on the definition of gastroesophageal reflux disease in the pediatric population. Arch Pediatr. 2010;17(11):1586-93.
10. Eichenwald EC, Cummings JJ, Aucott SW, Goldsmith JP, Hand IL, Juul SE, et al. Diagnosis and management of gastroesophageal reflux in preterm infants. Paediatrics. 2018; 142(1).
11. Zeevenhooven J, Browne PD, L'Hoir MP, de Weerth C, Benninga MA. Infant colic: mechanisms and management. Nat Rev Gastroenterol Hepatol. 2018;15(8):479-96.
12. Sarasu JM, Narang M, Shah D. Infantile colic: an update. Indian Paediatr. 2018; 55(11):979-87.

13. Daelemans S, Peeters L, Hauser B, Vandenplas Y. Recent advances in understanding and managing infantile colic. F1000Res. 2018;7.
14. Schreck Bird A, Gregory PJ, Jalloh MA, Risoldi Cochrane Z, Hein DJ. Probiotics for the treatment of infantile colic: a systematic review. Journal of pharmacy practice. 2017;30(3):366-74.
15. Wessel MA, Cobb JC, Jackson EB, Harris Jr GS, Detwiler AC. Paroxysmal fussing in infancy, sometimes called "colic". Pediatrics. 1954;14(5):421-35.
16. Savino F, Ceratto S, De Marco A, Cordero di Montezemolo L. Looking for new treatments of infantile colic. Italian J Pediatr. 2014;40(1):1-6.
17. Hjern A, Lindblom K, Reuter A, Silfverdal SA. A systematic review of prevention and treatment of infantile colic. Acta Paediatrica. 2020;109(9):1733-44.
18. Camilleri M, Park SY, Scarpato E, Staiano A. Exploring hypotheses and rationale for causes of infantile colic. Neurogastroenterol Motil. 2017;29(2):e12943.
19. Skonieczna-Żydecka K, Janda K, Kaczmarczyk M, Marlicz W, Łoniewski I, Łoniewska B. The effect of probiotics on symptoms, gut microbiota and inflammatory markers in infantile colic: a systematic review, meta-analysis and meta-regression of randomized controlled trials. J Clin Med. 2020;9(4):999.
20. Arias A, Bennison J, Justus K, Thurman D. Educating parents about normal stool pattern changes in infants. J Pediatr Health Care. 2001;15(5):269-74.
21. Lewis LG, Rudolph CD. Practical approach to defecation disorders in children. Pediatric annals. 1997;26(4):260-8.
22. Kramer EA, den Hertog-Kuijl JH, van den Broek LM, van Leengoed E, Bulk AM, Kneepkens CF, et al. Defecation patterns in infants: a prospective cohort study. Archives of Disease in Childhood. 2015;100(6):533-6.
23. Rajindrajith S, Devanarayana NM. Constipation in children: novel insight into epidemiology, pathophysiology and management. J Neurogastroenterol Motil. 2011;17(1):35.
24. Candy DC, Edwards D, Geraint M. Treatment of faecal impaction with polyethelene glycol plus electrolytes (PGE+ E) followed by a double-blind comparison of PEG+ E versus lactulose as maintenance therapy. J Pediatr Gastroenterol Nutr. 2006;43(1):65-70.
25. Koppen IJ, Benninga MA, Singendonk MM. Motility disorders in infants. Early Hum Dev. 2017;114:1-6.
26. Vandenplas Y, Alarcon P, Alliet P, De Greef E, De Ronne N, Hoffman I, et al. Algorithms for managing infant constipation, colic, regurgitation and cow's milk allergy in formula-fed infants. Acta Paediatrica. 2015;104(5):449-57.
27. Lewis LG, Rudolph CD. Practical approach to defecation disorders in children. Pediatr Ann. 1997;26(4):260-8.
28. Vriesman MH, Koppen IJ, Camilleri M, Di Lorenzo C, Benninga MA. Management of functional constipation in children and adults. Nat Rev Gastroenterol Hepatol. 2020;17(1):21-39.
29. Shava U, Yachha SK, Srivastava A, Poddar U, SenSarma M. Assessment of stool frequency and colonic transit time in Indian children with functional constipation and healthy controls. Indian Journal of Gastroenterology. 2018;37(5):410-5.
30. van den Berg MM, Benninga MA, Di Lorenzo C. Epidemiology of childhood constipation: a systematic review. Am J Gastroenterol. 2006;101(10):2401-9.

SECTION 3: Problems of Infant and Young Child Feeding Practices

18. **Anatomical Problems of Breast and Nipple**
    Veerendra Kumar, Srilaxmi AN, Ramaraju HE

19. **Barriers of Breastfeeding**
    Basavanthappa SP, Anita Nyamagoudar, Sudhakar Hegade

20. **Breastfeeding Difficulties**
    Madhu Pujar, Sowmya D, Durgappa H

21. **Practical Problems of Lactation**
    Swarna Rekha Bhat, Durgappa H

22. **"Not Enough Milk"**
    Ruchi Nanavathi, Medha Goyal, Durgappa H

23. **Breastfeeding Myths**
    Varsha CR, Ashok R Datar, Durgappa H, Anita Nyamagoudar

24. **Feeding During and After Illnesses**
    Sudhindrashayana R Fattepur, Shilpa C, Vinod H Ratageri

25. **Hypernatremic Dehydration in Infants**
    Sumana Nanjundachar, Prakash M Kabbur, Anita Nyamagoudar, Durgappa H

26. **Infant Milk Substitutes**
    Prathibha Rao, Srikanth BK, Pranam GM

27. **Bottle-feeding**
    Vikas Patil, Durgappa H, Vani KT, Arpita JS

28. **Feeding and Eating Disorders in Children**
    Suchetha S Rao, B Shantharam Baliga

CHAPTER 18

Anatomical Problems of Breast and Nipple

Veerendra Kumar, Srilaxmi AN, Ramaraju HE

"Baby feeds at the breast and not at the nipple"

INTRODUCTION

Early problems in lactation can have a profound effect on a child's health. The birthing and lactation experience should be pleasant and memorable for the right reasons. Anatomical problems of the breast and nipple can be devastating to the physical and psychological health of the mother and may contribute to poor neonatal outcomes. Clear knowledge of these problems among both the healthcare workers and prospective mothers can negate most of the lactation difficulties.

- *Breast developmental anomalies:*
  - *Underdevelopment of breasts:* Hypomania
  - *Overdevelopment of breasts:* Polymastia, Macromastia—Breasts may be large due to either increased sensitivity to the female hormones due to elevated levels of the hormones in the blood
  - Breast asymmetry (unequally sized breasts)[1]
- *Long nipple:* This may cause difficulties as the baby does not take the breast far enough back into the mouth, likely to suck only the nipple and not take the breast with lactiferous sinuses into the mouth. It is important to reassure the mother. Breast milk can be expressed in a baby's mouth or fed with the help of a cup.
- *Short nipple:* Usually short nipple does not interfere with breastfeeding. Baby will form a teat from the breast and nipple.
- *Abnormally large nipple:* In this case, if the baby is small then his/her mouth may not be able to get beyond the nipple and on to the breast. Lactation should be initiated by expressing milk.
- *Inverted nipple or flat nipple:* Flat and inverted nipples are common anatomical problems of breast and nipple encountered in 9% of primiparous women. Most cases of flat/inverted nipples will not cause any problems during breastfeeding.

Nipple inversion is defined as a state in which part of the nipple or the entire nipple is retracted below the surface of the areola. Inverted nipple can be congenital or acquired. Lactiferous duct developmental abnormality and fibrosis around the lactiferous ducts due to inflammation may be the causative factors.[2]

PINCH TEST

It is a test to diagnose flat and inverted nipples. Position the thumb and fore finger on the areola, about 2–3 cm behind the nipple. Pinch the fingers together and see what the nipple looks like:
- *Nipple stands out:* This is a normal nipple; it should be easy for the baby to latch and breastfeed.
- *Nipple stays flat:* This is a flat nipple; most babies can breastfeed easily but some may need help with latching.
- *Nipple pulls inward:* This is an inverted nipple; the baby will likely need some help to latch and breastfeed in the beginning.

Baby with normal suck can overcome mild inversion. Latching-on and breastfeeding become difficult with moderate-to-severe inversion of the nipple. Treatment and deep latch techniques can help with proper latching and breastfeeding.[3]

MANAGEMENT

Inverted and flat nipples are not always a problem as the baby attaches to the breast and not to the nipple.

Soon after delivery:
- Build confidence in the mother.
- Counsel and convince the mother that the baby sucks at the breast, not at the nipple.
- Let the baby explore the breast.
- Maintain skin to skin contact between mother and the baby.

The antenatal nipple manipulation in a flat or retracted nipple is not advised as it may induce premature labor. Most flat nipples and/or inverted nipples become elongated during pregnancy or childbirth. Before the feeds, the nipple can be grasped and rolled between the index and thumb to make the nipple erect.

When the above measures fail, following methods can be tried to treat flat or inverted nipples:
- Breast shells
- Breast pumps/syringing
- Nipple shield
- Surgery.

Breast Shells (La Leche)

Breast shells may help to draw out flat or inverted nipples. They gradually draw the nipple out with gentle pressure. With continued wearing, it corrects the inversion over several weeks. Breast shells are in two pieces and are made out of plastic. The inner piece has a hole that fits over the nipple. The pressure on the tissue around the nipple causes the nipple itself to protrude through the hole. Breast shells may be worn during the antenatal period. After birth, they can be worn for about half an hour before feedings to draw out the nipple. They should not be worn at night. The hardness of plastic may cause discomfort in some. Shells are not suitable for those who use them while lying down. It is difficult to use in women with large breasts.[4]

When clinically indicated, a nipple shield may facilitate breastfeeding mother–infant dyad, without the risk of decreased infant weight gain.[5,6] It is not an alternative solution to the inexperienced mother who needs extra support in the early process of learning to breastfeed.[6]

Breast Pump or Modified Syringe

A breast pump or modified syringe can be used immediately before breastfeeding to draw an inverted nipple. This makes latching easier for the baby **(Fig. 1)**. By applying uniform

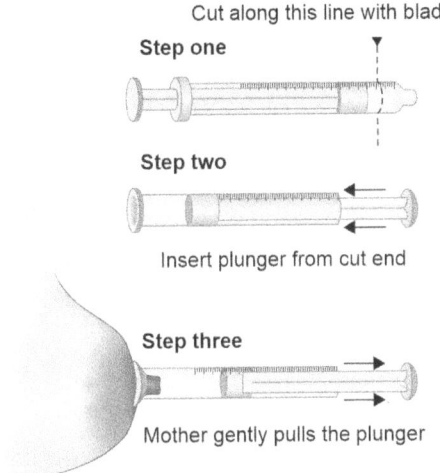

Fig. 1: Modifies syringe technique.

pressure from the center of the nipple these devices help to break the adhesions under the nipple.

Nirmala Kesaree syringe: Mothers with inverted nipples are helped to breastfeed with a modified 10-mL syringe. Mothers can breastfeed without any difficulty within a week. It is also shown to sustain sufficient breastfeeding.[7]

Nipple Shield

If other strategies are not working, a nipple shield could help the baby latch-on. Nipple shields should only be used with the guidance of a lactation expert to avoid improper usage that may lead to further problems.

Surgical Treatment

Very rarely corrective surgery may be needed. Further research is required to assess the psychological and breastfeeding benefits of the surgical procedure.[8-10]

NINE Procedure (No Incision Nipple Eversion): The advantages are—fast recovery, no scar mark, low recurrence rate, ability to breastfeed, not just an inverted nipple is corrected but a nipple can be created if nothing is there. The elaborative procedure can be watched using this video link - .https://youtu.be/8cjpvglQick

■ KEY MESSAGES

- Anatomical problems of the breast and nipple are the common hurdles for breastfeeding among primiparous women in the postpartum period.
- Antenatal breast examination is important to identify, anticipate and manage breastfeeding difficulties during the postpartum period.
- Antenatal manipulation of the nipple is not advised as it may induce premature labor.
- In most cases, flat and retracted nipples get elongated during pregnancy or delivery.

■ REFERENCES

1. Agbenorku P. Breast developmental anomalies: a review of the problem. Br J Med Med Res. 2012;(4):587-96.
2. Koyama S, Wu HJ, Easwaran T, Thopady S, Foley J. The nipple: a simple intersection of mammary gland and integument, but the focal point of organ function. J Mammary Gland Biol Neoplasia. 2013;18(2):121-31.
3. Alam M. Correction of Inverted Breast Nipple by Using Serdev Suture. Clin Surg. 2019;4:2590.
4. Alexander JM, Grant AM, Cambell MJ. Randomized controlled trial of breast shells and Hoffman's exercises for inverted and non-proctacile nipples. BMJ. 1992;304(6833):1030-2.
5. Chertok IR. Reexamination of ultra-thin nipple shield use, infant growth

and maternal satisfaction. J ClinNurs. 2009;18(21): 2949-955.
6. Kronborg H, Foverskov E, Nilsson I, Maastrup R. Why do mothers use nipple shields and how does this influence duration of exclusive feeding?. Matern Child Nutr. 2017;13(1):e12251.
7. Kesaree N, Banupurmath CR, Banupurmath S, Shamnuru K. treatment of inverted nipples using disposible syringe. J Hum Lact. 1993;9(1):27-9.
8. Pompei S, Tedesco M. A new surgical technique for the correction of the inverted nipple. Aesthetic Plast Surg. 1999;23(5):371-4.
9. Ritz M, Silfen R, Morgan D, Southwick G. Simple technique for inverted nipple correction. Aesthetic Plast Surg. 2005;29(1): 24-7.
10. Gould DJ, Nadeau MH, Macias LH, Stevens WG. Inverted nipple repair revisited: a 7-year experience. Aesthetic Plast Surg. 2015;35(2):156-64.

CHAPTER 19

Barriers of Breastfeeding

Basavanthappa SP, Anita Nyamagoudar, Sudhakar Hegade

"Breastfeeding is an opportunity for mother and baby."

■ INTRODUCTION

Breastfeeding was the best, is the best, and will remain the best as for as infant feeding is concerned. The effect of mass scale commercial propaganda by baby food companies has resulted in very disheartening and gloomy situation regarding infant feeding. Purchase of feeding bottles, bottle sterilizer, bottle warmer, animal milk, or milk formula is a huge financial burden for many Indian families. The added cost of hospitalization due to bottle-feeding needs no further mention. Exclusive breastfeeding (EBF) can save 8,500 crores INR in India alone annually.

It has been found that breastfed children have *at least six times greater chance of survival* in the early months than non-breastfed children, along with reduction in respiratory and diarrheal diseases. A global health journal series on child survival identified the promotion of EBF of infants during the first 6 months of life and continued breastfeeding to 12 months as the single most-effective preventive public health intervention for reducing the under-five mortality. EBF and early initiation to breastfeeding rates continue to remain low. It may be related to lack of the community awareness, education on the importance of breastfeeding, the risks of artificial feeding, inadequate information, and training programs of healthcare professionals on infant nutrition and breastfeeding.[1]

■ MAGNITUDE OF THE PROBLEM

Universally, the breastfeeding rate was on the decline for the last four decades. The percentages of infants younger than 6 months old who were exclusively breastfed were on an average about 40% in Asia. The numbers for rates of EBF are discouraging even among the developed countries. However in the last decade, >25 countries have demonstrated a rise in the rates of EBF at least by 20%.[2]

Barriers to Exclusive Breastfeeding[3-10]

- *Maternal factors:* Younger age, primigravida mother, exhaustive delivery, cesarean section, maternal separation/anesthesia, maternal illness—medical and psychological, local breast problems, lack of mother-baby-friendly environment.
- *Infant factors:* Too small, sick baby, hospitalized baby and baby with congenital anomalies

- *Family:* Nuclear family, lack of support, influence of family members
- *Healthcare professionals:* Lack of education/assistance and support
- *Peer pressure:* Negative influence
- *Advertising media:* Anticizing toward IMS (Infant Milk Substitutes) Act
- *Infant milk substitutes:* Easy availability
- *Environmental:* Embarrassment to feed in public
- *Return to work:* Stress, crèches unavailable at workplace
- *Miscellaneous:* Myths, lower socioeconomic status, mixed feeding

IMPACT OF BARRIERS ON BREASTFEEDING PRACTICES

Maternal Impact

The use of prelacteal feeds increases when breastfeeding is not initiated at birth. Mothers perceive breastfeeding as a challenge when they have not received antenatal counseling or have experienced any of the above challenges listed in the previous section.[5,8]

A research study conducted showed that the most significant self-reported factors for the discontinuation of EBF in the first month were the baby had trouble suckling and latching on (54%); sore nipples, cracked, and bleeding (37%); breasts were painful (29%); and breasts were overfull or engorged (24%). Perception of mothers that they did not have enough milk is also important factor for non-initiation or discontinuation for breastfeeding.[3,6]

Impact on the Infant

The infant's physiological status is also an important factor that determines the initiation of breastfeeding. Prelacteal feeds and mixed feeding lead increased risk of diarrheal and respiratory illness among infants, thereby increasing the rates of hospitalization. The microbiota of the infant which is determined by mother's own milk is disrupted by formula feeding. All the benefits of breastfeeding, which are considered rightly as child's way to healthy growth are missed among formula fed babies.[11]

Mixed feeding, especially giving water or other liquids, can also causes the supply of breast milk to decrease as the baby sucks less at the breast. Mixed feeding can leads to nipple confusion and preferential bottle-feeding by the baby. Supplementing breastfeeding with formula negatively affects breastfeeding. The infant's energy needs are satisfied by the supplement, which results in a reduction of the frequency and vigor of sucking by the infant at the breast. The consequent decrease in stimulation to the breast results in less milk production and therefore less available milk for the infant at the next feeding thus requires more supplementation for the infant to achieve satiety. Most mothers believe that formula milk is second best milk that her baby can get but health professionals should tell her that only her breast milk is the best for her baby.[11]

Impact on Society

The rates of breastfeeding will decline with each passing year if societal misconceptions are not addressed. The financial obligations of formula feeding are huge for mothers of lower socioeconomic status.

The media can impact and promote change in health behaviors. Given the strong presence of media in our society, the information presented in the media shapes beliefs, attitudes, and perceived norms. In fictional television programs, breastfeeding was portrayed as problematic, funny, and embarrassing. In contrast, bottle-feeding was present in all types of television programming, and problems or risks of bottle-feeding were rarely mentioned. Bottle-feeding representations in advertisements portrayed positive male involvement in parenthood. Most references to breastfeeding were verbal, and most references to bottle-feeding were visual.

WAYS TO OVERCOME BARRIERS OF BREASTFEEDING[12-14]

- Nurses and other healthcare professionals should acquire the knowledge and skill to provide breastfeeding information and support throughout the preconception, prenatal, and postpartum periods.
- All hospitals who are taking care of mothers and the babies should be associated with BFHI (Baby Friendly Hospital Initiative)
- Antenatal counseling for mothers regarding breastfeeding and antenatal breast examination and preparation of a mother for successful breastfeeding.
- Immediate Kangaroo Mother Care (iKMC) initiated soon after birth among stable babies can break all the barriers obstructing exclusive and successful breastfeeding.
- Lactation consultants or trained nurses provide timely practical help to mothers with local breast problems such as sore nipples, retracted nipple, breast abscess as well as poor milk secretion. Emphasizing the importance of colostrum and reassuring regarding its minimal quantity is essential to build mother's confidence.
- *The Maternity Benefits (Amendment) Act 2017* requires employer to provide nursing breaks of prescribed duration for new mothers in order to express breast milk for nursing child. This act increased the right to paid maternity leave for working women from 12 weeks to 26 weeks, the third highest in the world, but unfortunately the law applicable only to those who work in a company with at least 10 employees. In India, 84% of those women are working in unorganized sectors or for companies with fewer than 10 employees.
- Special scenarios such as maternal HIV, untreated Tuberculosis, COVID-19 infection, Hepatitis B infection and substance abuse need specific care of both mother and the newborn.
- Sustained community level, family level support: Raise awareness about the benefits of exclusive breastfeeding using mass media, such as television, radio, newspaper and magazines for encouraging this practice.
- Implementation of national health education campaigns that encourage women to breastfeed, especially during pregnancy by all primary healthcare nurses. Enhancement and development of policies, rules, regulations, legislation and laws that appropriately promote as well support breastfeeding.
- Establishment of human milk banks across the states (One per district) and sustained services at all of them can significantly increase the rates of exclusive human milk diet for infants.
- Quality Improvement Initiatives that target increasing the rates of EBF are the need of the hour, as part of implementation research.

KEY MESSAGES

- Exclusive breastfeeding is a chain of events that can be easily disrupted with maternal/infant/environmental factors.
- Immediate uninterrupted skin-to-skin contact between the mother and baby enhances the duration of breastfeeding practices.

- Educating the mothers on the benefits of breastfeeding and harmful effects of the formula feeding is important.
- Timely technical assistance and support to the mother is essential to enhance breastfeeding practices.
- And building the confidence in the mother is most important.

REFERENCES

1. Ahluwalia I, Morrow B, Hsia J. Why do women stop breastfeeding? Findings from the pregnancy risk assessment and monitoring system. Pediatrics. 2005;116:1408-12.
2. Breastfeeding. UNICEF. The global breastfeeding collectives.
3. Amir LH, Donath SM. Maternal diet and breastfeeding: a case for rethinking physiological explanations for breastfeeding determinants. Early Hum Dev. 2012;88(7):467-71.
4. Haider R, Kabir I, Hamdani JD, Habte D. Reasons for failure of breastfeeding counseling: mothers' perspective in Bangladesh. Bull World Health Organ. 1997;75(3):191-6.
5. Leung TF, Tam WH, Hung ECW, Fok TF, Wong GWK. Socio-demographic and atopic factors affecting breastfeeding intention to Chinese mothers. J Paediatr Child Health. 2003;39(6):460-4.
6. Majra JP, Silan VK. Barriers to early initiation and continuation of breastfeeding in a tertiary care institute of Haryana: A qualitative study in nursing care providers. J Clin Diagn Res. 2016;10:LC16-20.
7. Mandal B, Roe BE, Fein SB. The differential effects of full-time and part-time work status on breast feeding. Health Policy. 2010;97(1):79-86.
8. Noel-Weiss J, Rupp A, Cragg B, Bassett V, Woodend AK. Randomized controlled trial to determine effects of prenatal breastfeeding workshop on maternal breastfeeding self-efficacy and breastfeeding duration. J Obstet Gynecol Neonatal Nurs. 2016;35(5):616-24.
9. Rowe-Murray HJ, Fisher JR. Baby friendly hospital practices: cesarean section is a persistent barrier to early initiation of breastfeeding. Birth. 2002;29(2):124-31.
10. Hawkins SS, Dow-Fleisner S, Noble A. Breast feeding and the Affordable care Act. Pediatr Clin North Am. 2015;62(5):1071-91.
11. Yilmaz G, Caylan N, Karacan CD, Bodur I, Gokcay G. Effect of cup feeding and bottle feeding on breastfeeding in late preterm infants a randomized controlled study. J Hum Lact. 2014;30(2):174-9.
12. Protecting, promoting and supporting breastfeeding in facilities providing maternity and newborn services: implementing the revised Baby-friendly Hospital Initiative 2018. Geneva: World Health Organization and the United Nations Children's Fund (UNICEF); 2018.
13. WHO Immediate KMC Study Group; Arya S, Naburi H, Kawaza K, Newton S, Anyabolu CH, Bergman N, et al. Immediate "Kangaroo Mother Care" and survival of infants with low birth weight. N Engl J Med. 2021;384(21):2028-38.
14. The Maternity Benefits (Amendment) Act. No 6 of 2017. New Delhi. The 28th March, 2107/ Chaitra 7, 1939 (Saka).

CHAPTER 20

Breastfeeding Difficulties

Madhu Pujar, Sowmya D, Durgappa H

"Incorrect technique of breastfeeding is the root cause for most problems of breastfeeding".

INTRODUCTION

Breastfeeding difficulties are the common problems seen among lactating women. The recent prospective study of 552 mothers showed that around 72% of mothers experienced breastfeeding difficulties at 3 months of delivery and most problems of breastfeeding were reported within the first month of birth.[1] The problems of breastfeeding mentioned in **Box 1** are due to the *incorrect technique of breastfeeding*. Hence, timely skilled technical support and assistance are key to success **(Fig. 1)**. The common problems of breastfeeding include nipple pain, breast engorgement, plugged duct, mastitis, breast abscess, oversupply of milk, difficult deliveries, and galactoceles.

BOX 1: Problems associated with incorrect technique of breastfeeding.
- Cracked/sore nipple
- Breast engorgement
- Plugged duct
- Mastitis
- Breast abscess
- Cessation of breastfeeding
- Psychological stress among the mothers

NIPPLE PAIN (SORE/CRACKED NIPPLE)

It is one of the common reasons for premature cessation of breastfeeding among mothers in the postpartum period.[2] The most common cause for nipple pain is *incorrect positioning and latching on to the breast (90%)*.[3] The incidence of nipple pain and trauma varies in the literature between 34 and 96% in breastfeeding women.[4] The clinical picture

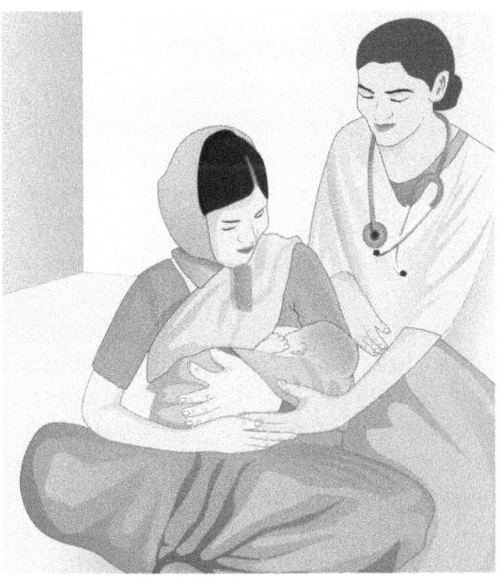

Fig. 1: Skilled practical assistance.

includes soreness of the nipple, sharp shooting pain, and redness, and is often associated with breast engorgement.

Management[2,5]

- *No topical agents are proven to be effective in relieving nipple pain.* Optimization of the technique of breastfeeding is the most effective way in relieving the nipple pain resulting from the incorrect technique of breastfeeding.
- Mothers can apply hindmilk over the sore nipple.
- Keep nipple exposed to air.
- Avoid frequent washing with soap.
- Frequent efficient breast milk removal is most important in preventing the further progression and recurrence of the problem.

In case of persistent pain in the nipples despite optimization of the technique of breastfeeding, one has to rule out other conditions causing nipple pain such as nipple infections, dermatitis of the nipple, ankyloglossia, and palatal anomalies in the baby.[6]

BREAST ENGORGEMENT

It is *overfilling* of the breast due to an imbalance between the production and drainage of breast milk. The common causes include delayed initiation of breastfeeding, improper latching, and inefficient breast milk removal, and this is one of the most common reasons for early cessation of lactation.[7]

Breast engorgement is a pathological condition characterized by bilateral enlargement of breasts, pain, discomfort in the breast, and flue like symptoms. It should be distinguished from physiological breast engorgement which occurs during 2-3 days of the postpartum period[8] in which secretary activation of the breast is triggered by delivery of the placenta (progesterone withdrawal) and subsequent rise in prolactin levels. Increased milk production and interstitial edema results invisibly larger, warmer, and slight discomfort in the breast which will usually resolve within a few days of delivery.[9]

Breast engorgement on other hand is discomforting and debilitating condition affecting 15-50% of women[10] and the prevalence may be even higher depending on the definition used. Any combination of pain, pyrexia, breast tension, and difficulty in breastfeeding should suggest breast engorgement. Another study from Swedish reported that 75% of mothers experienced symptoms of breast engorgement within 8 weeks of the postpartum period.[11] Hence, it is important to be vigilant of the mothers during the postpartum period.

Treatment[9,12-17]

- Psychological support to the mother is important.
- Relieve the discomfort with *gentle breast massage*.
- Apply *warm compresses* over the breasts which will facilitate the drainage of milk flow and reduces the pain.
- Express the breast milk around the areola so that this part of the breast becomes soft and easy for the baby to latch on.
- Attempt to *optimize the breastfeeding technique*, if still finding difficulty in latching, start expressing the breast milk from all the quadrants of the breast.
- Then apply *cold compresses* in between the feeding which will cause vasoconstriction and reduce edema.
- Green cabbage leaves application over the breast is beneficial.
- *Analgesics* may be considered in case of severe discomfort.
- It is important to keep "*regular complete emptying*" of the breast to prevent the recurrence of the condition.

PLUGGED DUCT

A plugged duct is inflammation and narrowing of the lactiferous duct resulting from *milk stasis*.[18,19] It usually presents between 3 and 6 weeks of the postpartum period. In one study, it was reported that two-thirds of lactating mothers experience plugged ducts at some point in time. If it is left untreated, may lead to the development of mastitis and breast abscess. The main cause for plugged ducts is due to inefficient breast milk removal. So, efficient management during lactation is the key to success.[20]

The clinical picture includes localized tender lump, and shooting pains, the overlying skin may become red and inflamed and the mother may have a mild fever. In some cases, white bleb may be seen on the tip of the nipple. Most cases of plugged duct resolve within 24–48 hours after the onset and prolonged blockage of the duct may lead to infective mastitis and even breast abscess.

Management[21]

- Provide psychological support to the mother.
- Gentle breast massaging is beneficial in relieving the discomfort.
- Apply warm compresses which will facilitate milk flow and reduce the pain.
- Frequent efficient emptying of the breast is most important in preventing further progression of the problem.

SIMPLE STEPS HAVE BEEN DESCRIBED IN THE RECANALIZATION OF PLUGGED DUCT[22]

- Preparation with 1 or 2 dry sterile towels
- Clean the plugged duct outlet
- Nipple manipulation
- Push and press the areola
- Push and knead the breast
- Check for residual milk stasis.

MASTITIS

Inflammation of the breast resulting from milk stasis due to inefficient breast milk removal.[18,19] The incidence of mastitis among breastfeeding mothers in different countries varies from 2 to 33%, with approximately an average 10%,[23] there are various risk factors for mastitis **Box 2**.

Pathogenesis

Inefficient breast milk removal is the root cause of the development of mastitis among mothers in the postpartum period. Mastitis results due to disruption of the breast microbiome. The factors interplaying in the development of mastitis include maternal nutrition, microbiota, antibiotics use, and manual expression of breast milk.[24]

The clinical picture includes sudden onset of high-grade fever (38–39°C), erythema, induration, pain and discomfort in the breast, and myalgia. If it is left untreated may lead to breast abscess.[19]

Etiology

The main causative agent of mastitis is a *Staphylococcus aureus* (90%) and in <10% of cases, gram-negative bacteria, *Proteus, klebsiella, Escherichia, Streptococcus epidermidis*, and *Enterococcus*[20].

BOX 2: The risk factors for mastitis.
- Sore nipple/cracked nipples
- Cleft lip/palate
- Latching difficulties
- Blocked Ducts
- Missed feeding
- Previous mastitis
- Primi mother
- Not using breast support

MANAGEMENT OF MASTITIS

The WHO has recommended four principles for the management of mastitis:[23]
1. *Supportive counseling:* This is the psychological support that helps to reduce the frustrating feelings in the mother.
2. Effective breast milk removal
3. Antibiotic therapy covering the *S. aureus*
4. Symptomatic treatment.

Management[19]

- *Supportive:* As it is frustrating and mothers look sick, it is important to provide psychological support.
- *Effective breast milk removal:* Encourage frequent breastfeeding for longer durations, if necessary, express by hand or pump.
- *Antibiotics:* Anti-*S. aureus* antibiotics; cloxacillin, cephalexin, cefadroxil, cefuroxime, and cefazolin. The duration of antibiotics should be 10–14 days.
- *Symptomatic therapy:* Analgesics ibuprofen, rest, plenty of oral fluids, and application of warm compresses.

BREAST ABSCESS

It always follows mastitis, resulting from milk stasis due to inefficient breast milk removal.[24] The incidence of breast abscess[25] ranges from 0.4 to 11%.[26] The highest incidence is reported in <12 weeks of the postpartum period.[27] In one study, it was reported that 3–11% of women having mastitis will develop breast abscess.[28]

Clinical pictures include fever, pain in the breast, myalgia, and swelling in the breast which is erythematous and tender.

Diagnosis

Ultrasound-guided aspiration to look for pus cells, gram staining, and culture sensitivity.

Management[25-29]

- Provide psychological support to the mother
- Incision and drainage is the most effective way to relieve the discomfort.
- Appropriate antibiotics covering the *S. aureus*.
- Analgesics—Ibuprofen is safe in relieving the pain.
- Good rest is essential.
- Adequate fluid intake is beneficial.
- Efficient emptying of the breast is critical to maintaining milk flow.

BREASTFEEDING AND DIFFICULT LABOR

It is not uncommon to see the delayed initiation of breastfeeding among mothers who have delivered babies by cesarean section or had exhaustive labour.[30] The delayed start of breastfeeding has a negative impact on the health of babies. Hence, breastfeeding should be supported among mothers and there is a need for training the healthcare professionals on optimal breastfeeding practices.

Ways to Overcome

- Ensure immediate skin-to-skin contact between mother and baby right from the time of birth of a baby which will activate the lactational reflexes.
- Practice the breast crawl method; immediately after delivery, place the baby on the upper abdomen of the mother so that the baby will crawl toward the breast and starts suckling.
- In case of exhaustive deliveries, the mothers can breastfeed the baby either in a leaning-back position or in a side-lying position which will also reduce the stress on the mother and baby.

OVERSUPPLY OF MILK

It is a condition where the supply of milk exceeds the demands of Infants. The infants often have difficulty handling the large amount of forceful milk secreted during the letdown reflex, leading to frequent choking episodes. Babies become irritable, cry excessively, and paradoxically may lose weight and the mother may subsequently develop breast engorgement.[31] To manage it effectively, relevant history and examination are important.

Management
- *Modifications of breastfeeding positions:* Feeding the baby in the upright position or lying back position reduces the risk of choking episodes.
- The mother can be asked to express an excess amount of milk and then allow the baby to suckle at the breast.
- *Scissor-hold method:* Ask the mother to scissor the breast with help of her fingers while breastfeeding the baby so that milk flow is controlled.
- *Modification of breastfeeding strategies:* Feed the baby on one side leaving the other breast for 3 hours and repeat the same to the other side, this will reduce the milk let-down reflex and thus may decrease the oversupply of milk.
- Medications like low-dose oral contraceptives may be tried in case of severe cases of oversupply of milk.

GALACTOCELE

Galactoceles are the milk retention cysts resulting from duct block. It presents as cystic painless swelling during pregnancy, lactation, and weaning. Initially, it contains milky fluid and which may later become thickened creamy, or oily as the fluid gets absorbed. Ultrasonography (USG) examination is diagnostic to distinguish galactoceles from other breast conditions such as adenomas, fibroadenomas, and breast abscesses. Aspiration of swelling confirms the diagnosis of galactoceles.[32]

Management
Intervention is needed only when it is bothering the mother. If she has symptoms, needle aspiration of the cyst or surgical excision is advised.

KEY MESSAGES

- Breastfeeding difficulties are a common hurdle among nursing mothers. The most common cause of nipple pain is "incorrect technique of breastfeeding".
- "Inefficient breast milk removal" is the root cause for most problems with breastfeeding.
- Timely technical assistance and support are critical in optimizing the technique of breastfeeding among mothers
- All the healthcare professionals involved in the services of maternal and child health need to undergo training on optimal infant and young child feeding practices.
- Change of attitude of healthcare professionals and society is critical.

REFERENCES

1. Gianni ML, Bettinelli ME, Manfra P, Sorrentino G, Bezze E, Plevani L, et al. Breastfeeding difficulties and risk for early breastfeeding cessation. Nutrients. 2019;11(10):2266.
2. Guille S, Sinclair M, Bunting B, Reid B, McCarron PA. Positioning and attachment interventions for nipple pain: a systematic review. Evidence-Based Midwifery. 2020; 30(3):293-306.

3. Kent JC, Ashton E, Hardwick CM, Rowan MK, Chia ES, Fairclough KA, et al. Nipple pain in breastfeeding mothers: incidence, causes, and treatments. Int J Environ Res Public Health.. 2015;12(10):12247-63.
4. Dennis CL, Jackson K, Watson J. Interventions for treating painful nipples among breastfeeding women. Cochrane Database of Systematic Reviews.2014;(12):CD007366.
5. Morland-Schultz K, Hill PD. Prevention of and therapies for nipple pain: a systematic review. J Obstet Gynecol Neonatal Nurs. 2005;34(4):428-37.
6. Amir LH, Baeza C, Charlamb JR, Jones W. Identifying the cause of breast and nipple pain during lactation. BMJ. 2021;374:n1628.
7. Sangar K. Engorgement of breast-potential problem in lactation. Nightingale Nursing Times. 2004;1(5):17-21.
8. Nikodem VC, Danziger D, Gebka N, Gulmezoglu AM, Hofmeyr GJ. Do cabbage leaves prevent breast engorgement? A randomized, controlled study. Birth. 1993;20(2):61-4.
9. Mangesi L, Zakarija-Grkovic I. Treatments for breast engorgement during lactation. Cochrane Database of Systematic Reviews. 2016(6).
10. Hill PD, Humenick SS. The occurrence of breast engorgement. J Hum Lactation. 1994;10(2):79-86.
11. Kvist LJ, Rydhstroem H. Factors related to breast abscess after delivery: A population-based study. BJOG. 2005;112(8):1070-4.
12. Zakarija-Grkovic I, Stewart F. Treatments for breast engorgement during lactation. Cochrane Database Syst Rev. 2020;9(9): CD006946.
13. Berens PD. Breast pain: Engorgement, nipple pain, and mastitis. Clin Obstet Gynecol. 2015;58(4):902-14.
14. Wong BB, Chan YH, Leow MQ, Lu Y, Chong YS, Koh SS, et al. Application of cabbage leaves compared to gel packs for mothers with breast engorgement: Randomised controlled trial. Int J Nurs Stud. 2017;76:92-9.
15. Siregar E, Hardjanti TS. Nonpharmacological treatments for breast engorgement: a systematic review. In Proceedings of the International Conference on Applied Science and Health. 2019;4:492-502.
16. Moon JL, Humenick SS. Breast engorgement: contributing variables and variables amenable to nursing intervention. J Obstet, Gynecol, Neonatal Nurs. 1989;18(4): 309-15.
17. Anderson L, Kynoch K, Kildea S, Lee N. Effectiveness of breast massage for the treatment of women with breastfeeding problems: a systematic review. JBI Evidence Synthesis. 2019;17(8):1668-94.
18. Yao Y, Long T, Pan Y, Li Y, Wu L, Fu B, et al. A five-step systematic therapy for treating plugged ducts and mastitis in breastfeeding women: a case–control study. Asian Nurs Res. 2021;15(3):197-202.
19. Pustotina O. Management of mastitis and breast engorgement in breastfeeding women. J Matern Fetal Neonatal Med. 2016;29(19):3121-5. .
20. Campbell SH. Recurrent plugged ducts. J Hum Lact. 2006;22(3):340-3.
21. Witt AM, Bolman M, Kredit S, Vanic A. Therapeutic breast massage in lactation for the management of engorgement, plugged ducts, and mastitis. J Hum Lact. 2016;32(1):123-31.
22. Zhao C, Tang R, Wang J, Guan X, Zheng J, Hu J, et al. Six-step recanalization manual therapy: a novel method for treating plugged ducts in lactating women. J Hum Lact. 2014;30(3):324-30.
23. World Health Organization. Section 13: Mastitis Causes and Management. Geneva: Department of Child and Adolescent Health and Development; 2000.
24. Mitchell KB, Johnson HM, Rodríguez JM, Eglash A, Scherzinger C, Widmer K, et al. Academy of Breastfeeding Medicine Academy of Breastfeeding Medicine Clinical Protocol# 36: The Mastitis Spectrum, Revised 2022. Breastfeed Med. 2022;17(5):360-76.

25. 29. Lam E, Chan T, Wiseman SM. Breast abscess: evidence-based management recommendations. Expert Rev Anti Infect Ther. 2014;12(7):753-62.
26. Dener C, İnan A. Breast abscesses in lactating women. World J Surg. 2003;27(2):130-3.
27. Merchant-Marchant DJ. Inflammation of the breast. Obstet Gynecol Clin. 2002;29(1): 89-102.
28. Cullinane M, Amir LH, Donath SM, Garland SM, Tabrizi SN, Payne MS, et al. Determinants of mastitis in women in the CASTLE study: a cohort study. BMC Fam Pract. 2015; 16(1):1-8.
29. Devereux WP. Acute puerperal mastitis: evaluation of its management. Am J Obstet Gynecol. 1970;108(1):78-81.
30. Prior E, Santhakumaran S, Gale C, Philipps LH, Modi N, Hyde MJ. Breastfeeding after cesarean delivery: a systematic review and meta-analysis of world literature. Am J Clin Nutr. 2012;95(5):1113-35.
31. Trimeloni L, Spencer J. Diagnosis and management of breast milk oversupply. J Am Board Fam Med. 2016;29(1):139-42.
32. Gada PB, Bakhshi G. Galactocele. In: StatPearls. Treasure Island (FL): StatPearls Publishing; 2023.

CHAPTER 21

Practical Problems of Lactation

Swarna Rekha Bhat, Durgappa H

"Breast feeding is not always easy, but it is always worth it"

INTRODUCTION

The most detrimental assumption we all make is that breastfeeding is a natural phenomenon and all mothers should be able to feed their babies but many mothers need help to do this. It is also a common assumption that if a neonate or infant is healthy, he/she should be able to take breastfeeds but they too need help. Understanding infant behavior is a very important step toward successful breastfeeding and counseling of the mother in this regard. It would be prudent to emphasize that breastfeeding is a "relational" (interconnected) activity between mother and baby and not just a nutritional activity. This section will be describing in brief sleep-wake cycles of neonate/infant, feeding behavior and some common feeding problems.

SLEEP-WAKE CYCLE

Understanding the sleep-wake pattern of normal neonates and infants is crucial to predict feeding behavior of neonates.

In the first few days of life, neonates may spend almost 16–18 hours sleeping.[1] Though demand feeding is the norm, in the first few days babies may have to be woken up to be fed. The average sleep time decreases to about 12–14 hours by 6 months, with duration of night-time sleep gradually increasing. Waking time between naps is about 45 minutes–1 hour initially and increases to about 3 hours by 6 months. The usual duration of naps is 1–2 hours but could be as short as 15–30 minutes in the initial few weeks. It is important that the mother is aware of her baby's sleep pattern so that she can plan the baby's feeding schedule.

Sleep in the neonatal period may be classified as quiet sleep, active sleep (mostly REM sleep), and transitional sleep and awake. In the neonatal period, quiet and active sleep each account for about 50% of sleep duration.

NORMAL FEEDING BEHAVIOR

A term infant has all the reflexes needed to take breastfeeds. Neonates and infants also have specific feeding skills which help them to express hunger and satiety **(Table 1)**. It is important for the mother to recognize these early cues and feed accordingly rather than deciding to feed as per clock or when breasts are full or stop feeding when breasts are empty.

Each neonate has a specific feeding behavior; again, it is important for the mother to recognize this. Most neonates latch

TABLE 1: Hunger and satiety cues in neonates and infants.

Hunger cues	Satiety cues
0–3 months	*0–3 months*
Opens and closes mouth	Slows or decreases sucking
Brings hands to face, roots and sucks at fingers, hands	Pushes away or arches
Makes sucking noises and action	Falls asleep
Flexes arms and legs, clenches hands	Extends arms and legs and fingers
Gets irritable and cries (late cue)	Turns head away from breast
4–7 months	*4–7 months*
Moves head toward breast	Releases nipples
Smiles, gazes at mother	Seals mouth
Makes cooing sound	• Turns head away from breast • Easily distracted

immediately when breast is offered and feed and suck vigorously till they are full and delatch by themselves. This behavior is easily understood and handled. However, some neonates and infants may take time to latch (even though they do not have any difficulty latching) may suck slowly and for a longer duration, may get easily distracted. Some neonates and infants may fall asleep during a feed and may need to be woken up.[2]

Neonates and infants may resort to *cluster feeding* (frequent feeds in short bursts) and this may be very frustrating for the mother. This is a normal response to hunger, but it could also mean the baby is tired, overstimulated, wanting attention, and insecure and can occur during "growth spurts". Growth spurts are time periods when neonates and infants feed frequently and this actually may help in increasing milk production. These are noticed to occur around 7–10 days, 2–3 weeks, 4–6 weeks and 3 months of age and could continue to occur till 6 months of age at periodic intervals. These are the most vulnerable time periods when mother may switch to other feeds as she feels breast milk is not sufficient.

Responsive feeding (RF) refers to a reciprocal relationship between an infant and the caregiver that is characterized by immediate response from the caregiver to the feelings of hunger and satiety of a baby through verbal or nonverbal cues.[3]

In simple words, RF refers to mothers feeding their babies in response to early hunger cues rather than feeding in response to crying which is a late response to hunger. Practicing RF is associated with increased chances of exclusive breastfeeding in the first 6 months. Hunger and satiety cues are enumerated in **Table 1** and it is important that the mother learns to recognize these.

"NORMAL" OR "PHYSIOLOGICAL" PROBLEMS ASSOCIATED WITH BREASTFEEDING AND SOLUTIONS[4]

This is referred to as physiological because these problems can occur in healthy normal neonates but sometimes may also occur due to pathological reasons. For example, choking can occur if the milk flow is too fast, but it can also indicate swallowing problem, cleft palate, etc.

No Latching Ability

One of the simplest reasons for not latching is prematurity. Often normal size late preterms are mistaken for term neonates and these neonates have difficulty latching. Babies may not latch if the positioning is not right.

Positioning the baby appropriately will help the baby to latch. They may not latch well if there are any breast issues such as engorged breasts for which the mother should express a little milk and then restart feeding. Not latching may also occur if the baby is not hungry, too sleepy, or tired.

Refusal to Feed

The more serious causes of refusal to feed will be dealt with in another section. A baby may refuse to feed if he/she is not hungry, is full, is too tired, or sleepy. They may refuse to feed if there are any distractions and sometimes neonates prefer to feed only on one side. Environmental factors such as change in routine, a different place, too much distraction, and even a change in mother's smell can result in the baby not wanting to feed. A nose block could also prevent a baby from feeding well. During positioning and attachment, the mother or the person assisting may touch the baby's occiput; this may prevent the baby from latching and feeding. Nipple confusion is another common reason for refusing to feed. This occurs if the baby is on bottle feeds or even paladai or spoon feeds in addition to breastfeeds as the method of feeding is different when different methods are used simultaneously.

Choking

The most common cause for choking is if the milk flow is too fast and the baby is unable to handle the fast flow of milk. The mother can use a scissor hold and control flow of milk, she can express milk and then feed or she can change the position (keep the baby more upright) so that baby does not choke. It could also occur if there is any oral abnormality like cleft palate or if the baby is sleepy or not alert because of any neurological problem and cannot swallow properly.

Falling Asleep While Feeding

The most likely cause is that the baby is full or too sleepy. Some neonates have a tendency to feed in short bursts, sleep, and then feed again. Again, it is important that the mother recognizes her baby's feeding behavior to address this issue. She needs to stop feeding and then refeed when the baby wakes up. When fed for a shorter time the baby may wake up earlier for a feed and this is quite normal.

Continuous Sucking

This could occur if milk flow is not adequate. It could also occur during cluster feeding and during growth spurts, in this situation it may help in improving milk secretion. Some babies suck continuously and this may not be for nutrition but as a soothing or calming behavior.

Not Sucking Well

Preterm and late preterm neonates may not suck well. As mentioned earlier a late preterm good weight baby may be mistaken for a term neonate. Sometimes normal neonates may not suck well if they are full or they are too sleepy or tired. It is best to stop feeding and retry after sometime. However, if this persists the baby may be having a more serious problem like, sepsis and CNS depression due to asphyxia.

Fussy or Crying during Feeding

There could be many reasons for this. Babies may fuss and cry while feeding if they are not hungry and do not want to feed. It could occur because of too little milk flow or too much of milk flow. It could also be because the baby wants to burp or pass gas or is feeling uncomfortable. If the baby makes fuss and cries during a feed, it is best to stop feeding, burp the baby, console, and restart to feed. It could also be due to "colic" related to the type of that food mother has eaten. Gastroesophageal reflux can cause excessive crying during a feed.

Nipple Biting

This could occur inadvertently once teeth have erupted or it could occur when an older baby is sucking vigorously because of hunger or because the feed has been delayed. This can precipitate a cracked nipple. The mother should recognize early hunger cues and should feed the baby accordingly. Too little flow of milk can also result in the baby biting the nipple. Sometimes, the baby may bite the nipple to decrease the flow in case there is too much milk-flow.

TABLE 2: Practical problems and solutions.

Common problems	Physiologic causes	Solutions
Inability to latch	• Preterm, late preterm • Improper positioning • Engorged breasts	• Needs assistance • Correct positioning • Express milk before feeding
Refusal to feed	• If baby is not hungry, is full or too sleepy • Environmental factors • If mother touches baby's occiput while feeding • Nipple confusion	• Discontinue feeding and retry after sometime • Always follow same routine, avoid distractions while feeding • Avoid touching the baby's occiput • Avoid multiple methods of feeding
Choking	Too much milk flow	Use scissor position to decrease flow
Falling asleep while feeding	Baby is satisfied, tired, or full	Wake up baby by tickling, if baby continues to sleep, stop feeding and feed again when baby is awake
Continuous sucking	Too little milk flow	Initiate measures to improve lactation
Not sucking well	• If baby is tired • Preterm, late preterm neonates	Should seek medical help if this persists
Fussy or crying during feed	• Not wanting a feed because baby is tired, sleepy • Too much or too little milk flow • Gastroesophageal reflux, need to burp, and colic	• Stop and reinitiate feeding after sometime • *Check on milk flow:* If too much use scissor technique, if too little express some milk into baby's mouth • Stop feeding, burp, and refeed
Nipple biting	• Could be normal • If milk flow is too much • If baby is very hungry or milk flow is less	If persists will need to check if milk flow is less and provide lactational support
Arching while feeding	If occiput is being touched Could be due to reflux, neurological problem	Avoid touching baby's occiput Consult doctor
Latching and relatching	• Could be playful or distracted • If initial latching not ok	• Avoid distraction • Check positioning and attachment

Arching the Back and Body while Feeding

This is more likely to occur if the baby has gastroesophageal reflux or has truncal hypertonia. This can also occur if the baby does not want to feed or his/her occiput is being held while positioning the baby for a feed.

Latching and Relatching

If the initial latch is not satisfactory the baby may try to relatch. Too much or too little milk flow can also cause this. If a baby is distracted or is just being playful the baby may latch and relatch.

SOLUTIONS TO COMMON FEEDING PROBLEMS

As mentioned earlier, the above problems can occur in normal neonates, hence while taking a feeding history it is important to ask what exactly the problem is, in order to address the issue. Often mothers or the nurse who is helping say that baby is "not feeding well". It is important to address the issue of positioning and attachment. But the micro issues of feeding also need to be addressed. One needs to identify if the problem is with latching, sucking, delatching, milk flow, drowsy state of the baby, long or too short duration of sucks, chokes during feeding, etc.

The mother should be helped to analyze the problem, understand the sleep pattern, and recognize hunger and satiety cues and should also be made to understand the role of environmental causes to these problems. Most of the solutions are simple and obvious once the problem is recognized **(Table 2)**. As a general measure, it is advisable not to force the baby to feed, instead mother should stop feeding, console the baby, and the mother also needs to calm herself. Further, she can try to establish relatch with proper positioning and avoid touching the occiput. Skin-to-skin contact can sometimes help to solve these problems.[5] If there is too much milk flow, mother can either express the milk or use a scissor hold. If the milk flow is less then squeeze some milk into the baby's mouth or feed on the other side. Mother should always keep herself hydrated as dehydration can make the mother more irritable. Follow the same routine, avoid distractions while feeding and most importantly allow the baby to decide when to feed and when to stop feeding.

KEY MESSAGES

- It is important for mother to understand her baby's sleep wake pattern and recognize hunger and satiety cues.
- Most problems mentioned above are due to physiologic reasons and can be rectified by simple measures.
- If these problems are persisting there may be an underlying pathologic cause and the mother must consult a doctor.

REFERENCES

1. Barbeau DY, Weiss MD. Sleep disturbances in newborns. Children. 2017;4:90-106.
2. Burns E, Fenwick J, Sheehan A, Schmied V. This little piranha': a qualitative analysis of the language used by health professionals and mothers to describe infant behaviour during breastfeeding. Mater Child Nutr. 2016;12:111-24.
3. Harbron J, Booley S, Najaar B, Day CE. Responsive feeding: Establishing healthy eating behaviour early in life. S Afr J Clin Nutr. 2013;26:S141-9.
4. Wight NE. Management of common breastfeeding issues. PCNA. 2001;48:321-44.
5. Svensson KE, Velandia MI, Mattheisen AT, Welles-Nyström BL, Widström AM. Effects of mother-infant skin-to-skin contact on severe latch-on problems in older infants: a randomized trial. Int Breastfeeding J. 2013;8:1-13.

CHAPTER 22

"Not Enough Milk"

Ruchi Nanavathi, Medha Goyal, Durgappa H

"Breastfeeding reminds us of the universal truth of abundance; the more we give out, the more we are filled up, and that divine nourishment—the source from which we all draw is, like a mothers breast, ever full and ever flowing".
—**Sarah Buckley**

INTRODUCTION

Breastfeeding is the most natural way to feed a newborn baby. Breastfeeding gives the little one the best start in life as breast milk is the only food and drink that the term baby needs in the first 6 months of life. Breastfeeding has been our Indian culture. Indian mothers are breastfeeding their babies since time immemorial. However, with changing lifestyles, breastfeeding rates have declined over the last few decades. Though our mothers start breastfeeding naturally, at the slightest problem encountered they do not hesitate to shift to alternative milk. The concern of "not enough milk" is a common cause of worry in many breastfeeding mothers. However, almost often it is a not a problem requires simple measures. But if inadequately managed, this simple problem has deep implications in the form of stopping breastfeeding in the first few weeks after delivery and resorting to quick solutions such as formula feeds or animal milk.

"Not enough milk" is also referred to as insufficient milk or low milk flow. Not enough milk is the most common reason for the premature cessation of breastfeeding. In the majority of cases, there is no identifiable cause that is found for insufficient milk secretion and it is simply because of "perception of insufficient milk secretion". The most common cause for low milk flow is infrequent and incomplete emptying of the breast and rarely due to other underlying reasons.

The approach to this issue is scientifically based on understanding the physiology of lactation. The problem can be easily circumvented in the first place if lactation is adequately managed with knowledge of the principles of lactation but unfortunately, many clinicians are unequipped with an adequate understanding of the physiology and recommend supplementation; it proves to be counter-productive and can further lead to insufficient milk. Formula feeding may appear as a better alternative as it is seemingly less time-consuming and mothers are coupled with a belief that formula can provide a nutritionally equivalent substitute to mothers' milk.

UNDERSTANDING THE "GOLDEN PHYSIOLOGY" OF LACTATION[1]

Lactation is the physiologic completion of the reproductive cycle. The breasts develop throughout pregnancy and prepare to take over the role of fully nourishing the infant. There are two stages in the initiation of lactation—(1) secretory differentiation and (2) secretory activation. During these stages, the mammary epithelial cells differentiate into lactocytes with the capacity to synthesize unique milk constituents (secretory differentiation) followed by initiation of copious milk secretion (secretory activation). This physiologic adaptation of the mammary gland is supported by the presence of a lactogenic hormone complex which includes estrogen, progesterone, prolactin, and metabolic hormones such as insulin and cortisol. All this preparation is kept inactive by a tight balance of inhibiting hormones. In the first few hours and days of postpartum, the breast responds to changes in hormonal milieu due to the withdrawal of placental and luteal hormones (mainly progesterone) and importantly to the stimulus of the newborn infant's suckling to produce and release milk. The depression of prolactin-inhibitory factors and/or stimulation of prolactin-releasing factors during the first 4 days postpartum is reflected by the *"coming in"* of milk **(Fig. 1)**. In a non-nursing mother, the prolactin levels drop to normal in 2 weeks, independent of any intervention implying the need for timely supporting lactation before it progresses to complete lactation failure. The oxytocin reflex is nature's way to support lactation and encourage milk release in a mother simply by seeing, touching, hearing, smelling, or thinking about her infant.

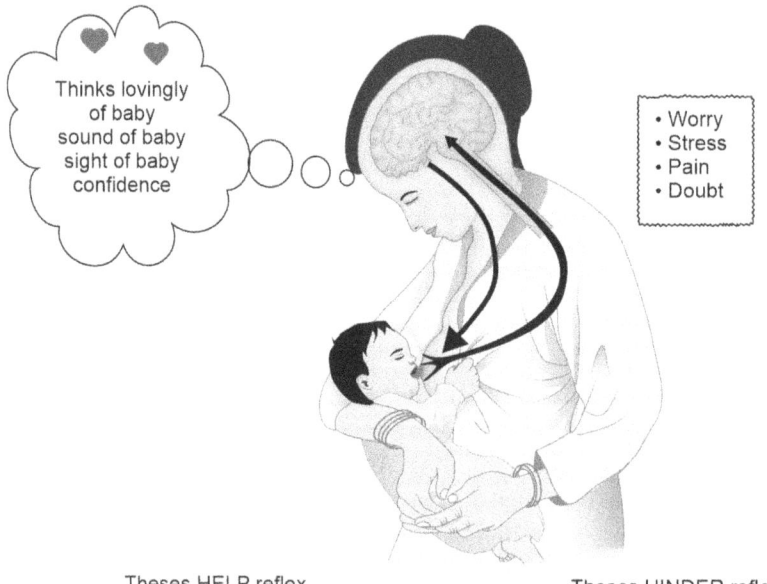

Fig. 1: Factors influencing breast milk secretion.

FACTORS INFLUENCING BREAST MILK SECRETION

Factors influencing breast milk secretion shown in the **Figure 1**.

APPLICATION OF PHYSIOLOGY FOR A SUCCESSFUL LACTATION

The common causes hampering the prolactin reflex include improper positioning and attachment while breastfeeding, infrequent feeding, prolonged separation of the mother-baby dyad, prelacteal feeds, top feeding with formulas or water, and use of feeding bottles and pacifiers. Nipple soreness and breast engorgement further increase the chances of an unsuccessful lactation. Hence identifying and rectifying any such trivial-looking practices that prevent proper stimulation and emptying of the breast goes a long way in establishing successful lactation.[1,2]

An important point to understand about lactation physiology is that secretory activation usually begins 30–40 hours after delivery. Hence, the colostrum available during the first 24–48 hours after birth is of small volume and represents milk already secreted in the ducts and not a rapid synthesis of milk. Term newborns have significant stores and can mobilize energy from these stores and also can utilize alternative energy substrates.

APPROACH TO AN ISSUE OF "NOT SUFFICIENT MILK"

A detailed history is the first vital step in identifying the risk factors of insufficient milk syndrome. Mothers feel that there is not enough milk in clinical situations such as frequent crying or waking up of the baby, baby sucking for a short time, irritable baby, little milk on expression, small size breast, empty/sagging breast on palpation, and cracked nipples/malformed nipples. It is essential to differentiate between primary lactational failure and delayed lactogenesis based on the history as the management is entirely different.[2,3]

- *Primary lactation failure:* It is caused by the factors affecting mammogenesis leading to insufficient breast tissue. These include hypoplastic breasts, breast surgery such as mastectomy, breast reduction or cyst removal, severe systemic illnesses, and Sheehan's syndrome caused due to by postpartum hemorrhage leading to pituitary ischemia/infarction results in lack of/absence of prolactin.
- *Delayed lactogenesis:* This is mainly related to factors leading to inadequate breast stimulation.
- *Neonatal factors:* Prematurity, low birth weight, birth asphyxia, craniofacial defects (cleft palate), critical congenital heart disease, and illness requiring intensive care.
- *Maternal factors:* Stress during delivery, maternal-infant separation, cesarean delivery, delayed initiation of feeding, inadequate breast emptying, local breast problems (flat, sore nipples, engorgement, and retracted nipples), inappropriate positioning and technique, sociocultural issues (discontinuation of feeds due to minor ailments), scheduled feeding, anxiety, excessive maternal fatigue, lack of knowledge of breastfeeding, maternal obesity, type 1 diabetes, and rarely maternal psychiatric disorders (postpartum psychosis), ingestion of certain drugs/hormones, and occasionally retained placenta. Mothers who had faced difficulties in breastfeeding their first children are more prone to complain about milk insufficiency.

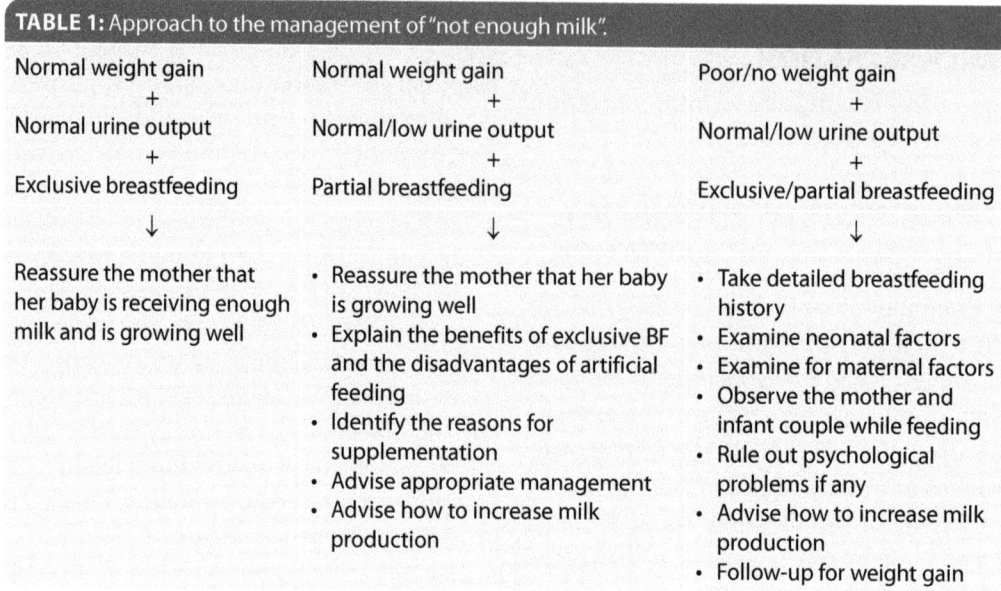

TABLE 1: Approach to the management of "not enough milk".

Normal weight gain + Normal urine output + Exclusive breastfeeding ↓	Normal weight gain + Normal/low urine output + Partial breastfeeding ↓	Poor/no weight gain + Normal/low urine output + Exclusive/partial breastfeeding ↓
Reassure the mother that her baby is receiving enough milk and is growing well	• Reassure the mother that her baby is growing well • Explain the benefits of exclusive BF and the disadvantages of artificial feeding • Identify the reasons for supplementation • Advise appropriate management • Advise how to increase milk production	• Take detailed breastfeeding history • Examine neonatal factors • Examine for maternal factors • Observe the mother and infant couple while feeding • Rule out psychological problems if any • Advise how to increase milk production • Follow-up for weight gain

- *Environmental factors:* Inadequate support and guidance from healthcare professionals, inadvertent marketing of commercial formulas, and early introduction of bottle-feeds and pacifiers.

Examination of the Mother-infant Couple

Examination of the infant to rule out any of the above-mentioned neonatal factors and examining the mother for local breast and nipple problems is crucial. It is always rewarding to observe the mother-infant couple while breastfeeding about positioning and attachment at the breast (latching on). The most common cause of sore, cracked nipples, is incorrect positioning and ineffective latch-on. These painful feeding sessions can cause a lactating mother to skip, postpone, or limit nursing sessions. Rarely, tongue tie can cause severe nipple pain and inadequate milk supply as the infant is not able to draw the teat effectively into the mouth and that leads to nipple trauma. For a new lactating mother, latch-on difficulties are frustrating and may feel like a rejection to her and doubt her milk sufficiency.

MANAGEMENT

It is important to distinguish between a mother whose milk production is low and a mother who feels her milk production is low although she is receiving enough milk. Early recognition and treatment of breastfeeding problems offer the best chance of resolving lactation difficulty before developing complications from insufficient milk. Counseling and reassurance to the mothers are the cornerstone in managing the problem of low milk production as most of the time it is the perception of the mother and not a reality. The assistance from a skilled caregiver will enable her to learn the science and art of feeding her baby. The approach to the management of "not enough milk" is summarized in **Table 1**.

- *Management of the neonatal factors:* These mothers need strong support and

encouragement. She should be made aware that her small sick baby needs her milk to get better faster. The mother should be taught to express milk either manually or using pumps at least 8–10 times a day to keep up the milk supply till her preterm or sick baby can suck efficiently at the breast. This expressed milk is then fed to the baby through a feeding tube or using a spoon, cup, or paladar special feeders as applicable.
- *Correct techniques of breastfeeding:* Teaching these mothers the fundamentals of the correct technique reduces physical discomfort during feeding, improves infant attachment to the breast, and improves lactation. She can observe masseter muscle during suckling and sounds of swallowing. Various positions such as cradle, cross-cradle, football, etc., can be taught to the mother using written material or by one-on-one bedside assistance as per the case.
- *Management of local breast and nipple problems* should be taken care of appropriately.
- *Galactagogues* are medications that are believed to assist initiation, maintenance, or augmentation of maternal milk production. The efficacy of metoclopramide in enhancing milk production in women with inadequate milk supply has been reported. Domperidone has also been used for its effect on increasing prolactin and increasing milk production.

PREVENTION OF LOW MILK PRODUCTION[1,2,4]

Prenatal Measures

- *Prenatal breastfeeding education:* The decision to breastfeed is influenced by diverse factors. Counseling expectant mothers and addressing their concerns at prenatal visits go a long way toward lactation success.
- *Prenatal breast examination:* Examination of breast and nipple-areola complex helps to assess lactation potential and provides an opportunity for timely detection of any problems. Women who report little or no prenatal breast enlargement are likely to have insufficient lactation. Flat nipples or inverted nipples do not preclude successful breastfeeding. Most infants learn to nurse from any nipple configuration, provided a mother is given proper guidance in correct positioning and latch-on. True inverted nipples are rare and gently stretching to evert them can be taught before delivery. Mostly breastfeeding is unrelated to breast appearance except in conditions such as tubular breast deformity, hypoplastic breasts, or any prior breast irradiation. Prior breast surgery involving periareolar breast incision can sever milk ducts or disrupt innervation. Excisional biopsy or drainage of breast abscess through a periareolar incision increases the risk of milk insufficiency.

Postnatal Measures

- *Breastfeeding practices:* This includes early initiation of breastfeeding, encouragement for breast crawl, continuous rooming-in, cue-based demand feeding, and avoiding prelacteal or supplemental feeds. The time of first breastfeeding and frequency on day 2 have been correlated with milk volume by day 5. Hospitals should comply with baby friendly hospital initiative (BFHI) guidelines.
- *Breastfeeding support:* Family should be counseled regarding their important role in breastfeeding by nurturing and encouraging new mothers and providing

help with household duties and infant care at home.
- *Breastfeeding education:* The mother should be convinced regarding the following aspects:
  - Breast milk is the only food and drink that her newborn baby needs in the first 6 months of life for optimal physical, mental, and social development.
  - The preferred pattern of optimal nutrition is unrestricted breastfeeding *ad libitum* (not by the clock), usually leading to 10 or more feedings per day.
  - Every mother has the natural capacity to produce enough milk for her baby. The size of the breast does not correlate with her ability to produce milk.
  - Milk volume varies between 2 and 20 mL per feeding in the first 3 days and the volume of milk increases over time over the first 2 weeks, starting at <100 mL/day and increasing to about 600 mL/day at 96 hours.
  - Mother should follow baby's *hunger cues* which include increased alertness at feeding times, rooting, mouthing movements, sucking fingers/hands, and crying (a late hunger sign). Feeding a crying or irritable baby is challenging and could be counterproductive at times.
  - The infant usually nurses for about 10–15 minutes per feeding in the first few days. Breastfed infants consume 50% of feed in 2 minutes and 80-90% in 5 minutes. Some infants are satisfied in 8-10 minutes and others take 30 minutes to consume the same volume. The duration of feeding should be guided by the infant's response and not by time.
  - An exclusively breastfed baby passing pale yellow-colored urine six to eight times a day is suggestive of adequate milk intake.
  - Many signs that she takes as an indication of poor milk supply does not indicate such a situation in reality.
  - *Signs of early satiety:* Sounds of swallowing decrease and stop, non-nutritive suckling occurs in brief bursts, arms and legs relax, and the infant falls asleep and releases the nipple.
  - *Signs of successful lactation:* Dripping of milk from the opposite breast, dripping at sight or thought of the infant, no pain while breastfeeding, and adequate weight in the baby.
  - Adequate rest is important as maternal fatigue can be a cause of lactation insufficiency.
  - *Harmful practices for breastfeeding:* Scheduled feeding, infrequent feeding, and omitting of night feeds and bottle-feeding. Feeding on schedule results in fewer feeds than on-demand and less frequent feeds directly lead to insufficient milk.

Mothers want to do their best for their babies. As neonatal caregivers, it is our fundamental duty to provide practical information and necessary support to enable mothers to continue nursing their babies and support nature's way of nourishing young infants. Let's help the baby to navigate the course from birth to breast. It is said, "God could not be everywhere so he made mothers".

KEY MESSAGES

- Perception of insufficient milk secretion (PIMS) is the most common reason for premature cessation of lactation.

- Infrequent ineffective emptying of the breast is the most common reason for low milk flow.
- Frequent efficient breast milk removal is the effective way to maintain adequate milk secretion.

REFERENCES

1. Lawrence RA, Lawrence RM. Breastfeeding: A Guide for the Medical Profession, 8th edition. Philadelphia: Elsevier; 2015.
2. Neifert MR. Clinical aspects of lactation. Promoting breastfeeding success. Clin Perinatol. 1999;26(2):281-306.
3. Gussler JD, Briesemeister LH. The insufficient milk syndrome: a biocultural explanation. Med Anthropol. 1980;4(2):145-74.
4. Howard CR, Howard FM, Lanphear B, Eberly S, deBlieck EA, Oakes D, et al. A randomized clinical trial of pacifier use and bottle-feeding or cupfeeding and their effect on breastfeeding. Pediatrics. 2003;111(3):511-8.

CHAPTER 23

Breastfeeding Myths

Varsha CR, Ashok R Datar, Durgappa H, Anita Nyamagoudar

"Breastfeeding is a natural 'safety net' against the worst effects of poverty".
—*James P Grant*

INTRODUCTION

Breastfeeding is the foundation on which infant nutrition and growth is built. It is not an exaggeration to call mother's milk the "Elixir of life". Every baby needs to be breastfed for optimum growth and development. But, a big hurdle in the establishment and continuation of breastfeeding are the myths surrounding it.

A new mother is bombarded with information both correct and incorrect. With the advancement of technology and flooding of information on social media, mothers are exposed to both myths and facts. There is also influence of elders in the family.

Healthcare workers have an important task of dispelling these myths. Here are a few common myths in our country India followed by the relevant facts.

- *Myth:* Colostrum should not be fed to the baby.
  Fact: Colostrum is the first milk secreted after delivery. It is watery and yellowish in color. It has high levels of immunoglobulin, lactoferrin, lyzozymes, lactalbumin, fats that carry important vitamins and polyunsaturated fatty acids (PUFAs). It is considered as the first vaccine a neonate receives. It is the ideal first feed for a newborn and no newborn should be deprived of colostrum.

- *Myth:* Newborns need to be given prelacteal feeds like sugar water, honey, cow's milk, etc.
  Fact: Babies do not need any prelacteal feeds. The assumption that prelacteals help babies to establish breastfeeding is false. In fact, babies may refuse to breastfeed after consuming prelacteals (as they are high in sugar and easily delivered to the baby's mouth without sucking).

  Breast milk provides complete nourishment to the baby. Babies do not require water if exclusively breastfed till 6 months. Prelacteal feeds may lead to infections in the newborns with serious consequences like sepsis. Honey can contain spores of bacteria that produce "Botulinum toxin" leading to "botulism" in infants.[1]

- *Myth:* First time mothers or mothers who have undergone C-section cannot produce enough breast milk in the first few days.
  Fact: Most women are capable of producing milk for their newborns soon after delivery, be it vaginal or cesarean (C)-section. C-section is not a contraindication to

breastfeeding. But, it is a painful experience for mother and can interfere with feeding. Hence, such mothers need to be supported by counseling and assistance during feeding.[2] Mother and baby should be roomed-in and breastfeeding initiated irrespective of the mode of delivery.

- *Myth:* A mother who is underweight or has comorbidities like heart or kidney ailments cannot produce milk.
  Fact: This assumption is incorrect. All mothers are capable of breastfeeding and should be encouraged to do so. Mothers with diabetes can have delayed lactation. Some other causes of inadequate lactation are severe systemic maternal illness, postpartum depression, and intake of drugs that inhibits lactation. These physical reasons are rare and the most common causes are social and psychological. Thus, mothers and the family members need constant guidance and counseling for establishment and continuation of exclusive breastfeeding in these situations.[3]
- *Myth:* Breastfeeding should be stopped if mother is taking any medication or has an infection.
  Fact: Mothers with most illnesses can continue to breastfeed their babies except rare occasions like open tuberculosis or HIV (if she chooses not to). There are many benefits to continuing breastfeeding during illness.
  A woman's body makes antibodies against her infections, which go into the breast milk and which can help to protect the baby from the infection. Stopping breastfeeding leaves the baby exposed to all the hazards of artificial feeding. Most drugs are safe with breastfeeding and a mother should be advised accordingly by the physician/pediatrician.

Maternal use of nicotine, alcohol, ecstasy, amphetamines, cocaine, and related stimulants has been demonstrated to have harmful effects on breastfed babies. Mothers should be encouraged not to use these substances and given opportunities and support to abstain.

- *Myth:* Nipples have to be washed before each feed.
  Fact: This is not necessary. Washing the nipple before each feed interferes with lubrication of areola and can easily lead to discontinuity in the skin of areola and nipple. Mother has to maintain good personal hygiene and take a clean bath every day.
- *Myth:* Women with small breasts cannot produce enough milk.
  Fact: Size of the breasts does not dictate the quantity and quality of the breast milk.
- *Myth:* Baby should be fed every 2 hours by the clock.
  Fact: During the initial few days after birth babies require frequent feeding every 1 or 2 hours till feeding is well established. Once the mother becomes comfortable with her baby and understands her baby's sleep-wake pattern and breastfeeding needs, she can feed her baby on demand. It can range from 1 to 3 hours. This may not apply to very low birth weight (VLBW) babies or newborns with other morbidities. These babies need feeding at prescribed intervals as directed by the healthcare worker.
- *Myth:* If the baby is feeding frequently or for longer periods of time then milk is inadequate and the baby needs to be fed formula/cow's milk.
  Fact: The adequacy of breastfeeding is assessed by weight gain, urine output, stool output, and sleeping pattern. Mothers need to be made aware that

babies differ in their feeding patterns and there are babies who take frequent short feeds or who cluster feed (prolonged hours of feeding). If the baby is gaining weight well then inadequate milk is improbable.

- *Myth:* If the mother's breasts are not engorged and leaking milk then her milk supply is inadequate.
  Fact: This is a false assumption. Some mothers may not experience this in spite of producing adequate milk.
- *Myth:* Twin babies always require formula milk.
  Fact: A mother is capable of having enough lactation for her twins. Twins and high multiples tend to have lower birth weights and gestation and breastfeeding is essential. It is not always necessary to supplement twin babies with formula milk.[4] Mothers need support and counseling to establish and maintain breastfeeding of twins as it is both physically and emotionally challenging.
- *Myth:* Mother's diet needs to be restricted during breastfeeding. Drinking more water will dilute the breast milk; hence, water intake should be restricted.
  Fact: A breastfeeding mother should consume a wholesome and well-balanced diet rich in macronutrients (proteins, fats, and carbohydrates) and micronutrients (minerals and vitamins) with enough fiber.[5]

The above misconception leads to nutritional deficiencies in the mother and also affects the baby's growth in severe cases. A recent study has established thiamine deficiency as the cause of severe pulmonary hypertension in infants whose mothers were fed only polished rice during lactation.[6] A well-balanced diet is of paramount importance for the health of a lactating mother and her infant. Healthcare workers must make it a routine practice to give nutritional guidance to the new mother and dispel myths.

- *Myth:* Exercising makes breast milk sour.
  Fact: This is untrue. A mother should maintain a healthy physical activity routine as soon as she gets clearance from her obstetrician.
- *Myth:* It is not necessary to exclusively breastfeed till 6 months.
  Fact: Breast milk is a complete food for the infant till 6 months of age. In a healthy baby vitamin D3 is the only supplement recommended. Early complementary feeding before 6 months is unnecessary and may expose the baby to infections.
- *Myth:* Modern formula milk is as good as breast milk.
  Fact: Industrially manufactured formula milk at present cannot match the benefits of breast milk. It is rich in immunoglobulins and living cells and this cannot be replicated in a laboratory.[7] Beyond somatic growth, breast milk as a biologic fluid has a variety of other benefits, including modulation of postnatal intestinal function, immune ontogeny, and brain development. Breastfeeding leads to bonding between the mother and her infant which is the best mode of early stimulation for optimal neurological development.
- *Myth:* A mother should stop breastfeeding if the baby has diarrhea.
  Fact: A mother should continue to breastfeed her child during a bout of diarrhea.

A sick baby may refuse food and other liquids but will continue to breastfeed. Thus, breastfeeding will be an important source of nutrition and hydration during the time of illness.

- *Myth:* Refrigerated expressed breast milk cannot be used.
  Fact: Expressed breast milk can be refrigerated and used up to 4 days at 4°C and for 6 months if frozen at −18°C or lower. Once thawed it should be used within 1 or 2 hours. Freshly expressed or pumped milk can be kept at room temperature for up to 4 hours.[8]
- *Myth:* Every mother and baby adapt to breastfeeding instinctively.
  Fact: Though breastfeeding is a natural process not all mothers and babies can establish breastfeeding smoothly. Each mother needs guidance and support from a healthcare worker or an experienced family member to establish breastfeeding.

Issues like retracted nipples, cracked nipples, admission of baby to neonatal intensive care unit (NICU), feeling of not having enough milk, postpartum blues, etc. can cause hindrance to establishment and continuation of breastfeeding.

The importance of early and exclusive breastfeeding cannot be emphasized enough. The mother should be counseled and all her queries answered patiently. Healthcare workers have to instill confidence in her and other caregivers about breastfeeding. It is our duty as healthcare professionals to make sure that myths do not become be hurdles to breastfeed.

KEY MESSAGES

- Brest feeding is a natural instinct to be protected, promoted and supported.
- Effective communication and counseling to breastfeeding woman and family members are most important to prevent deviations from the breastfeeding norms.

REFERENCES

1. Abdulla CO, Ayubi A, Zulfiquer F, Santhanam G, Ahmed MA, Deeb J. Infant botulism following honey ingestion. BMJ Case Rep. 2012;2012:bcr1120115153.
2. Banapurmath CR, Ramachandrappa S, Guruprasad G, Biradar SB. Is Cesarean Section a Barrier to Early Initiation of Breastfeeding? Indian Pediatr. 2013;50:1062-3.
3. Pitre S, Raju R, Pardeshi P, Jogdeo B. Factors responsible for lactation failure among mothers. nat j advan res. 2016;2(4):27-31.
4. Flidel-Rimon O, Shinwell ES. Breastfeeding twins and high multiples. Arch Dis Child Fetal Neonatal Ed. 2006;91(5):F377-80.
5. Kominiarek MA, Rajan P. Nutrition Recommendations in Pregnancy and Lactation. Med Clin North Am. 2016;100(6):1199-215.
6. Sastry UMK, Jayranganath M, Kumar RK, Ghosh S, Bharath AP, Subramanian A, et al. Thiamine-responsive acute severe pulmonary hypertension in exclusively breastfeeding infants: a prospective observational study. Arch Dis Child. 2021;106(3):241-6.
7. Martin CR, Ling P, Blackburn GL. Review of Infant Feeding: Key Features of Breast Milk and Infant Formula. Nutrients. 2016;8(5):279.
8. Centers for Disease Control and Prevention. (2022). CDC guidelines and recommendations for breast feeding. Proper Storage and Preparation of Breast Milk. [online] Available from: https://www.cdc.gov/breastfeeding/recommendations/handling_breastmilk.htm [Last accessed November, 2023].

24. Feeding During and After Illnesses

Sudhindrashayana R Fattepur, Shilpa C, Vinod H Ratageri

"When Gut Is Functional Use It"

INTRODUCTION

Infectious diseases like pneumonia (15%), diarrhea (8%), malaria (5%), and newborn sepsis (7%) are the major causes of mortality globally in children younger than 5 years of age (under-fives), and principally in the regions of sub-Saharan Africa (SSA) and Southern Asia as per the recent the United Nations International Children's Emergency Fund (UNICEF) reports.[1]

Nutrition-related factors contributed to 45% of under-five deaths (UNICEF 2019). Global evidence has established the serious implications of malnutrition on a child's physical and brain development; in turn, this has an adverse impact on cognitive development, and the overall productivity and economic development of a nation. The World Bank states, A 1% loss in adult height due to childhood stunting is associated with a 1.4% loss in economic productivity.[2] The adverse impact of undernutrition on brain structure and development cannot be corrected later in life and can lead to cognitive deficits and compromised learning abilities.[3] Needless to say that nutrition during the first 2 years of life is the most crucial one as it determines the adult height[4] as shown in **Figure 1**.

Illness reduces appetite and increases nutrient requirements, while inadequate intake of food (quantity or quality) makes the body more susceptible to illness.[5] A sick child needs more nourishment so that he can fight infections without using up the nutrient reserves of the body.[6]

VICIOUS CYCLE OF ILLNESS AND MALNUTRITION

Disease-related malnutrition comes down to three interlinked aspects: (1) increased nutritional requirements (such as during an illness or after a trauma), (2) reduced nutritional intake (due to pain, loss of interest, or side effects of treatment), and (3) increased nutritional losses (due to malabsorption or diarrhea) which in turn lead to more infections.[7] Evidence suggests that 50% of critically ill children admitted to intensive care are prone to malnutrition due to increased metabolic rate from their illnesses.[8] Thus, nutrition during illness especially critical illness is very important to break this cycle, as shown in **Figure 2**. The critically ill needs to receive constant optimal feeding to facilitate recovery especially breast milk since it is rich in immune components and nutrients.[8]

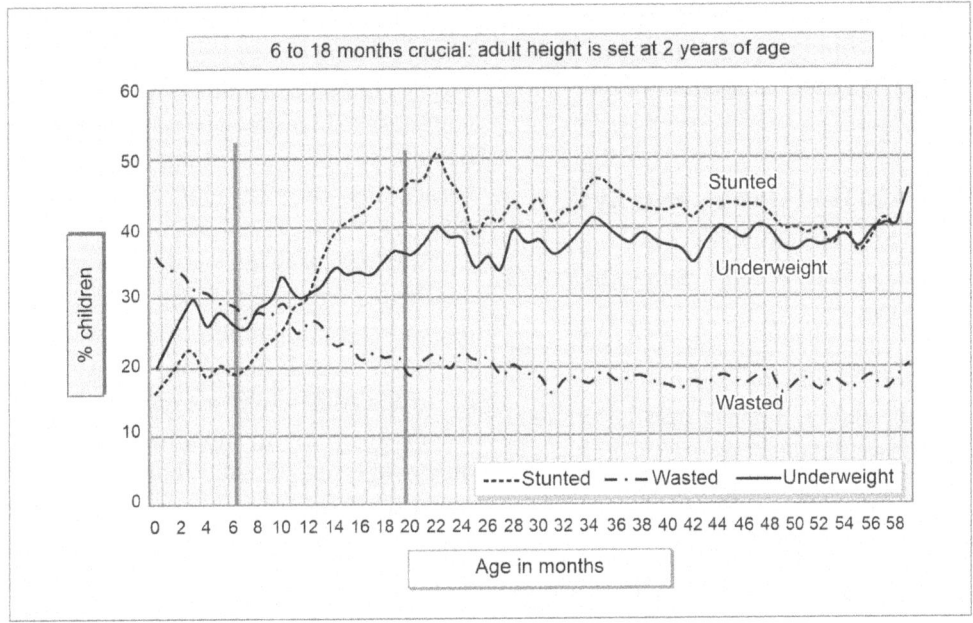

Fig. 1: Height at 2 years determines the productivity and income.
Source: National Family Health Survey, 4 2015–16.

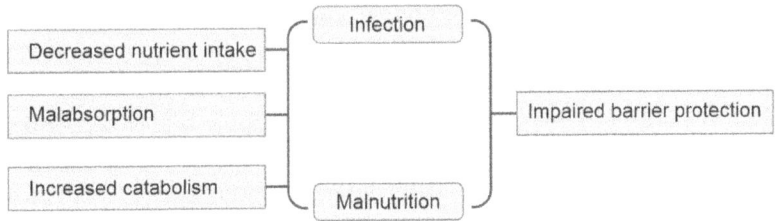

Fig. 2: The vicious cycle of infection and malnutrition.

WHAT ARE THE CAUSES FOR DECREASED ENTERAL INTAKE BY YOUNG INFANTS DURING ILLNESS?

It is observed that illness is a common cause of poor feeding for children below 6 months of age or above 6 months of age. The most common causes are:

Loss of Appetite

- When children fall sick, they may refuse to eat or feed mainly due to loss of appetite as commonly seen in adults also.
- This leads to poor rates of exclusive breastfeeding (EBF) as well as complementary feeding.
- Following recovery from illness, children regain the lost appetite.

Feeding Practices and Beliefs

- There is a common belief in the community that certain food items should not be given to a child during illness or after the illness.
- Families prefer to give light or easy-to-digest food irrespective of appetite.

- Often such food is not sufficient to fulfill the needs of the child during and after illness and may hamper the growth of the child.[9]

A Guide to Halt this Vicious Cycle

The steps to be followed during the acute phase of illness for a child <6 months would be as follows:
- If the child is very ill, s/he might reduce or completely stop the intake of breast milk or if the child is not very sick, yet irritable, then the child might want to be frequently breastfed. Moreover, the child will be thirsty particularly when s/he has a fever.
- In such circumstances, breastfeeding will be the most acceptable food for the child. Mothers should try to breastfeed more often. This will help to quench the child's thirst as well as provide nourishment.
- Steps to be followed after illness would be to breastfeed more frequently as the child will be hungrier. Demand feed should be ideal. If the mother has been breastfeeding her child regularly, she will be able to produce more milk as per demand.

Importance of breastfeeding for children above 6 months: Some mothers continue breastfeeding children till the child is about 2 years of age, but some may stop breastfeeding early. When a child at this age falls sick, s/he usually finds it comfortable to breastfeed even if s/he does not want to take complementary feeding. Breast milk is a wholesome food for the child and also a safe source of water, so it becomes very convenient for the mother as well to breastfeed when the child is sick. If a child falls sick after s/he has stopped breastfeeding, the mother cannot restart breastfeeding, and it can become difficult to manage to feed the child. Sometimes, such mothers may resort to bottle-feeding to comfort the child, and this can be dangerous. In this way, a mother who continues to breastfeed her child until 2 years has the advantage of being able to provide breast milk when her child falls sick during this age.[9]

Nutrition and its role in critical illness are being increasingly recognized. Hence, it becomes very much important to maintain adequate nutrition during the admission of critically ill children during and after discharge from the hospital. Though the quality of evidence is low, based on observational studies the recommendations are very strong as net benefits outweigh the harms.

GENERAL GUIDELINES DURING ILLNESS AND AFTER RECOVERY

During Illness

Ensure continued feeding and increase fluid intake, e.g., for a child under 6 months old breastfeed more frequently and longer at each feed, for a child 6–24 months old, ensure the child is breastfed more frequently and for longer duration at each feed, increase overall fluid intake, and offer other foods too. Give frequent, small nutrient-dense feeds that are soft, varied, and the child's favorite foods. Mashed or soft foods can be given if the child has trouble swallowing (do not dilute foods or milk). It is important to feed the child slowly and patiently, we need to encourage the child to eat but not force them.

During Recovery

Increase the amount of food after recovery from acute illness until the child regains weight and starts growing well. Feed frequently with an extra meal every day or snacks, and make sure, the child's increased hunger is met.

Quantity of the feeds: During illness emphasize continued feeding. Through this period of acute illness ailing children either reject or eat only small quantities of food offered to them. Do not withhold foods or liquids. However, during the period of recovery, children often have a good appetite and will be keen to eat more food than usual. Ensure the child eats more at every meal, and give an extra "meal" each day (or extra snacks in between meals) for at least 2weeks post-recovery. Any breastfed child should be breastfed frequently. Give plenty of fluids once every 1–2 hours for children who are not exclusively breastfed. Avoid sodas or artificially sweetened fruit juices, but give tender coconut water, rice water, yogurt, boiled water, or other nutritious foods.

In addition to rehydrating the child give a complete diet as soon as possible. The mother should be encouraged for breastfeeding. Optimal feeding during illness and recuperation is measured by the amount of food and liquids given to the child during illness.

Type of feeds: Breastmilk is the perfect food during and after illness and it is energy-rich, nutrient-rich, and hygienic. Sick children continue to breastfeed even when they are not taking other food or animal milk. If a sick breastfed baby is unable to suck properly, the mother should express milk and continue to feed the child with a spoon and/or cup. Ensure both the mothers and babies are kept together whenever hospitalizing breastfed children.

Energy and nutrient-rich foods: Children aged 6 months of age and above need energy and nutrient-rich foods, during and after illness, to regain strength, e.g., meat, poultry, fish, eggs, and milk whenever possible. This can also be achieved by adding dry milk powder to porridges or adding groundnuts/extra fat.

As an ailing child cannot absorb food well, he/she should be fed more often than usual. This can be achieved by frequent small feeds.

Breastfeeding in hospitalized children: Prospective studies on the association between breastfeeding and mortality in hospitalized children for diarrhea revealed a strong protective effect against mortality, fewer hospitalizations for neonatal fever, fewer investigations, and less invasive therapy and its complications. Breastfeeding particularly when exclusive and prolonged protects against severe morbidity and would result in lower rates of hospitalizations due to respiratory and diarrheal diseases. Increasing awareness of mothers about breastfeeding benefits to children, mothers, and society at large would promote breastfeeding and improve EBF and continued feeding.[10-15]

GENERAL RECOMMENDATION FOR FEEDING PRACTICES

During Illness

Give frequent small feeds. If a breastfed infant is too weak to suckle, the mother can express her milk and feed it with a spoon and cup. Encourage the older child to eat; be patient yet persistent. Offer foods that the child likes, to overcome a lack of appetite. Hold the child on your lap or keep him or her in a propped-up position (Do not feed a child lying down this can cause choking.). In case a child vomits the food, wait for 10 minutes then continue offering fluids or food. Never force a child to eat.

During Recuperation

As the child's appetite returns the child may seem hungry and responsive, with emphasis on frequent feeds. Give an extra meal every day or extra snacks for 2 weeks. Remember that recuperation takes time. Give special attention to feeding and this should continue for 2 or more weeks following an illness. Feeding during convalescence is vital to help the child "catch up" from nutritional losses. Older infants and young children continue to require energy and nutrient-dense food such as meat, liver, fish, eggs, milk, and oil to meet the requirements for catch-up growth. Extra feeds are crucial until the child has regained any weight loss and is on a normal growth curve again. The rule of thumb is to give a child an extra meal every day for at least 2 weeks.

Local customs and taboos: These include beliefs about withholding food/liquids. The most common belief is that all food including breast milk should be withheld during illness, especially diarrheal diseases. When a child has diarrhea, many believe in "resting the gut" or withholding milk. Mothers may be advised to delay feeding, dilute foods, or avoid giving milk. Withholding of food or liquids is less common during acute respiratory illness, malaria, or measles than during diarrheal episodes. It is common to come across both diseases and foods being classified as either "hot" or "cold". For example, "cold" foods typically include rice, curd, yogurt, and citrus fruits. These are considered appropriate during diarrhea. Their intake may be restricted during a cough or an illness with a rash. Foods such as ginger, honey, lentils, egg, and meats are thought appropriate during those illnesses and are considered hot foods.

BEST FEEDING PRACTICES DURING DIFFERENT ILLNESSES[16]

Diarrheal diseases: For an infant under 6 months old, continue breastfeeding during rehydration whenever the child wants.

Infants above 6 months (Foods during diarrhea): A child with diarrhea should be fed a normal diet as soon as possible. For better digestion, foods should be well cooked and mashed without much dilution. Fermented foods are also easy to digest. Fats and oils provide energy. For nonvegetarians, meat, fish, or egg should be given, if available. Potassium-rich foods such as bananas are very beneficial. A diet consisting of bananas and pectin is known to significantly reduce the amount of stool and vomiting. Persistent diarrhea or watery diarrhea that lasts for >2 weeks is related to about 45% of deaths. It is prudent to remember that antibiotics are not effective in all diarrheal diseases. The attention of the family must be given to feeding the child over many days. Children with persistent diarrhea are habitually given food that is too watery. Mothers need to know the importance of giving small, energy, and nutrient-rich feed at least six times a day. A child with persistent diarrhea may have some trouble digesting lactose in animal milk. Yogurt, if available, should be given in place of any animal milk usually taken by the child, or else the usual milk can be mixed with cereal. Milk should not be diluted. Breast milk does not cause lactose tolerance. A child with persistent diarrhea should be breastfed frequently.

Acute respiratory infection (pneumonia): Even mild ARI may cause a stuffy nose or cough, creating problems for breastfeeding. Feeding while coughing may put a child of any age at risk of aspiration of food. Patience, time, and confidence on the part of the mother are crucial for breastfeeding. If a breastfed child is unable to suckle properly, expressed milk should be fed with a cup and spoon. Give small feeds slowly with the child sitting up in a propped-up position.

Measles: The child may have severe diarrhea in addition to respiratory problems and high fever. Child may have a sore mouth. Keep the child hydrated. Advise parents to give soft and mashed foods that are non-spicy. The child should be given a vitamin A supplement.

Human immunodeficiency virus (HIV)/ Acquired immunodeficiency syndrome (AIDS): For infants <6 months on full replacement feeding. As part of determining what method of feeding is acceptable, feasible, affordable, sustainable, and safe (AFASS), the mother may have elected not to breastfeed her child during the first 6 months of life, or to discontinue breast milk after 6 months. Lack of breastfeeding makes the child vulnerable to frequent illness. Provider should counsel on hygienic preparation of milk/formula. During diarrhea, give yogurt-based drinks if possible. Mix animal milk with cereal, do not dilute the milk.

For the symptomatic child: A symptomatic child may have 50–100% greater energy requirements. The child may suffer frequently from thrush, fever, diarrhea, or vomiting. A child's medications may cause loss of appetite or changes in taste that make it difficult to eat. If a child is breastfeeding, continue breastfeeding. Feed frequently to ensure adequate intake. If a child has thrush, avoid spicy, salty, or sticky foods, or strong citrus fruits and juices that may irritate mouth sores. Avoid sugary foods; these encourage yeast. During recuperation from an illness, give energy-dense and micronutrient-rich foods.

KEY MESSAGES

- Infections are common illnesses causing significant morbidity and mortality in children.
- Feeding during and after illnesses has a positive impact on the growth and development of babies.
- Optimal nutrition during and after illnesses breaks the vicious cycle of infections and malnutrition.

REFERENCES

1. UNICEF. (2019), United Nations Inter-agency Group for Child Mortality Estimation (UN IGME). Levels and Trends in Child Mortality: Report 2019—Estimates developed by the United Nations Inter-agency Group for Child Mortality Estimation. [online] Available from www.unicef.org/reports/levels-and-trends-child-mortality-report-2019. [Last accessed November, 2023].
2. Vir SC, Suri S, Observer Research Foundation. (2021). The 5th National Family Health Survey of India: A Sub-National Analysis of Child Nutrition. ORF Occasional Paper No. 315, May 2021. [online] Available from: https://www.orfonline.org/wp-content/uploads/2021/05/ORF_OccasionalPaper_315_NFHS5-ChildNutrition.pdf [Last accessed November, 2023].
3. Kar BR, Rao SL, Chandramouli BA. Cognitive development in children with chronic protein energy malnutrition. Behav Brain Funct. 2008;4:31.
4. International Institute for Population Sciences (IIPS) and ICF. (2017). National Family Health Survey (NFHS-4), 2015-16: India. Mumbai: IIPS. [online] Available from: https://dhsprogram.com/pubs/pdf/FR339/FR339.pdf. [Last accessed November, 2023].
5. World Bank. (2006). Repositioning Nutrition as Central to Development: A Strategy for Large Scale Action. Washington, DC. [online] Available from: https://openknowledge.worldbank.org/handle/10986/7409. [Last accessed November, 2023].
6. Ministry of Women and Child Development Food and Nutrition Board, Government of India (2004). Indian National Guidelines on Infant and Young Child Feeding, vol. 26: Government of India; 2004. [online] Available from: https://wcd.nic.in/sites/default/files/nationalguidelines.pdf [Last accessed November, 2023].

7. Katona P, Katona-Apte J. The interaction between nutrition and infection. Clin Infect Dis. 2008;46(10):1582-8.
8. Abukari AS, Acheampong AK. Feeding the critically ill child in intensive care units: a descriptive qualitative study in two tertiary hospitals in Ghana. BMC Pediatr. 2021;21(1):395.
9. Ministry of Women and Child Development, Government of India. (2018). Poshan Abhiyaan, Feeding during illness. [online] Available from: https://womenchild.maharashtra.gov.in/upload/uploadfiles/files/NNM-ILAmodule-14-Feeding_During_Illness.pdf. [Last accessed November, 2023].
10. Sachdev HPS, Kumar S, Singh KK, Puri RK. Does Breastfeeding Influence Mortality in Children Hospitalized with Diarrhoea? J Trop Pediatr. 1991;37(6):275-9.
11. GafariAsl M, Fadakar Sogheh R, Ghavi A, Ahmad Shear barfi M. Related factors to continued breastfeeding in infants. J Holist Nurs Midwifery. 2014;24(2):1-8.
12. Netzer-Tomkins H, Rubin L, Ephros M. Breastfeeding Is Associated with Decreased Hospitalization for Neonatal Fever. Breastfeed Med. 2016;11:218-21.
13. Paricio Talayero JM, Lizán-García M, Otero Puime A, Benlloch Muncharaz MJ, Beseler Soto B, Sánchez-Palomares M, et al. Full breastfeeding and hospitalization as a result of infections in the first year of life. Pediatrics. 2006;118(1):e92-9.
14. Tiewsoh K, Lodha R, Pandey RM, Broor S, Kalaivani M, Kabra SK. Factors determining the outcome of children hospitalized with severe pneumonia. BMC Pediatr. 2009;9:15.
15. Quigley MA, Kelly YJ, Sacker A. Breastfeeding and hospitalization for diarrheal and respiratory infection in the United Kingdom Millennium Cohort Study. Pediatrics. 2007;119(4):e837-42.
16. Vikaspedia [Internet]. New Delhi: Ministry of Electronics and Information Technology; © 2022. (2022). Feeding Infants and Young Children During and After Illness. [online] Available from: https://vikaspedia.in/health/child-health/nutrition/feeding-infants-and-young-children-during-and-after-illness#:~:text=1.During%20illness&text=Breastfeed%20more%20frequently%20and%20longer%20at%20each%20feed%2C%20increase%20fluid,not%20dilute%20foods%20or%20milk. [Last accessed November, 2023].

CHAPTER 25: Hypernatremic Dehydration in Infants

Sumana Nanjundachar, Prakash M Kabbur, Anita Nyamagoudar, Durgappa H

"Breast milk is best, breastfeeding education is a must"

INTRODUCTION

Hypernatremia: Serum sodium levels >145 mEq/L is defined as hypernatremia. Some authors use a cut-off value above 150 mEq/L as hypernatremia. Dehydration/excessive weight loss is said to occur with a loss of >10% of birth weight within the first week of life.

Due to the contraction of extracellular volume and normal diuresis, neonates tend to lose about 10% of body weight in the first week of life. Thereafter, regaining birth weight occurs by the 10th day of life. Rapid weight loss or weight loss >10% is an indication for hospitalization. Neonatal hypernatremic dehydration occurs most commonly during the first 2–3 weeks of life.

Fluid and electrolyte balance can be a challenge due to physiological changes after birth such as:
- Fluid shifts between vascular compartments
- Growing needs of the newborn
- Solute handling by maturing kidneys
- Increased surface area of skin-to-weight ratio.

Infants above 36 weeks have enough kidney maturation to maintain sodium homeostasis.[1] In these infants, major causes of hypernatremia are water loss over sodium (hypernatremic dehydration), sodium intake exceeding sodium loss (salt poisoning),[2] or inadequate intake of breast milk in exclusively breastfed infants. The common risk factors for hypernatremic dehydration in infants include: inadequate breastfeeding, low birth weight, twin babies, primiparous women and hot environment **(Box 1)**.

Inadequate breastfeeding leads to hypernatremic dehydration in infants. When a mother-infant breastfeeding interaction is interrupted or inadequate, human milk

BOX 1: Risk factors of hypernatremic dehydration.
- *Maternal:*
  - Primigravida
  - Cesarean section
  - Faulty feeding
  - Gestational diabetes mellitus
  - Delayed lactogenesis stage II
  - Inability to breastfeed
- *Neonatal:*
  - Poor sucking efforts in a preterm/LBW baby
  - Septicemia/critically ill newborn
  - Cleft palate/craniofacial disorders
  - Twins
- *Environmental:*
  - Hot climates

(LBW: low birthweight)

TABLE 1: Sodium content in different type of milk.

Type of milk	Sodium in mmol/L
Colostrum	22 ± 12
Transitional milk	13 ± 3
Mature milk	7 ± 2

production is decreased, and this decline mitigates the physiologic decline in breast milk sodium levels leading to hypernatremic dehydration (Table 1). Inadequate breastfeeding is associated with raised breast milk sodium levels.

Adequate milk intake depends on the:
- Normal mammary development (mammogenesis)
- Unimpeded initiation of lactation (lactogenesis)
- Sustained ongoing milk synthesis (galactopoiesis)
- Effective milk removal.

Effective milk removal depends on the:
- Feeding technique
- Milk-ejection reflex
- Frequency and duration of feeding.

It is also important to note that improper formula preparation leads to hypertonic fluid administered to the infant along with other risk factors. Mothers need to be taught the correct techniques of expression of breastmilk by hand. Electric pumper donor milk should be made available to the mother, in case of an infant is not able to breastfeed effectively or the infant is separated from the mother. It is noted through unpublished data that high environmental temperatures are associated with elevated sodium levels in breastfeeding infants, implicating the probable association of high sweating and external loss of water in neonates. Exclusively breastfed infants are unlikely to have gastrointestinal (GI) infections and diarrhea. If the infant is given formula, there is a likely chance of gastroenteritis leading to excess water loss compared to sodium, leading to hypernatremia. It is important to note that babies fed with adequate fluid resuscitation respond well indicating intravascular volume depletion as the underlying pathology.

The bottom line is that adequate milk flow in the mother reduces the sodium content of breast milk.

CLINICAL FEATURES

It is estimated that 10% of breastfed infants develop hypernatremia[11] and 33% of breastfed infants with weight loss exceeding 10% have hypernatremia.[12,13] Clinically, it can be difficult to recognize breastfeeding-associated hypernatremia.

Most of the babies present with jaundice, fever, and other signs of sepsis such as lethargy, and poor feeding, and some of them may present with apnea, bradycardia, oliguria, inadequate stooling; rarely with acute renal failure, seizures, and cardiovascular collapse.[7] On examination, babies may have poor tone, lethargy with poor perfusion, weak pulses, sunken anterior fontanel, doughy feel to the skin, dry mucous membranes, tachycardia, and weight loss.

DIFFERENTIAL DIAGNOSIS

- Sepsis
- Meningitis
- Intracranial hemorrhage
- Congenital heart disease
- Inborn errors of metabolism
- Mineralocorticoid axis abnormality.

LABORATORY DIAGNOSIS

Obtain baseline serum electrolytes, complete blood cell count, glucose, calcium, and serum bilirubin, urea, and creatinine. The mother should hand-express the breast milk for sodium level analysis. Neurosonogram or MRI may be required depending on the availability of resources when the patients present with seizures or altered consciousness. Obtain consent and perform a lumbar puncture, blood culture, and urine culture as indicated based on age and presenting symptoms. The serial sodium levels during the transition of enteral feeds are to be estimated.

Measurement of serum and urine osmolality can be tested if the underlying etiology is not clear.

TREATMENT

There are no consensus guidelines on the type of intravenous (IV) fluid, quantity of fluid, or transition toward enteral feeds during the management of hypernatremic dehydration.

Once the diagnosis of hypernatremia is made based on a serum sodium level of ≥150 mEq/L, all infants should be hospitalized for IV rehydration and re-establishment of enteral feeding and breastfeeding. Hypernatremia correction protocol must be strictly followed, aiming for a sodium correction over 24–48 hours. After the admission of the baby, obtain investigations, place an IV catheter or a central IV access as clinically indicated, and begin IV fluids immediately. The degree of dehydration should be assessed based on clinical features and the weight difference during discharge and re-admission time. If details of weight are not available, then a bedside clinical decision has to be taken to treat with IV fluids.

GENERAL PRINCIPLES

In the setting of significant (moderate to severe) hypovolemia, fluid resuscitation with isotonic fluid to restore intravascular volume and tissue perfusion takes precedence over correction of the hypernatremia. However, overzealous fluid resuscitation is associated with cerebral edema. The next step is to correct hypernatremia. Lowering the sodium concentration too rapidly may lead to neurologic injury, hence, frequent clinical examinations and estimation of sodium levels are necessary.

Treatment involves two phases: In the emergent phase (intravascular volume restoration), by giving 10–20 mL of normal saline/kg, and during the rehydration phase, where the sum of remaining free water deficit and usual maintenance needs is administered over the next 48 hours.

- *Mild dehydration:* The baby is lethargic with less frequent urination and stooling with mild weight loss. These babies can be managed by ORS, maternal education, and encouragement to continue to breastfeed. A day observation until the baby can take an adequate amount of breast milk or the next breastfeeding alternative plus re-establishment of urine output is important. A follow-up should be planned.
- *Moderate and severe dehydration:* Admit the baby to intensive care if such a facility is available. Place an IV catheter or a central line depending on the clinical severity. Give NS bolus 10 cc/kg as required and begin 10% with 0.5 NS as described below.
- *Seizures:* Manage as above with fluid resuscitation and call a pediatric neurologist, if available. Manage seizures as per your institution or Indian Academy of Pediatrics guidelines.
- *Anuria:* If the baby is presented with anuria and shock, manage fluid resuscitation as above and consult a pediatric nephrologist

as available. Consider transferring the baby to the nearest tertiary care center for further renal failure management. Pass urinary catheter and avoid any nephrotoxic medications.

Calculating the free water deficit—use one of two common approaches:
1. Free water deficit in milliliters = Current total body water × [(current plasma Na/140) − 1]. Estimated total body water (TBW) as 60% of the child's weight in kilograms (0.6 L/kg). *Example:* 3 kg infant with a plasma sodium of 160, the free water deficit is: (0.6 L/kg) × (3 kg) × [(160/140) − 1] = 0.26 L or 260 mL.
2. Free water deficit in milliliters = (4 mL/kg) × (weight in kg) × (desired change in plasma Na). This approach uses the estimate that 4 mL/kg of free water will lower plasma sodium by approximately 1 mEq/L. Example: 3 kg infant described above with plasma sodium elevated 20 mEq/L above desired, water deficit would be: (4 mL/kg) × (3 kg) × (20 mEq/L change) = 240 mL. Consider only 3 mL/kg when serum Na is as high as in ≥190 mEq/L.[18]

The variation in free water needed between the two calculations is generally clinically negligible. Use the formula as clinically indicated. Provide on-going and maintenance fluids along with the above fluids. The fluid correction should occur over 24 hours with half of the correction occurring over the first 8 hours and the remainder over the next 16 hours. Longer correction times are indicated when dehydration is moderate (Na >160 mEq/L) to severe (Na ≥175 mEq/L) hypernatremia.[10]

Prescribed fluid: Normal saline (0.9% saline) is isotonic in patients with normal plasma sodium; however, it is a hypotonic fluid for children with hypernatremia, thus it is used as an initial rehydration fluid for hypernatremic hypovolemia.[19] Enteral fluids including oral rehydration therapy are also typically hypotonic. For neonates up to a month of age, use D10% with 0.5 NS. After a month of age, consider D5 with 0.5 NS. Adjust dextrose concentration as per serum glucose concentration and whether the baby can tolerate enteral feeds. Hypernatremia is commonly accompanied by hyperglycemia and hypocalcemia. Insulin to treat hyperglycemia is not recommended, since it can increase brain idiogenic osmole content. Correct hypocalcemia with calcium supplementation.[7]

Rate of correction: For children with chronic hypernatremia (plasma sodium ≥150 mEq/L for >24 hours) or those with acute severe hypernatremia (plasma sodium >160 mEq/L), rate of correction *should not* exceed a fall of sodium >0.5 mEq/L/h (i.e., 10–12 mEq/L/day)[20,21] unless in accidental sodium loading, a relatively rapid correction of the condition is usually safe.[7] A frequent check on serum sodium (preferably in the next 1–4 hours) during the initial phase of stabilization is crucial to ensure an appropriate decline in serum sodium levels. The rate of fluid administration should be adjusted rather than changing the fluid in the majority of cases.

TREATMENT OF SPECIFIC ETIOLOGIES

Treatment of sepsis/meningitis/faulty feeding/lactation failure should be addressed simultaneously.

In the meantime, encourage the mother to continue to pump BM, provide an electric pump if available or encourage her to hand express BM every 2–3 hours, and consult a lactation consultant as available. Once the infant can take enteral feeds, begin discharge education for the family on the continuation of breastfeeding, arrange follow-ups and provide financial support to the needy families.

Unfortunately, physicians receive limited education and awareness of breastfeeding complications during their training. Hypernatremia and hyperbilirubinemia in isolation or combination can disrupt the blood–brain barrier leading to encephalopathy, in turn, leading to more lethargy, poor intake, and worsening dehydration leading to short-term and long-term neurologic complications.[32-34] Lactation consultants play a key role in education and support in breastfeeding, especially in primiparous mothers who choose to exclusively breastfeed.[36] All healthcare providers dealing with cases of hypernatremia dehydration must be fully trained to assess and treat affected infants. Regular assessments and analyses of the readmission rates should be part of the hospital's ongoing quality improvement projects.[37] Jaundice is a common clinical sign of insufficient lactation and serum sodium measurement should be part of the management of hyperbilirubinemia.[38,39] It is important to educate and counsel all mothers especially primiparous mothers, by physicians and nurses at the time of discharge, provide written information on breastfeeding, and arrange all follow-ups.

COMPLICATIONS

- Acute kidney injury: May need dialysis
- Hyperbilirubinemia
- Cerebral edema
- Intracranial hemorrhage
- Hydrocephalus
- Cerebral venous thrombosis
- Gangrene
- Long-term neuroimpairment
- Mortality.

In short, education for breastfeeding must begin in the prenatal period by the obstetricians and should continue in the neonatal period through discharge, and education on adequate fluid intake by lactating mothers, especially in warmer months of the year. Awareness should also include education about hypernatremic dehydration due to inadequate breastfeeding, maintaining euthermia at home, avoiding the bundling of the babies, monitor urine output by caregivers. All breastfed babies must be followed up by a healthcare professional between 3 and 5 days after discharge with weight checks, assessment of general well-being including hydration status, jaundice, and elimination patterns; encouragement and assess breastfeeding. Hypernatremia must be treated judiciously with hospital admission, avoiding a sudden drop in sodium levels, providing supplemental donor breast milk or formula as per availability, arrange to follow-ups including neurodevelopmental as indicated based on the extent of hypernatremia. Overall family support by the treating physician team is needed along with NGO/government involvement to undertake preventive measures. Long-term follow-up studies are necessary to assess the neurodevelopmental outcomes of babies affected by hypernatremic dehydration.

KEY MESSAGES

- Hypernatremia can be a serious disorder in breastfed newborn.
- It can mimic sepsis and other neonatal conditions.
- Early recognition and treatment are the key to success.

- Support lactation through all available resources.
- Educate healthcare providers and families on effective breastfeeding.

REFERENCES

1. Al-Dahhan J, Haycock GB, Chantler C, Stimmler L. Sodium homeostasis in term and preterm neonates. I. Renal aspects. Arch Dis Child. 1983;58(5):335-42.
2. Dysart KC. (2018). Neonatal Hypernatremia. Merck Manuals. [online] Available from: https://www.msdmanuals.com/professional/pediatrics/metabolic,-electrolyte,-and-toxic-disorders-in-neonates/neonatal-hypernatremia [Last accessed November, 2023].
3. Lavagno C, Camozzi P, Renzi S, Lava SA, Simonetti GD, Bianchetti MG, et al. Breastfeeding-Associated Hypernatremia: A Systematic Review of the Literature. J Hum Lact. 2016;32(1):67-74.
4. Choukair MK. Fluids and electrolytes. In: Siberry GK (ed). The Harriet Lane Handbook, 15th edition. London: Mosby Publishers; 2000. pp. 232-3.
5. Rowland TW, Zori RT, Lafleur WR, Reiter EO. Malnutrition and hypernatremic dehydration in breast-fed infants. JAMA. 1982;247(7):1016-7.
6. Roddey OF Jr, Martin ES, Swetenburg RL. Critical weight loss and malnutrition in breast-fed infants. Am J Dis Child. 1981;135(7):597-9.
7. Gleason C, Juul S. Avery's Diseases of the Newborn, 10th edition. Netherlands: Expertconsult.com, Elsevier; 2018.
8. Abu-Salah O. High breast milk sodium concentration resulting in neonatal hypernatraemic dehydration. East Mediterr Health J. 2001;7:841-3.
9. Peters JM. Hypernatremia in breast-fed infants due to elevated breast milk sodium. J Am Osteopath Assoc. 1989;89:1165-70.
10. Karthikeyan G, Modi N. Neonatal hypernatremia due to high breast milk sodium. Indian Pediatr. 2003;40:72-3; 73-5.
11. International Institution of Population Sciences, Mumbai, India, Paswan B, Singh SK. (2017). National Family Health Survey (NFHS-4: 2015-2016). [online] Available from: https://dhsprogram.com/pubs/pdf/fr339/fr339.pdf [Last accessed November, 2023].
12. Marchini G, Stock S. Thirst and vasopressin secretion counteract dehydration in newborn infants. J Pediatr. 1997;130:736-9.
13. Dewey KG, Nommsen-Rivers LA, Heinig MJ, Cohen RJ. Risk factors for suboptimal infant breastfeeding behavior, delayed onset of lactation, and excess neonatal weight loss. Pediatrics. 2003;12:607-19.
14. Kaplan JA, Siegler RW, Schmunk GA. Fatal hypernatremic dehydration in exclusively breastfed newborn infants due to maternal lactation failure. Am J Forensic Med Pathol. 1998;19:19-22.
15. Ergenekon E, Unal S, Gücüyener K, Soysal SE, Koç E, Okumus N, et al. Hypernatremic dehydration in the newborn period and long-term follow up. Pediatr Int. 2007;49(1):19-23.
16. Morris-Jones PH, Houston IB, Evans RC. Prognosis of the neurological complications of acute hypernatraemia. Lancet. 1967;2:1385-9.
17. Finberg L. Infant dehydration. Wis Med J. 1995;94:600.
18. Finberg L, Kiley J, Luttrell CN. Mass accidental salt poisoning in infancy: a study of a hospital disaster. JAMA. 1963;184:90.
19. Colle E, Ayoub E, Raile R. Hypertonic dehydration (hypernatremia): the role of feedings high in solutes. Pediatrics. 1958;22:5-12.
20. Macaulay D, Blackhall MI. Hypernatraemic dehydration in infantile gastroenteritis. Arch Dis Child. 1961;36:543-50.
21. Oddie S, Richmond S, Coulthard M. Hypernatraemic dehydration and breastfeeding: a population study. Arch Dis Child. 2001;85:318-20.
22. Moritz ML, Manole MD, Bogen DL, Ayus JC. Breastfeeding-Associated Hypernatremia:

Are We Missing the Diagnosis? Pediatrics. 2005;116(3):e343-7.
23. Dennery PA, Seidman DS, Stevenson DK. Neonatal hyperbilirubinemia. N Engl J Med. 2001;344:581-90.
24. Weil WB, Wallace WM. Hypertonic dehydration in infancy. Pediatrics. 1956;17:171-83.
25. Freed GL, Clark SJ, Sorenson J, Lohr JA, Cefalo R, Curtis P. National assessment of physicians' breast-feeding knowledge, attitudes, training, and experience. JAMA.1995;273:472-6.
26. Behrman RE, Kliegman RM, Jenson HB. Nelson's Textbook of Pediatrics, 17th edition. Philadelphia, PA: WB Saunders; 2004. pp. 157-67.
27. Wennberg RP, Johansson BB, Folbergrova J, Siesjo BK. Bilirubin-induced changes in brain energy metabolism after the osmotic opening of the blood-brain barrier. Pediatr Res. 1991;30:473-8.
28. Moritz ML, Ayus JC. Disorders of water metabolism in children: hyponatremia and hypernatremia. Pediatr Rev. 2002;23:371-80.
29. Cooper WO, Atherton HD, Kahana M, Kotagal UR. Increased incidence of severe breastfeeding malnutrition and hypernatremia in a metropolitan area. Pediatrics. 1995;96:957-60.
30. Scott JX, Raghunath Gnananayagam JE, Simon A. Neonatal hypernatraemic dehydration and malnutrition associated with inadequate breastfeeding and elevated breast milk sodium. J Indian Med Assoc. 2003;101:318-21.
31. American Academy of Pediatrics, Subcommittee on Hyperbilirubinemia. Management of hyperbilirubinemia in the newborn infant 35 or more weeks of gestation. Pediatrics. 2004;114:297-316.
32. El-Bayoumi MA, Abdelkader AM, El-Assmy MM, Alwakeel AA, El-Tahan HM. Normal saline is a safe initial rehydration fluid in children with diarrhea-related hypernatremia. Eur J Pediatr. 2012;171(2): 383-8.
33. Ellis D, Kaye RD, Bontempo FA. Aortic and renal artery thrombosis in a neonate: recovery with thrombolytic therapy. Pediatr Nephrol. 1997;11:641-4.
34. Fang C, Mao J, Dai Y, Xia Y, Fu H, Chen Y, et al. Fluid management of hypernatraemic dehydration to prevent cerebral edema: a retrospective case-control study of 97 children in China. J Paediatr Child Health. 2010;46:301-3.
35. Manganaro R, Mami C, Marrone T, Marseglia L, Gemelli M. Incidence of dehydration and hypernatremia in exclusively breast-fed infants. J Pediatr. 2001;139:673-5.
36. Kahn A, Brachet E, Blum D. Controlled fall in natremia and risk of seizures in hypertonic dehydration. Intensive Care Med. 1979; 5:27-31.
37. Molteni KH. Initial management of hypernatremic dehydration in the breastfed infant. Clin Pediatr. 1994;33:731-40.
38. Arora S, McJunkin C, Wehrer J, Kuhn P. Major factors influencing breastfeeding rates: mother's perception of father's attitude and milk supply. Pediatrics. 2000;106(5):E67.
39. Gartner LM, Lee KS. Jaundice in the breastfed infant. Clin Perinatol. 1999;26:431-45, vii.

CHAPTER 26

Infant Milk Substitutes

Prathibha Rao, Srikanth BK, Pranam GM

> *"Thinking that baby formula is as good as breast milk is believing that thirty years of technology is superior to three million years of nature's evolution."*
> —**Christine Northrup**

INTRODUCTION

Breastfeeding must be promoted and supported globally as the norm for all babies worldwide. There are very few genuine contraindications to breastfeeding and very few women who are unable to breastfeed. Despite this, global breastfeeding rates are far lower than needed to optimize the health of both the mother and the baby. The data from the United Nations Children's Fund (UNICEF) and the World Health Organization (WHO) in 2018 suggests only 41% of all babies under 6 months are exclusively breastfed, far short of the global target of 70% for 2030.[1] Common reasons for women giving up breastfeeding or using supplemental formula are anxieties around insufficient milk supply,[2] returning to work, and lack of sleep. Mothers must be counseled that supplemental formula will potentially harm by reducing breast milk supply and must be actively discouraged. There are however some instances when breast milk substitute is required either to replace or supplement breast milk, for medical reasons, and on occasions when mothers are unable to or choose not to breastfeed. This chapter will discuss the types and composition of infant formulae, indications, disadvantages, and risks of breast milk substitutes (BMS). It will also describe the role of Pediatricians in regulating the use of BMS.

LEGISLATION

The international code of marketing of breast milk substitutes "The Code" is an international health policy framework, that was established in 1981 by the World Health Assembly (WHA), the decision-making arm of the WHO. It aimed to reduce mortality and improve health outcomes in children globally by promoting breastfeeding and preventing the marketing of breast milk substitutes which threatened to reduce breastfeeding rates in children. In the West, breastfeeding is officially recommended for at least 6 months but in developing countries, it is encouraged and practiced for much longer, often up to 2 years and beyond. There is evidence that breastfeeding up to and beyond the age of 2 years reduces child mortality. The Code, therefore, applies globally to all milk substitutes used in children until the age of 3 years.

Most countries have some form of legislation against the advertisement of artificial milk, and related products to the public and health workers. It also regulates the production, quality, safety, composition, and sale of formula milk, but the efficacy and implementation of these measures vary widely, with tragic consequences at times. The data from the "Global Breastfeeding Collective Scorecard—2019", produced by UNICEF and WHO found that only 18% of all the countries had fully implemented the code of marketing of breast milk substitutes. In India, the Infant Milk Substitutes, Feeding Bottles, and Infant Foods (IMS) Act was introduced in 1992 and further amended in 2003. This act bans all forms of promotion of food products marketed to children up to the age of two and restricts the sponsorship of infant formula companies to healthcare professionals.

COMPOSITION OF INFANT FORMULAE

There are three main categories of infant formulae, i.e., (1) Cow's milk-based, (2) soya-based, and (3) specialized formulae; and they vary in nutritive and calorific value, taste, and cost.[3,4]

Cow's milk is the base for most standard infant formulae used by healthy full-term infants and is modified to mimic the composition of human milk as far as possible. The average calorie content is 60–70 kcal/100 mL; lactose being the main carbohydrate component. Blended vegetable oils usually contribute to the fat content and most milks have added long-chain polyunsaturated fats, believed to boost visual function and developmental outcomes although evidence of clinical benefits of fortification is limited.[5]

Whey and casein are the main proteins, in variable proportions. Many formulae also contain prebiotics and/or probiotics. Despite the ongoing quest by formula milk companies to devise the "ideal" formula, nothing can match the unique, adaptable, bioactive, and immunological properties of human milk.

There are a large number of special formulae including:
- Lactose-free infant milk (containing glucose as the carbohydrate source)
- "Comfort" milk containing starch for reflux
- Preterm formulae, and postdischarge preterm formulae with increased total energy, protein, and fat content **(Table 1)**
- Extensive hydrolysates and amino acid formulae for babies with cow's milk protein intolerance.

Soya formulae are widely used but not recommended for infants under 6 months of age due to phytoestrogen content and cross-reactivity with cow's milk protein.

Breast milk fortifier[7] is widely used in neonatal units in Europe and the USA. It is made from extensively hydrolyzed cow's milk protein (with no added fat) and added to expressed breast milk for babies of <34 weeks and 1,500 g birth weight, once they are tolerating full enteral feeds. Typically, two sachets of breast milk fortifier (BMF) added to

TABLE 1: Comparison of the nutrient content of different commercially available formula milk.[6]

Nutrient/100 mL	Term formula	Preterm formula	Postdischarge formula
Total energy (kcal)	68	80	73
Protein (g)	1.4	2.4	1.9
Fat (g)	3.6	4.3	4.0
Carbohydrate (g)	7.3	8.6	7.6
Calcium (mg)	50	140	80
Phosphorus (mg)	30	75	50

100 mL of expressed breast milk will increase the calorie value from 67 to 82, and protein content from 1.6 to 2.7. It is also fortified with vitamins and minerals.

Formulations

- They are in powder form (which needs to be made up) and premade ready-to-feed solutions, which are sterile. The latter is more expensive.
- Pasteurized full-fat cow's milk may be given to babies over 12 months of age but is not recommended for younger babies.
- Goat's milk, rice milk, almond milk, and oats milk are not recommended for infants under the age of 1 year.

INDICATIONS FOR USE OF BREAST MILK SUBSTITUTES[8]

Specific Conditions in the Infant Where Breast Milk Cannot be Used and a Specialized Formula Must Be Used Instead

These infants will ideally be under the care of a specialist and receive specific dietetic input. Examples include:

- *Classical galactosemia:* The galactose-free formula is required.
- *Maple syrup urine disease:* A special formula free of leucine, isoleucine, and valine is needed.
- *Phenylketonuria:* Phenylalanine-free milk, with additional breast milk under supervision.

Situations where Breast Milk Remains the Best Option but the Temporary Addition of Formula is Justified

- *Preterm and very low birth weight infants:*[9] Expressed breast milk is the first choice, is safer, better tolerated, and associated with a significant reduction in necrotizing enterocolitis. However, breast milk on its own may be insufficient to sustain catch-up growth in infants <32 weeks of gestation. Therefore, some cases may require supplementation with artificial low birth weight formula or calorie supplements. In Western countries, breast milk fortifier is widely used to optimize the calorific and nutrient value of expressed breast milk, once babies are on full enteral feeds.[7]
- *Infants at risk of hypoglycemia (growth-restricted infants; infants of diabetic mothers):* Breastmilk is ketogenic and protects against the deleterious consequences of hypoglycemia; however, if there is a delay in the establishment of lactation or blood glucose levels remain low despite breastfeeding or the provision of expressed breast milk, temporary use of formula may be justified.
- Infants with hypernatremic dehydration occur in babies in the first week of life in association with >10% weight loss and delays in establishing lactation. It is more likely in firstborn and/or borderline preterm babies. These infants are recognized based on excess weight loss and may not be symptomatic. If the sodium is >150 mEq and weight loss is over 12%, we offer enhanced lactation support and temporary use of the formula for not >24–48 hours until breastfeeding is established.
- Infants with persistent or severe growth faltering due to inadequate lactation.

Maternal Conditions that Justify Permanent Avoidance of Breastfeeding

Maternal human immunodeficiency virus (HIV)—provided replacement feeding is safe, affordable, and sustainable.

Maternal Conditions that Justify Temporary Avoidance of Breastfeeding and Use of Appropriate Breast Milk Substitute

- Maternal postpartum psychosis
- Acute, severe maternal illness, i.e., sepsis; severe debilitation
- *Herpes simplex virus type 1:* If the mother has active lesions on the breast direct contact should be avoided until the lesions have healed.
- *Maternal medications:* Cytotoxic chemotherapy; lithium and carbimazole.[10] For the vast majority of medications, mothers may be on, the amounts excreted in breast milk are likely to be too small to be significant; however, pharmacological advice should be sought.
- *Infants with persistent breast milk jaundice:* Interruption of breastfeeds is not recommended but where bilirubin levels are unusually high, temporary cessation of breast milk and replacement with a formula for 48–72 hours, rapidly brings down bilirubin levels and establishes the diagnosis. Anecdotal evidence suggests once breastfeeding is resumed. Bilirubin levels do not usually rise.

Maternal Conditions Where Breastfeeding Can Continue, with Monitoring

- Mastitis; breast abscess
- Maternal tuberculosis
- Hepatitis B (provided the infant is fully vaccinated)
- Hepatitis C.

Mothers on Illicit Drugs (Opioids, Cocaine, and Amphetamines)

Breastfeeding is still the best choice, enhances bonding and reduces withdrawal symptoms. However, the risk to babies from long-term exposure through breast milk needs to be emphasized and mothers actively supported to give up their drug habit.

RISKS AND DISADVANTAGES OF BREAST MILK SUBSTITUTES (FIG. 1)

Short-term Risks

- Increased incidence of infection (otitis media, gastroenteritis, and respiratory tract infections); Global mortality from pneumonia and diarrhea is significantly higher in formula-fed infants[1]
- Feed intolerance; reflux
- Cow's milk protein intolerance, presenting as non-immunoglobulin E (non-IgE)-mediated allergy (diarrhea, vomiting, discomfort and excess crying, cow's milk colitis, eczema, and wheeze) or IgE-mediated immediate hypersensitivity and anaphylaxis.[11] Note, that the most common cause of anaphylaxis globally is cow's milk. These symptoms can occur even in breastfed infants whose mothers ingest dairy products, illustrating the highly allergenic potential of the cow's milk protein. It has been found that a single formula feed has the potential to significantly alter bowel flora and trigger symptoms of intolerance.
- Infections caused by lack of hygiene, improper storage of milk, or contamination of feeding bottles.
- Increased risk of hypernatremia, if feeds are not correctly made up and excess scoops of milk powder are added to feeds.
- Increased risk of necrotizing enterocolitis in preterm infants.
- Any regular use of the supplemental formula will reduce breast milk production.

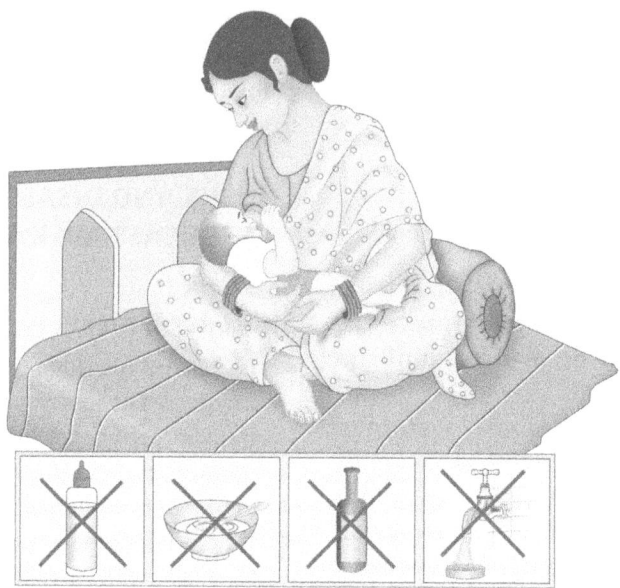

Fig. 1: Risks of artificial feeding.

- "Nipple confusion" caused by the use of artificial teats with formula supplement leading to refusal of breastfeeds

Long-Term Risks of Feeding Breast Milk Substitutes to the Infant

- Increased incidence of type 1 and type 2 diabetes
- Increased incidence of obesity
- Increased risk of asthma and atopic dermatitis
- Lower neurodevelopmental scores
- Overall increase in childhood mortality[1,12]
- Increased risk of sudden infant death syndrome.

Risks to the Mother for not Breastfeeding

- Increased risk of breast and ovarian cancer[1,13]
- Increased risk of obesity, retention of pre-pregnancy weight, and metabolic syndrome
- Expenses.

ROLE OF HEALTH PROFESSIONALS

Pediatricians, pediatric nurses, and midwives have a professional and ethical responsibility to promote exclusive breastfeeding and discourage the inappropriate use of formula except in situations where medically indicated. We can make a valuable contribution to promoting safe infant feeding practices in the following ways:

- Ensure adequate education of trainees, midwives, and healthcare workers with particular reference to baby-friendly principles.
- Discourage the use of formula on postnatal wards unless strictly indicated; when given it must be for a brief period while lactation support is provided to the mother.
- Avoid any endorsements or gratuities by baby milk companies.
- Lead an example by encouraging our staff with babies to breastfeed and

facilitate the expression of breast milk in the workplace.
- Appropriate counseling of mothers in the antenatal period about the benefits of breastfeeding and the risks and disadvantages of artificial milk in an objective and unbiased way.
- Ensure we have all the facts before making decisions to use BMS. This is particularly relevant for women on medications, the vast majority of which do not contraindicate breastfeeding.
- Ensure mothers are supported to practice strict hygiene and correct practices while making up the feeds.

KEY MESSAGES

- Breastfeeding is an unparalleled way of feeding method for the optimal health of infants and young children.
- Breastmilk substitute use is associated with an increased risk of contamination, infections, and malnutrition in children.
- The preparation of infant feed should be done under good hygienic conditions.
- Breastmilk substitute use is associated with a negative impact on the environment and economy of the family.

REFERENCES

1. Victora CG, Bahl R, Barros AJD, França GVA, Horton S, Krasevec J, et al. Breastfeeding in the 21st century: epidemiology, mechanisms, and lifelong effect. Lancet. 2016;387(10017):475-90.
2. Lewallen LP, Dick MJ, Flowers J, Powell W, Zickefoose KT, Wall YG, et al. Breastfeeding support and early cessation. J Obstet Gynecol Neonatal Nurs. 2006;35(2):166-72.
3. Martin CR, Ling P-R, Blackburn GL. Review of Infant Feeding: Key Features of Breast Milk and Infant Formula. Nutrients. 2016;8(5):279.
4. Koletzko B, Baker S, Cleghorn G, Neto UF, Gopalan S, Hernell O, et al. Global standard for the composition of infant formula: recommendations of an ESPGHAN coordinated international expert group. J Pediatr Gastroenterol Nutr. 2005;41(5):584-99.
5. Martin CR, Dasilva DA, Cluette-Brown JE, Dimonda C, Hamill A, Bhutta AQ, et al. Decreased postnatal docosahexaenoic and arachidonic acid blood levels in premature infants are associated with neonatal morbidities. J Pediatr. 2011;159(5):743-49.e1-2.
6. Morgan JA, Young L, McCormick FM, McGuire W. Promoting growth for preterm infants following hospital discharge. Arch Dis Child Fetal Neonatal Ed. 2012;97(4):F295-298.
7. Lucas A, Fewtrell MS, Morley R, Lucas PJ, Baker BA, Lister G, et al. Randomized outcome trial of human milk fortification and developmental outcome in preterm infants. Am J Clin Nutr. 1996;64(2):142-51.
8. World Health Organization. (2009). Acceptable medical reasons for the use of breast-milk substitutes. [online] Available from: https://www.who.int/publications/i/item/WHO_FCH_CAH_09.01 [Last accessed November, 2023].
9. World Health Organization. (2011). Guidelines on optimal feeding of low birth-weight infants in low- and middle-income countries [online]. Available from: https://www.who.int/publications/i/item/9789241548366 [Last accessed November, 2023].
10. Drugs and Lactation Database (LactMed). Bethesda (MD): National Library of Medicine (US); 2006.
11. Lifschitz C, Szajewska H. Cow's milk allergy: evidence-based diagnosis and management for the practitioner. Eur J Pediatr. 2015; 174(2):141-50.
12. Sankar MJ, Sinha B, Chowdhury R, Bhandari N, Taneja S, Martines J, et al. Optimal breastfeeding practices and infant and child mortality: a systematic review and meta-analysis. Acta Paediatrica. 2015; 104(S467):3-13.
13. Unicef.org. Breastfeeding: A Mother's Gift, for Every Child. [online] Available from: https://www.unicef.org/nutrition/index_24824.html [Last accessed November, 2023].

CHAPTER 27

Bottle-feeding

Vikas Patil, Durgappa H, Vani KT, Arpita JS

"Bottles fill his stomach, but breastfeeding fills his soul".
—**Diane Wiessinger**

INTRODUCTION

Bottle-feeding is widely prevalent worldwide, which is associated with negative impacts on breastfeeding practices, the health of mother and baby, and ecological economics. Recent studies have shown that bottle-fed infants have an increased risk of nipple confusion, breastfeeding difficulties, malnutrition, infections, gastroesophageal reflux, tooth decay, jaw developmental problems, neurodevelopmental, and behavioral problems. In addition, it also has negative impacts on the economy and environment of the nation.[1]

HISTORICAL ASPECT OF BOTTLE-FEEDING

There is evidence that artificial feeding methods for newborn infants have been used to supplement or complement breastfeeding since the beginning of recorded history. The nipple was invented in Sweden in the late 16th century and the idea of giving foods other than human breast milk became more common in the last part of the 18th century, these foods were given by finger, spoon, or papboats. The use of milk by other mammals was described by Underwood in 1784. Bottles and rubber nipples that resemble those in use today were introduced in the 1830s. Artificial nipples and bottles were most commonly used for feeding.[1]

MAGNITUDE

The prevalence of bottle-feeding is rising in both developed and developing countries of the world. Globally, 62% of infants <6 months and 41% at 2 years of age are bottle-fed.[2] A study from Central Ethiopia reported that the prevalence of bottle-feeding among infants was 19.6%.[3] Another study from Uttarakhand, India reported that 53% of infants were partially or fully bottle-fed,[4] indicating effective and early interventions are required to prohibit bottle-feeding in children.

REASONS FOR BOTTLE-FEEDING

There are various reasons for bottle-feeding among children. The common factors influencing bottle-feeding in infants include working mothers, urbanization, high-income group mothers, cesarean section, use of pacifiers, education of mothers, and an older child with an age group between

6 and 23 months. In addition, the hesitancy of mothers to breastfeed in a public place, false perception of insufficient milk secretion, workplace stress, and influence of advertising media on the use of infant milk substitutes were reported.[4]

PROBLEMS ASSOCIATED WITH BOTTLE-FEEDING

Bottle-fed babies have a higher risk of morbidity and mortality which is explained by the absence of anti-infective factors in the infant milk substitutes, risk of contamination, and infections associated with bottle-feeding.

THE EFFECTS OF BOTTLE-FEEDING ON CHILDREN

Otitis Media

Bottle-feeding and otitis media: Bottle-feeding is associated with an increased risk of otitis media compared to breastfed infants. Breastfed infants have a lower risk of acute otitis media (AOM) which is explained by the presence of ant-infective factors such as human milk oligosaccharide (HMO), immunoglobulins, and microbiota formation in the Eustachian tube and negative pressure generated during breastfeeding prevents the pooling of saliva into the Eustachian tube which is missing in bottle-fed babies.[5]

Lower Respiratory Tract Infection

Bottle-fed infants have a higher risk of respiratory infections. A recent meta-analysis has shown that bottle-fed infants have a 3.6-fold increased risk of hospitalizations for lower respiratory infections compared with breastfed babies which were attributed to lack of anti-infective factors, improper sterilization techniques, and storage of milk for longer duration.[6,7]

Gastrointestinal Infections

Bottle-feeding is associated with an increased risk of diarrheal diseases in children. Recent studies have found that bottle-fed infants had a 1.7–2.8 times increased risk of gastrointestinal infections and diarrhea.[8,9] The most severe form of infection reported in preterm and low birth weight and bottle-fed babies is necrotizing enterocolitis.

Obesity and Metabolic Disease

Bottle-feeding is associated with metabolic syndromes. Studies have shown that bottle-fed infants have a 1.6 times higher risk of metabolic disorders;[10,11] type 2 diabetes, hypertension, cardiovascular diseases, and dyslipidemia during their adulthood. Passive feeding is the most important risk factors for obesity.

Neurodevelopmental Problems

Formula feeding has a negative impact on the neurodevelopment of children. Studies have reported that formula-fed infants have modestly lower intelligence quotient. Recent studies have demonstrated that breastfed infants have better neuro-development, sleep pattern and psychosocial development compared to top-fed babies.[10]

Oromandibular Problems

Tooth decay, jaw development problems, and malocclusion occur in bottle-fed infants due to a direct trophic effect of altered sucking mechanics on the growing facial bones of the infant and there is an increased prevalence of non-nutritive sucking in bottle-fed infants.[11,12]

Nipple Confusion

Nipple confusion is a common problem associated with bottle-feeding. Bottle-feeding leads to difficulty in latching to the breast and even a single bottle-feed is sufficient to cause nipple confusion. As bottle-feeding is a passive process, makes infants more comfortable and avoid breastfeeding.[1]

Sudden Infant Death Syndrome

Studies have shown sudden infant death syndrome (SIDS) to be more common in bottle-fed infants even when risk factors were avoided.[13]

Allergic Disorders

The risk of asthma and atopic dermatitis is increased in bottle-fed infants. In a meta-analysis, a 1.7-fold increased risk of developing asthma was found among bottle-fed infants.[14]

Effects on the Mothers

Early weaning and lack of breastfeeding are associated with health risks for the mother. Short-term effects are breast engorgement, breast abscess, loss of lactational amenorrhea, etc. Important long-term adverse effects observed are breast cancer, ovarian cancer, and impaired glucose tolerance and lipid metabolism.[14,15]

Effects on the Environment

Bottle-feeding also contributes to the destruction of the ecosystem mainly through deforestation, soil erosion, climatic changes, and waste resources, while breastfeeding is a renewable resource.[16]

Effects on the Economy

Top feeding has a negative impact on the economy. It has been estimated that globally, 302 billion dollars of economic loss occurs due to lower intelligence associated with not breastfeeding optimally.[17] The list of problems of bottle-feeding are enumerated in **Table 1**.

If the mother and family members are not willing to change the bottle-feeding behavior then the following advice needs to be given to prevent the risk of contamination and infections.

TABLE 1: Problems of bottle-feeding.

Infants and children	• Otitis media • Lower respiratory tract infections • Diarrhea • Undernutrition • Obesity • Jaw development problems • Teeth decay • Nipple confusion • Allergic reactions • Sudden infant death syndrome • Neurodevelopment problems • Gastroesophageal reflux disorders

Mother	• Short term:
	  – Baby and mother bonding
	  – Breast engorgement
	  – Breast abscess
	  – Loss of lactational amenorrhea
	• Long term:
	  – Breast cancer
	  – Ovarian cancer
	  – Impaired glucose tolerance
	  – Lipid metabolism

Environment	• Deforestation • Greenhouse effect • Global warming • Ecological imbalance
Economy	Negative impacts on the economy of the nation

CLEANING, STERILIZING, PREPARATION, AND STORING TECHNIQUES[18]

Cleaning

- *Step 1:* Wash your hands with soap and water and dry them using a clean cloth.
- *Step 2:* Wash all feeding and preparation equipment thoroughly in hot soapy water. Use a clean bottle and teat brush to scrub inside and outside of bottles and teats to make sure that all remaining feed is removed from the hard-to-reach places.
- *Step 3:* Rinse thoroughly in safe water.

Sterilizing

Cleaned equipment can be sterilized with a pan and boiling water by the following method:
- Fill water in a large pan
- Place the cleaned feeding and preparation equipment into the water. Make sure that the equipment is completely covered with water and that no air bubbles are trapped.
- Cover the pan with a lid and bring it to a rolling boil, making sure the pan does not boil dry.
- Keep the pan covered until the feeding equipment is needed.

Preparation of a Bottle-feed

- Clean and disinfect the surface on which feed is to be prepared.
- Wash your hands with soap and water, and dry them with a clean or disposable cloth.
- Boil portable water. If using an automatic kettle, wait until the kettle switches off. If using a pan to boil water, make sure the water comes to a rolling boil.
- Taking care to avoid scalds, pour the appropriate amount of boiled water into a cleaned and sterilized feeding bottle. The water should be no cooler than 70°C, hence do not leave it for >30 minutes after boiling.
- Add the exact amount of formula to the water in the bottle. Mix thoroughly by gently shaking or swirling the bottle.
- Immediately cool to feeding temperature by holding the bottle under cold running tap water, or by placing it in a container of cold or iced water. So that you do not contaminate the feed, make sure that the level of the cooling water is below the lid of the bottle.
- The external surface of the bottle is to be dried with a clean or disposable cloth.
- Check the temperature of the feed by dripping a little onto the inside of your wrist. It should feel lukewarm, not hot. If it still feels hot, cool it for some more time before feeding.

STORAGE OF BOTTLE-FEEDS

It is safest to prepare a fresh feed each time one is needed and to consume it immediately. This is because prepared feeds provide ideal conditions for bacteria to grow—especially when kept at room temperature. If you need to prepare feeds in advance for use later, they should be prepared in individual bottles, cooled quickly, and placed in the refrigerator (no higher than 5°C). Throw away any refrigerated feed that has not been used within 24 hours.

REWARMING OF REFRIGERATED BOTTLE-FEEDS

Take out the feeding bottle from the refrigerator just before it is needed. Rewarm for not >15 minutes. Feeds can be rewarmed by placing them in a container of warm water, making sure the level of the water is below the top of the cup. Occasionally shake or swirl the bottle to make sure that it heats evenly. Throw away any rewarmed feed that has not been consumed within 2 hours.

POSITIONS FOR BOTTLE-FEEDING THE BABY

The baby should be in a semiupright position and support their head. Do not feed the baby in a lying down position as this may cause middle ear infections. To prevent swallowing of air as they suck, tilt the bottle so that the formula fills the neck of the bottle and covers the nipple.

WAYS TO OVERCOME BOTTLE-FEEDING

- Antenatal education on the benefits of optimal infant feeding practices is important
- Early initiation of breastfeeding and skilled practical assistance and support is crucial
- Discourage prelacteal feeds used in newborn
- Protect the mother and baby from infant milk substitutes
- Strictly implementing the Infant Milk Substitutes, Feeding Bottles, and Infant Foods (IMS) Act in prohibiting the use of infant formula is essential.

KEY MESSAGES

- The prevalence of bottle-feeding is on the rise worldwide.
- Bottle-feeding has a negative impact on the growth, development, and health of children.
- It is associated with an increased risk of morbidity and mortality among children.
- Has a negative impact on ecology and economics.

- Effective antenatal counseling on the benefits of optimal infant feeding practices is important.
- Educate the mothers on the harmful effects associated with bottle-feeding.
- Discourage the use of prelacteal feeds.
- Implementing a stringent law is essential to protect, promote, and support breastfeeding practices.

REFERENCES

1. Dowling DA, Thanattherakul W. Nipple confusion, alternative feeding methods, and breast-feeding supplementation: State of the science. Newborn and infant nursing reviews. 2001;1(4):217-23.
2. World Health Organization. Breastfeeding. [online] Available from: https://www.who.int/health-topics/breastfeeding#tab=tab_1 [Last accessed November, 2023].
3. Kebebe T, Assaye H. Intention, magnitude and factors associated with bottle feeding among mothers of 0-23 months old children in Holeta town, Central Ethiopia: a cross sectional study. BMC Nutr. 2017;3:53.
4. Rathaur VK, Pathania M, Pannu C, Jain A, Dhar M, Pathania N, et al. Prevalent infant feeding practices among the mothers presenting at a tertiary care hospital in Garhwal Himalayan region, Uttarakhand, India. J Family Med Prim Care. 2018;7(1):45-52.
5. Stuebe A. The Risks of Not Breastfeeding for Mothers and Infants. Rev Obstet Gynecol. 2009 Fall;2(4):222-31.
6. Bachrach VR, Schwarz E, Bachrach LR. Breastfeeding and the risk of hospitalization for respiratory disease in infancy: a meta-analysis. Arch Pediatr Adolesc Med. 2003;157(3):237-43.
7. Chien PF, Howie PW. Breast milk and the risk of opportunistic infection in infancy in industrialized and non-industrialized settings. Adv Nutr Res. 2001;10:69-104.
8. Kramer MS, Chalmers B, Hodnett ED, Sevkovskaya Z, Dzikovich I, Shapiro S, et al. Promotion of Breastfeeding Intervention Trial (PROBIT): a randomized trial in the Republic of Belarus. JAMA. 2001;285(4):413-20.

9. Horta BL, Bahl R, Martinés JC. Evidence on the long-term effects of breastfeeding: systematic review and meta-analyses. Geneva: World Health Organization; 2007. pp. 1-57.
10. Anderson JW, Johnstone BM, Remley DT. Breast-feeding and cognitive development: a meta-analysis. Am J ClinNutr. 1999;70(4):525-35.
11. Abreu LG, Paiva SM, Pordeus IA, Martins CC. Breastfeeding, bottle feeding and risk of malocclusion in mixed and permanent dentitions: a systematic review. Braz Oral Res. 2016;30:1806-83242016000100401.
12. Straub WJ. Malfunction of the tongue: Part I. The abnormal swallowing habit: Its cause, effects, and results in relation to orthodontic treatment and speech therapy. Am J Orthod. 1960;46(6):404-24.
13. McVea KL, Turner PD, Peppler DK. The role of breastfeeding in sudden infant death syndrome. J Hum Lact. 2000;16(1):13-20.
14. Ip S, Chung M, Raman G, Chew P, Magula N, DeVine D, et al. Breastfeeding and maternal and infant health outcomes in developed countries. Evid Rep Technol Assess (Full Rep). 2007;153:1-186.
15. Stuebe AM, Rich-Edwards JW. The reset hypothesis: lactation and maternal metabolism. Am J Perinatol. 2009;26(1):81-8.
16. Smith JP. A commentary on the carbon footprint of milk formula: harms to planetary health and policy implications. Int Breastfeed J. 2019;14:49. https://doi.org/10.1186/s13006-019-0243-8.
17. Weimer J. Breastfeeding: Health and Economic Issues. Food Review. 1999;22(2):31-5.
18. World health Organization. (2007). Safe preparation, storage and handling of powdered infant formula: guidelines. [online] Available from: https://www.who.int/publications/i/item/9789241595414 [Last accessed November, 2023].

CHAPTER 28

Feeding and Eating Disorders in Children

Suchetha S Rao, B Shantharam Baliga

"Today more than 95% of all chronic diseases are caused by food choices, toxic food ingredients, nutritional deficiencies, and lack of physical exercises".
—Mike Adams

INTRODUCTION

Most of the parents report that their child is under eating, overeating, or a fussy eater. Refusal to eat is the most common complaint from the mother. Approximately 25-45% of children with normal development and 80% of children with developmental delay experience some type of feeding problem.[1] Act of eating results in the intake of nutrients and also contributes to learning. Eating has an impact not only physical growth of the child but also on the emotional and psychosocial development. In the first stage consisting from birth to 3 months, the infant learns self-regulation and organization. In the second stage (3-7 months), the infant and parent develop an attachment, and the infant develops basic trust and self-soothing. In the third stage (7-36 months), child emotionally separates from the parent and discovers autonomy and independence.[2] In children feeding occurs in the context of the child-caregiver dyad. Any disruption in this interaction will increase the risk of feeding disorders.

There is no consensual definition of pediatric feeding disorder. The proposed definition is based on the World health organization's International Classification of disability, functioning, and health, recommendation. Thus pediatric feeding disorder is defined as impaired oral intake which is not age-appropriate and is associated with nutritional, medical, feeding skill, and/or psychological dysfunction.[3,4] The diagnostic and statistical manual for mental disorders, fifth edition (DSM-V) assists clinicians with diagnostic criteria for various eating disorders. The terminology eating disorder has been changed to feeding and eating disorder in DSM-V.[4]

TYPES OF FEEDING AND EATING DISORDERS

Feeding disorders are of three types, i.e., organic, behavioral, and a combination of both.[5,6] Most feeding problems are temporary and can be resolved if recognized and addressed early. Untreated feeding problems can persist and evolve into eating disorders in adolescents and adults.[6,7] Differentiating transient feeding difficulties from clinically significant feeding disorders is very essential for optimizing a child's health and development. Children with feeding disorders require a multiprofessional approach and management will involve family-centered models.[8] Clinical features and management of common feeding disorders are addressed in this chapter.

COMMON FEEDING AND EATING DISORDERS

Anorexia Nervosa

Anorexia nervosa (AN) is characterized by fear of becoming fat or engaging in behavior to avoid weight gain and disturbance in the way one experiences body image. AN is more common in females than in males, various studies report different ratios, the common reported ratio being 10:1. Median age of onset of AN is 12.3 years.[9,10]

DSM-V Diagnostic Criteria[4]

- Restriction of energy intake relative to requirements, leading to significantly low body weight in the context of age, sex, developmental trajectory, and physical health (less than minimally normal/expected).
- Intense fear of gaining weight or becoming fat or persistent behavior that interferes with weight gain.
- Disturbance in the way in which one's body weight or shape is experienced, undue influence of body weight or shape on self-evaluation, or persistent lack of recognition of the seriousness of the current low body weight.

Specify if:
- *Restricting type:* During the last 3 months, the individual has not engaged in recurrent episodes of binge eating or purging behavior.
- *Binge-eating/purging type:* During the last 3 month, the individual has engaged in recurrent episodes of binge eating or purging behavior.

Specify if:
- *In partial remission:* After full criteria for AN were previously met, Criterion A (low body weight) has not been met for a sustained period, but either Criterion B (intense fear of gaining weight or becoming fat or behavior that interferes with weight gain) or Criterion C (disturbances in self-perception of weight and shape) is still met.
- *In full remission:* After full criteria for AN were previously met, none of the criteria has been met for a sustained period.

Management

- *Behavioral therapy:* Family-based treatment (FBT) is considered the golden standard for the treatment of adolescents with AN. FBT adopts an agnostic stance regarding the etiology of AN. FBT focuses on the family plays a pivotal role through which adolescents can achieve recovery. Parents are assigned the key responsibility of restoring the child to wellness and siblings play a supportive role. The FBT consists of three phases; the first phase focuses on refeeding and weight restoration, the next phase on gradually returning responsibility to the adolescent, and the final phase on establishing a healthy adolescent identity.[11]
- *Cognitive behavioral therapy (CBT):* CBT has been one of the leading treatments in AN and is used as an FBT alternative. CBT has been found effective to prevent relapses after inpatient hospitalization.[11]
- *Pharmacotherapy:* In the acute phase of AN, common comorbid features of

anxiety and depression were observed, hence antidepressant medications were considered beneficial. Research has revealed a paucity of the benefits of these drugs. First-generation antipsychotics have failed to show weight gain or improvement in the symptoms. Atypical antipsychotic, olanzapine represents a promising pharmacological agent to promote modest weight gain in AN in adults.[11]

Bulimia Nervosa

Bulimia nervosa (BN) is characterized by binge eating episodes, extreme measures to compensate for fear of weight gain due to overeating, and body image concerns. The typical onset of BN is in late adolescence. BN may be associated with medical and psychological comorbidities.[12]

DSM-V Diagnostic Criteria[4]

- Recurrent episodes of binge eating. An episode of binge eating is characterized by the following:
  - Eating, in a discrete period (e.g., within any 2-hour period), an amount of food that is larger than what most individuals would eat in a similar period under similar circumstances.
  - A sense of lack of control over eating during the episode (e.g., a feeling that one cannot stop eating or control what or how much one is eating).
- Recurrent inappropriate compensatory behaviors to prevent weight gain, such as self-induced vomiting; misuse of laxatives, diuretics, or other medications; fasting; or excessive exercise.
- The binge eating and inappropriate compensatory behaviors both occur, on average, at least once a week for 3 month.
- Self-evaluation is unduly influenced by body shape and weight.
- The disturbance does not occur exclusively during episodes of AN.

Specify if:
- *In partial remission:* After full criteria for BN were previously met, some, but not all, of the criteria, have been met for a sustained period.
- In full remission: After full criteria for BN were previously met, none of the criteria has been met for a sustained period.

Specify current severity:
- The minimum level of severity is based on the frequency of inappropriate compensatory behaviors (see later). The level of severity may be increased to reflect other symptoms and the degree of functional disability.
  - *Mild:* An average of 1–3 episodes of inappropriate compensatory behaviors per week
  - *Moderate:* An average of 4–7 episodes of inappropriate compensatory behaviors per week
  - *Severe:* An average of 8–13 episodes of inappropriate compensatory behaviors per week
  - *Extreme:* An average of 14 or more episodes of inappropriate compensatory behaviors per week

Management

- *Psychotherapy:* CBT and interpersonal therapy have been tried extensively in adult BN and have shown promising results. There are limited randomized control trials of psychotherapy in adolescents. Current treatment guidelines recommend family-based treatment for adolescent BN (FBT-BN) which empowers the parents to recover their adolescents.

Cognitive behavioral therapy adapted for adolescents (CBT-A) is another alternative when FBT-BN is not acceptable or parents are not available.[13]

- *Pharmacotherapy:* Psychotherapy is the mainstay of treatment in BN. Pharmacotherapy will be considered if psychotherapy is unavailable or ineffective. For adults, various drugs have been tested but there are limited trials available for pharmacotherapy for adolescent BN. Fluoxetine 60 mg/day has shown benefits and is acceptable for adolescent BN.[13]

Avoidant or Restrictive Food Intake Disorder

This disorder is characterized by the avoidant or restrictive type of food intake due to various underlying etiologies. The presentations include low interest in food and eating, avoidance related to sensory issues, and fear-related avoidance or restriction. This disorder results in insufficient intake of a particular food group or micronutrients. These children may be underweight, normal, or overweight hence this disorder may go unnoticed.[14]

DSM-V Diagnostic Criteria[4]

- An eating or feeding disturbance (e.g., apparent lack of interest in eating or food, avoidance based on sensory characteristics of food; concern about aversive consequences of eating) as manifested by persistent failure to meet appropriate nutritional and/or energy needs associated with one (or more) of the following:
  - Significant weight loss (or failure to achieve expected weight gain or faltering growth in children)
  - Significant nutritional deficiency
  - Dependence on enteral feeding or oral nutritional supplements
  - Marked interference with psychosocial functioning
- The disturbance is not better explained by a lack of available food or by an associated culturally sanctioned practice.
- The eating disturbance does not occur exclusively during anorexia nervosa or BN, and there is no evidence of a disturbance in the way in which one's body weight or shape is experienced.
- The eating disturbance is not attributable to a concurrent medical condition or not better explained by another mental disorder. When eating disturbance occurs in the context of another condition or disorder, the severity of the eating disturbance exceeds that routinely associated with the condition or disorder and warrants additional clinical attention.

Management

Oral nutritional supplementation and medical supervision of refeeding are recommended. In severely malnourished children, tube feeding may be warranted. Intensive behavioral intervention has been used for children. Cognitive-based therapy and family-based therapy have been found effective for adolescents with avoidant or restrictive food intake disorder (ARFID).[14]

Binge Eating Disorder

Binge eating disorder (BED) is the most common disorder with a prevalence of 1–3% in the general population. Children with BEDs have a high prevalence of physical and psychiatric comorbidities.[2,15]

DSM-V Diagnostic Criteria[4]

- *Criteria 1:* Recurrent episodes of binge eating. An episode of binge eating is characterized by both of the following:

- Eating in a discrete period (within 2 hours), an amount of food that is larger than what most people would eat in a similar period under similar circumstances
- A sense of lack of control over eating during the episode
* *Criteria 2:* Episodes of binge eating are associated with more than and equal to three of the following:
  - Eating more rapidly than normal
  - Eating until uncomfortably full
  - Eating a large quantity of food even when not physically hungry
  - Eating alone due to embarrassment of how much one is eating
  - Feeling disgusted with oneself, guilty, and depressed afterward
* *Criteria 3:* Marked distress regarding binge eating present.
* *Criteria 4:* The binge eating episode occurs at least 1 day a week for 3 months.
* *Criteria 5:* Binge eating is not associated with regular use of inappropriate compensatory behavior (e.g., purging, fasting, and excessive exercise) and does not occur exclusively during an episode of AN or BN.

Management

Cognitive-behavioral therapy and family-based therapy have been adopted for adolescents with BED. Pharmacotherapy has a limited role, a small number of trials have reported the efficacy of topiramate and lisdexamfetamine in BED.[15]

Pica

Pica is characterized by eating non-nutritive and non-food items such as clay, raw starches, paper, chalk, clothes, baby powder, and more. Many factors have been implicated in the etiology of pica. Risk factors for developing this disorder include stress, child neglect, cultural factors, nutritional deficiencies such as iron and zinc deficiency, and underlying mental health problems.[16]

DSM-V Diagnostic Criteria[4]

- Persistent eating of non-nutritive and non-food substances for at least more than a month
- The eating of non-nutritive and non-food substances is inappropriate for the developmental level of an individual which lasts for more than a month
- This eating behavior is not a part of culturally supported or socially normative practice
- When this occurs in the context of an underlying medical condition or mental disorder it is severe and warrants additional attention.

Management

Assessment for neglect, mental illness, and developmental delay is essential. Iron, zinc, and other nutritional supplements should be provided if deficiency is identified. Strategies to decrease exposure to a craved substance are important. Behavioral and aversive therapies are found helpful in patients with mental disabilities.[16]

Rumination Disorder

Rumination disorder often occurs in infants and young children and children with developmental disabilities. The exact cause of rumination disorder is not known. Physical illness, severe stress, child neglect, and abnormal relation between the mother and the child may be contributing factors. It may be the way for the child to gain attention.[17]

DSM-V Diagnostic Criteria[4]

- Repeated regurgitation of food for 1 month or more. Regurgitated food may be rechewed, swallowed, or spit out.
- The repeated regurgitation cannot be attributed to gastrointestinal or other medical conditions.
- The eating disorder does not occur exclusively during AN, BN, or BED.
- If the eating disorder occurs in the context of another mental illness or neurodevelopmental disorder, they are sufficiently severe to warrant additional medical attention.

Management

Physical examination and laboratory tests are required to rule out gastrointestinal conditions. Treatment of rumination disorder focuses mainly on changing a child's behavior. Encouraging more interaction between the mother and child during feeding, changing the child's posture during and after feeding, reducing distraction during feeding, and making feeding a more relaxed and pleasurable experience are some of the approaches found useful. Distracting the child when they begin rumination and aversive conditioning, placing something bad tasting when they begin to regurgitate food have also been tried methods.[17]

Picky Eating

Picky eating or fussy eating is a common behavioral problem in early childhood.[5] There is no universal definition for picky eater, the most commonly accepted definition was proposed by Dove et al. Picky eaters are the children who consume an inadequate variety of foods through rejection of food that are familiar (as well as unfamiliar) to them. Alternative definitions include mention of strong food preferences, restriction of vegetable intake, special methods of food preparation, provision of food different from that of caregivers, and disruption of daily routine that are problematic to the child as well as to the family.[5] Peak prevalence of picky eating occurs at 3 years. Factors that are predictive of a child becoming a picky eater can occur during 3 phases: before and during pregnancy, in the first year of life reflecting early feeding practices, and in the second year of life. Picky eating can be due to factors in the child, in the parent/caregiver, and factors involving child-parent interaction.[5] Picky eating can cause stress to parents and have a negative impact on family relations, hence healthcare providers need to identify picky eaters and give appropriate advice to caregivers. For most children, this behavior tends to resolve spontaneously with increasing social exposure but in some, it may be embedded leading to eating disorders during adolescence or adulthood.[18]

Management

Ways to overcome picky eating behaviour include:
- Do not threaten the babies to eat and feed the babies with patience.
- Avoid monotonous nontasty food items and try variety of tasty food items.
- Improve palatability and taste by adding jaggery and ghee.
- Encourage finger feeding and praise them when they eat enough, and offer food to other neighbor children.
- Avoid junk and processed foods.
- Avoid diversions during feeding the baby.

Food Neophobia

Food neophobia is defined as persistent reluctance to eat new foods, unwillingness to taste newly introduced flavors, or unknown consistency food. A combination of biological, environmental, and psychological factors contributes to food neophobia. The incidence of food neophobia is highest between 2 and 6 years of age.[6] Early taste exposures, fetal and neonatal may determine later taste preferences. During breastfeeding, depending on the food chosen by the mother, an infant is exposed to various taste experiences which contribute to the acceptance of new foods later. A child's reluctance to eat certain food may be contributed to the late introduction of new foods into the diet. Parents imposing their taste preferences on the infants may be an additional contributing factor. Neophobic food behavior has a significant impact on the quality of diet in the future.[19]

Management

The management of children with feeding neophobia includes several different factors: Meals should be given in small amounts and at fixed times, the food item should be offered to the child repeatedly but without applying pressure, attempts should be made to leave the food item within the child's reach without necessarily offering it to them, and the new product should be given in the company of familiar products using the food chaining method. Food chaining is a method helpful in feeding therapy for patients with eating disorders. Initially, the food item should be based on products known to the child but in a different way than before (e.g., changing the shape of pasta) or changing the form of administration (e.g., cutting fruit instead of blending). These products are treated as already known to the patient, but it is necessary to gradually change the routine and start introducing various forms of their administration.[20,21]

KEY MESSAGES

1. Approximately 25–45 % of children with normal development experience some type of feeding problem.
2. Feeding disorders can be organic, behavioral, or a combination of both.
3. Most feeding problems are temporary and can be resolved if recognized and addressed early.
4. Children with feeding disorders require a multiprofessional approach and management will involve family-centered models.

REFERENCES

1. Bryant-Waugh R, Markham L, Kreipe RE, Walsh BT. Feeding and eating disorders in childhood. Int J Eat Disord. 2010;43(2):98-111.
2. Goday PS, Huh SY, Silverman A, Lukens CT, Dodrill P, Cohen SS, et al. Pediatric Feeding Disorder: Consensus Definition and Conceptual Framework. J Pediatr Gastroenterol Nutr. 2019;68(1):124-9.
3. Amoretti MC. Do Feeding and Eating Disorders Fit the General Definition of Mental Disorder? Topoi. 2021;40(3):555-64.
4. American Psychiatric Association. Feeding and eating disorders. Diagnostic and Statistical Manual of Mental Disorders. Washington, DC: American Psychiatric Association; 2013.
5. Were FN, Lifschitz C. Complementary feeding: Beyond nutrition. Ann Nutr Metab. 2018;73(Suppl 1):20-5.
6. Kerzner B, Milano K, MacLean WC, Berall G, Stuart S, Chatoor I. A practical approach to classifying and managing feeding difficulties. Pediatrics. 2015;135(2):344-53.
7. Treasure J, Duarte TA, Schmidt U. Eating disorders. Lancet. 2020;395(10227):899-911.
8. Bryant-Waugh R. Feeding and Eating Disorders in Children. Psychiatr Clin North Am. 2019;42(1):157-67.
9. Norris ML, Apsimon M, Harrison M, Obeid N, Buchholz A, Henderson KA, et al. An examination of medical and psychological

morbidity in adolescent males with eating disorders. Eat Disord. 2012;20(5):405-15.
10. Swanson SA, Crow SJ, Le Grange D, Swendsen J, Merikangas KR. Prevalence and correlates of eating disorders in adolescents. Results from the national comorbidity survey replication adolescent supplement. Arch Gen Psychiatry. 2011;68(7):714-23.
11. Muratore AF, Attia E. Current Therapeutic Approaches to Anorexia Nervosa: State of the Art. Clin Ther. 2021;43(1):85-94.
12. Hay PJ, Claudino AM. Bulimia nervosa: online interventions. BMJ Clin Evid. 2015; 2015:1009.
13. Hagan KE, Walsh BT. State of the Art: The Therapeutic Approaches to Bulimia Nervosa. Clin Ther. 2021;43(1):40-9.
14. Bourne L, Bryant-Waugh R, Cook J, Mandy W. Avoidant/restrictive food intake disorder: A systematic scoping review of the current literature. Psychiatry Res. 2020;288:112961.
15. McCuen-Wurst C, Ruggieri M, Allison KC. Disordered eating and obesity: associations between binge eating disorder, night eating syndrome, and weight-related co-morbidities. Ann N Y Acad Sci. 2018;1411(1):96.
16. Advani S, Kochhar G, Chachra S, Dhawan P. Eating everything except food (pica): A rare case report and review. J Int Soc Prev Community Dent. 2014;4(1):1.
17. Murray HB, Juarascio AS, Di Lorenzo C, Drossman DA, Thomas JJ. Diagnosis and Treatment of Rumination Syndrome: a Critical Review. Am J Gastroenterol. 2019 (114);562-78.
18. Taylor CM, Emmett PM. Picky eating in children : causes and consequences. Proc Nutr Soc. 2020;78(2):161-9.
19. Łoboś P, Januszewicz A. Food neophobia in children. Pediatr Endocrinol Diabetes Metab. 2019;25(3):150-4.
20. Fraker C, Fishbein M, Walbert L, Cox S. Food Chaining: The Proven 6-Step Plan to Stop Picky Eating, Solve Feeding Problems, and Expand Your Child's Diet. Boston, MA, USA: Da Capo Press; 2007.
21. Zucker NL, LaVia MC, Craske MG, Foukal M, Harris AA, Datta N, et al. Feeling and body investigators (FBI): ARFID division—An acceptance-based interoceptive exposure treatment for children with ARFID. Int J Eat Disord. 2018;52:466-72.

SECTION 4: Breastfeeding in Special Circumstances

29. **Feeding in Infants with Cleft Lip and Palate**
    Mallikarjuna Honnali Bannajji, Suvarna P Reddy, Durgappa H

30. **Breastfeeding and Maternal Infections**
    Mallanagouda M Patil, Neelamma Patil, Durgappa H

31. **Breastfeeding and Metabolic Disorders**
    Prathik Bandiya, Mahesh Kamate

32. **Breastfeeding during Emergency**
    G Guruprasad, Chaitali Raghoji, Durgappa H

33. **Nursing Strike**
    Shashidhar A, Durgappa H, Anish B Samaga

34. **Relactation and Induced Lactation**
    Shobha C Banapurmath, CR Banapurmath

CHAPTER 29

Feeding in Infants with Cleft Lip and Palate

Mallikarjuna Honnali Bannajji, Suvarna P Reddy, Durgappa H

"No parent is ever prepared in advance to become the parent of a special child".
—Barsch

INTRODUCTION

Craniofacial anomalies are the common congenital defects encountered in infants. No mother is mentally prepared to handle special child immediately after birth. Infants with clefts invariably will have feeding difficulties. So, it is important to diagnose craniofacial anomalies antenatally and provide adequate knowledge and education to mothers and care takers regarding the optimal feeding practices and surgical interventions so that adequate nutrition is ensured to the baby.

ANATOMICAL ASPECTS

Clefts are formed due to failure of fusion of embryonic components of face, median nasal processes, lateral nasal processes, and maxillary processes in the midline. The severity of cleft lip may range from a simple notch in the upper lip to complete opening in the lip, extending into floor of the nasal cavity involving the alveolus of incisive foramen. The cleft palate may involve the soft palate extending partially or completely through hard and soft palate. If it is submucosal cleft, it may not be detected immediately and may remain subtle with no corresponding signs and symptoms.[1]

Out of total cases, combined cleft lip and palate account for 50%, isolated cleft lip and palate are 20% and 30%, respectively, and cleft lip extending to the alveolus occurs in 5% of cases.[2] The majority of cases are unilateral; however, 10% of clefts are bilateral.[3]

MAGNITUDE OF THE PROBLEM

Globally, the prevalence of cleft lip and palate ranges from 0.8 to 2.7 cases per 1,000 live births.[4] In India, the incidence of cleft lip is around 1.3 per 1,000 live births and cleft palate is 0.23 per 1,000 live births[5] and approximately 28,600 infants are born with cleft lip and palate every year. The incidence is higher in southern states due to higher consanguinity.[6]

The basic problem in babies with cleft lip and palate: The success of breastfeeding depends upon the size and type of cleft and maturity of the infant.[7] Cleft lip and palate often interferes with breastfeeding process. Infants with clefts lip have difficulty in sealing up of lip around the breast and infants with cleft palate have difficulty in generating suction and compression of breast tissue between the tongue and palate due to anatomical gap between oral and nasal cavity.[8,9]

IMPACTS ON BREASTFEEDING PRACTICE

The immediate concern for the baby is optimal nutrition. The cleft lip and palate have negative impact on breastfeeding practices in infants. Studies have shown that breastfeeding rates were significantly lower in infants having cleft lip and palate compared to those infants without clefts. So, it is important to optimize the feeding practices in these babies.[8]

PROBLEMS ASSOCIATED WITH CLEFT LIP AND PALATE

Problems associated with cleft lip and palate include difficulty in latching, recurrent nasal regurgitation, choking, excessive air swallowing, inability to extract milk, prolonged feeding, fatigue, failure to thrive, anemia, speech and hearing problems and psychological stress among the mothers (Box 1).[10-12] The detailed sequence of events are illustrated in **Flowchart 1**.

MANAGEMENT OF INFANTS WITH CLEFT LIP AND PALATE

Diagnosis

It is an essential to have routine antenatal ultrasound examinations to look for craniofacial anomalies. In addition, counsel the mothers and care takers on optimal feeding practices for the baby.

The Management of Cleft Lip and Palate

The multidisciplinary approach is required including the team of plastic surgery, oral and faciomaxillary surgery, dentistry, orthodontics, Otolaryngology, Genetics, nutrition and child development to address the clinical problems that accompany the clefts.

> **BOX 1:** Problems associated in infants with cleft lip and palate.
> - Ineffective sucking
> - Prolonged feeding
> - Fatigue
> - Failure to thrive
> - Anemia
> - Excessive air swallowing
> - Recurrent nasal regurgitation
> - Aspirations
> - Recurrent otitis media
> - Speech and hearing
> - Dentition
> - Jaw developmental problems
> - Psychological stress
> - Breastfeeding failure
> - Infant and mother bonding

The various feeding methods found to be helpful for feeding the baby include modifications of feeding positions, feeding devices, prosthesis, and surgical repairs.

Modifications of Feeding Positions

Infants with Cleft Lip

Infants with cleft lip do not have major feeding problems. They need some modifications in positions during breastfeeding. If the cleft is unilateral, adopt *football* position or *straddle position* to feed the baby.

Football/Straddle method: In this method, position the baby with cleft toward the breast, this will allow the cleft to be tucked into breast tissue and makes it easier for the infant to suckle. Further support to infant's cheek decreases the width of the cleft which simultaneously increases the closure around the nipple (**Fig. 1**). In all these methods, it is important to hold the baby in "upright position" and this allows milk flow down and this helps in preventing choking. In incorrect position, milk may enter respiratory airways. The breastfeeding would be more difficult in

Flowchart 1: Elements of the feeding difficulty and their inter-relationship in infants with cleft palate.[8]

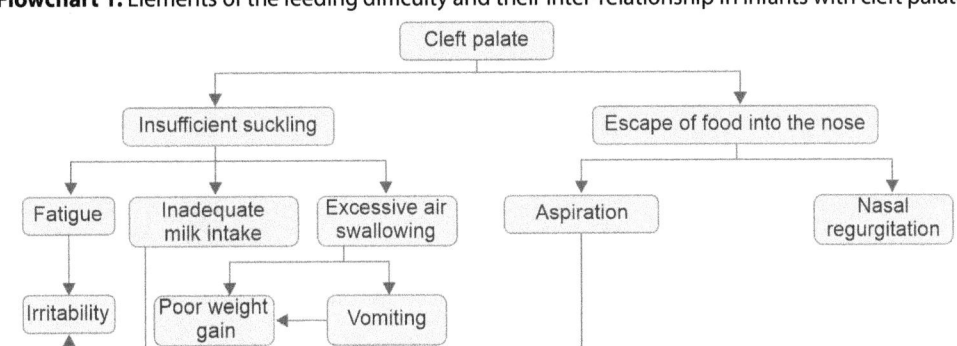

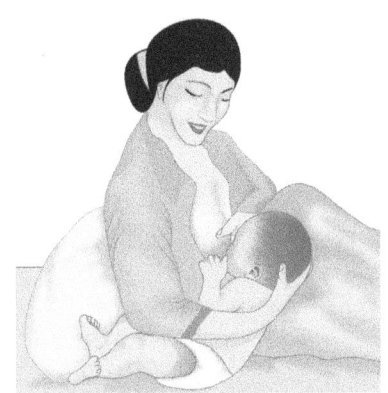

Fig. 1: Football/Straddle method.

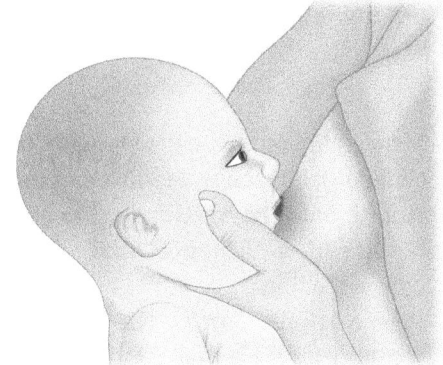

Fig. 2: Dancer hand position.

babies having bilateral cleft lip due to inability to form "airtight seal" around the nipple. In such circumstances, Dancer hand position is recommended.

Dancer hand position: It is recommended in bilateral CL. In this method, the hand slides under the breasts with three fingers support the breast, with forefinger and thumb forming U-shape to support the baby's chin **(Fig. 2)**. This helps the baby to press the nipple and areola between the gums. In conditions where there is failure to thrive, one can switch over to specially designed bottles as nutrition cannot be compromised.[12]

Babies with Cleft Palate

In most cases, the infants are unable to latch well on to the breast as there is inefficient suction. If it is not possible to provide optimal nutrition, one can try with special bottles. There are various specially designed bottle and teats.

Devices: The specially designed feeding bottles and nipples:

- *Hebarman feeder (Medela special needs feeder):* The nipple has one-way valve that allows the milk to enter baby's mouth when nipple is squeezed and flow can also be adjusted **(Fig. 3)**.

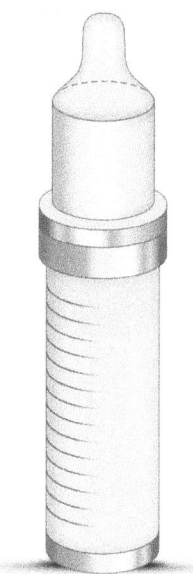

Fig. 3: Hebarman feeder.

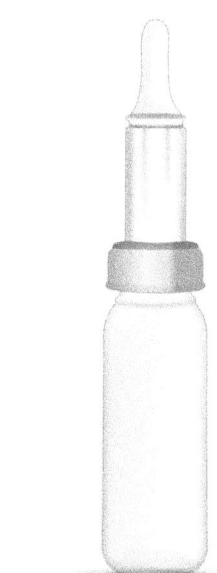

Fig. 4: Mead–Johnson cleft palate nursery bottle.

- Mead–Johnson cleft palate nursery bottle (Enfamil): It is soft squeezable bottle with stiff nipple **(Fig. 4)**. Gently squeeze the bottle with a pulsing rhythm while the baby is feeding.
- *Pigeon nipple/bottle:* The nipple has soft and hard part with one way valve. The soft side sits on the baby's tongue and makes it easy to suck on it **(Fig. 5)**.
- These are made up of soft squeezable plastic to help draw milk from the bottle with very little pressure. A long nipple to press against tongue with Y cut in the tip of the nipple is recommended. It is important to keep the baby in "upright" position with the head in one hand and bottle in another hand.
- *Cup and spoon feeding:* It is always safe to feed the babies with cup and spoon as it requires minimal effort to sterilize compared to bottles.[7,12-14]
- Before the surgical repair of Cleft Palate, baby needs to be completely weaned from bottle-feeding because of the reason that

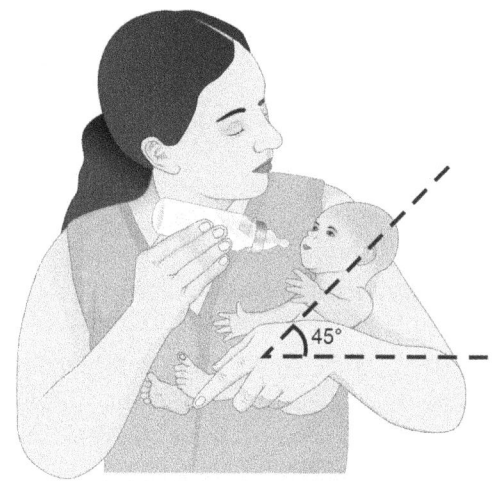

Fig. 5: Pigeon nipple/bottle.

bottle nipple may rub against the sutures and breakdown the repair. A long-handed spoon with a flat bowl may be used to feed the babies in the postoperative period.[7]
- *Prosthesis:* Feeding obturators are passive devices designed to provide a normal counter for infant of cleft alveolus and palate. This separates the oral and nasal cavity and provides a surface to oppose

the nipple. The use of obturators has been a major controversy.

There are two schools of thoughts:
- First one advocates its advantages that they help in feeding, facilitate lip and palate repair, and facial growth.
- Other school of thought claims its disadvantages—impression taking process is cumbersome for the infant and sterilization and maintenance of hygiene is another issue.[7]

Surgical repair: It is important to follow the "rule of 10" for infants before taking for surgical repair. The Rule of 10 includes—Hb:10 g, 10 weeks of age, and 10 lbs of weight. Cleft lip repair and soft palate lengthening is done at 3 months of age and palate repair is done at 9 months of age along with initiation of speech therapy.

KEY MESSAGES

- No mother is mentally prepared to handle the special child.
- Antenatal diagnosis and appropriate counseling regarding optimal feeding practices is essential.
- Babies with cleft lip and palate invariably have feeding difficulties.
- Modifications of feeding positions and use of appropriate devices are helpful.
- Frequent burping is important to prevent regurgitation.
- Feeding under good hygienic conditions is most important.
- Periodic growth monitoring is essential.
- Motivate the mothers to register the babies with clefts under international free intervention projects like smile train where cleft repair is done with free of cost.

REFERENCES

1. Sadler TW. Langman's Medical Embryology, 13th edition. Philadelphia: Wolters Kluwer; 2016. p. 297-9.
2. Mulliken JB. Repair of bilateral complete cleft lip and nasal deformity—State of the art. Cleft Palate Craniofac J. 2000;37:342-7.
3. Wolf LS, Glass RP. Feeding and Swallowing Disorders in Infancy: Assessment and Management. Tucson, AZ: Therapy Skill Builders; 1992.
4. Conway H, Wagner KJ. Incidence of clefts in New York City. Cleft Palate Craniofac J. 1996;33:284-90.
5. Young G. Cleft lip and palate. (1998). UTMB Department of Otolaryngology Grand Rounds. www.utmb.edu/otoref/Grnds/Cleft-lip-palate-9801/Cleft-lip-palate-9801.htm. [Last accessed November, 2023].
6. Reddy SG, Reddy RR, Bronkhorst EM, Prasad R, Ettema AM, Sailer HF, et al. Incidence of cleft lip and palate in the state of Andhra Pradesh, South India. Indian J Plastic Surg. 2010;43:184-9.
7. Reid JA, Reilly S, Kilpatrick NM. Breastmilk consumption in babies with clefts. Presented at the 63rd Annual Meeting of the American Cleft Palate-Craniofacial Association, Vancouver, BC, Canada, 2006.
8. Sree Devi E, Sai Sankar AJ, Manoj Kumar MG, Sujatha B. Maiden morsel - feeding in cleft lip and palate infants. J Int Soc Prev Community Dent. 2012;2(2):31-7.
9. Reid J, Reilly S, Kilpatrick N. Sucking performance of babies with cleft conditions. Cleft Palate Craniofac J. 2007;44:312-20.
10. Reid J. A review of feeding interventions for infants with cleft palate. Cleft Craniofac J. 2004;41(3):268-78.
11. Trenouth MJ, Campbell AN. Questionnaire evaluation of feeding methods for cleft lip and palate neonates. Int J Pediatr Dent. 1996;6:241-4.
12. Saunders ID, Geary L, Flemming P, Gregg TA. A simplified feeding appliance for the infant with a cleft lip and palate. Quintessence Int. 1989;20:907-10.
13. Reilly S, Reid J, Skeat JS; Academy of Breastfeeding Medicine Clinical Protocol Committee. ABM Clinical Protocol #17: Guidelines for breastfeeding infants with cleft lip, cleft palate, or cleft lip and palate. Breastfeed Med 2007 Dec;2(4):243-50.
14. Jindal MK, Khan SY. How to feed cleft patient? Int J Clin Pediatr Dent. 2013;6:100-3.

CHAPTER 30

Breastfeeding and Maternal Infections

Mallanagouda M Patil, Neelamma Patil, Durgappa H

"Mother's milk is soul food for babies. The babies of the world need a lot more soul food".
—Ina May Gaskin

INTRODUCTION

Breastfeeding is the cornerstone for the optimal growth, development, and survival of infants and young children. It is nutritious, safe, sustainable, and available all time needing no preparation or storage, playing a vital role in the prevention of major childhood illnesses, i.e., diarrhea, pneumonia, and malnutrition which are the most common conditions causing morbidity and mortality among children across the world.[1]

There is often a dilemma among mothers with infections regarding infant feeding practices. Though breastfeeding is safe in most maternal infections, appropriate preventive measures need to be taken to reduce the risk of transmission of infections from mothers to babies. Common maternal infections include human immunodeficiency virus (HIV), hepatitis B, hepatitis C, coronavirus disease-2019 (COVID-19), H1N1, herpes simplex virus (HSV), varicella, cytomegalovirus (CMV), and pulmonary tuberculosis (TB) **(Table 1)**.[1,2]

MATERNAL INFECTIONS AND RECOMMENDATIONS

Mother Living with HIV and Breastfeeding

The risk of transmission of HIV infection from mother to baby through breastfeeding varies from 5 to 15%. With the appropriate preventive measures: Antiretroviral (ARV) drugs tenofovir (TDF), lamivudine (3TC) or emtricitabine (FTC), and efavirenz (EFZ) to mother and nevirapine prophylaxis to infant can reduce the risk of transmission to <0.5%.[3]

Recommendations

Feeding an infant born to a mother living with HIV can be challenging and often distressing for the mother and family members. The options for infant feeding methods should be offered to mothers and caretakers with appropriate education. Informed, patient-centered, and balanced decisions should be taken after weighing the risks over benefits for the good health of the mother and baby. Ideally, whenever it is *acceptable, feasible,*

CHAPTER 30: Breastfeeding and Maternal Infections

TABLE 1: Maternal infections and risk of transmission via breastfeeding.

Maternal infections	Risk of transmission via BM	Recommendations
HIV[1-4]	5–15%	• AFASS-replacement therapy • If no, EBF with maternal ARV drugs + nevirapine prophylaxis to baby
Hepatitis B[5-11]	Negligible	EBF + hepatitis B vaccine + immunoglobulins <12 hours of delivery
Hepatitis C[12,13]	Negligible	EBF
COVID-19[14-20]	Negligible	EBF + hand and respiratory hygiene
H1N1[21,22]	Negligible	EBF + hand and respiratory hygiene
HSV[23-25]	Negligible	EBF unless lesions are on the breast
Varicella[26,27]	Negligible	EBF unless lesions are on the breast
CMV[28-33]	CMV DNA is detectable in the BM of about 95% of CMV-seropositive mothers	No recommendations against breastfeeding for CMV-positive mother
Tuberculosis[34,35]	Negligible	EBF + INH prophylaxis + B_6 to infants + respiratory hygiene

(AFASS: acceptable, feasible, affordable, sustainable, and safe; ARV: antiretroviral; BM: breast milk; CMV: cytomegalovirus; COVID-19: coronavirus disease-2019; DNA: deoxyribonucleic acid; EBF: exclusively breastfeed; HIV: human immunodeficiency virus; HSV: herpes simplex virus; INH: isoniazid)

Note:
- If the mother is diagnosed with HIV in the first trimester—maternal antiretroviral therapy (ART) + infant nevirapine prophylaxis for 6 weeks.
- If the mother is diagnosed with HIV beyond the first trimester—maternal ART + infant nevirapine prophylaxis for 12 weeks.
- If the maternal viral load is >1,000 copies—maternal ART + infant nevirapine prophylaxis for 12 weeks + start zidovudine/lopinavir at 2nd week for 6 weeks.
- If the maternal viral load is <1,000 copies—maternal ART + infant nevirapine prophylaxis for 12 weeks.[1,2]
- If preterm < 28 weeks of gestation exposed to varicella—immunoglobulin to the newborn.[27]

affordable, sustainable, and safe (AFASS), one should always recommend replacement therapy for the baby. Mothers/caretakers need to be given appropriate information on the method of preparation of infant food, hygiene, and optimal feeding method.

If replacement feeding is not feasible, then one can advise exclusive breastfeeding for 6 months and thereafter; complementary feeding along with breastfeeding for 12 months, under the cover of triple therapy (ARV drugs) for the mother and nevirapine prophylaxis for the infant. Sustained adherence to ARV drugs is crucial throughout breastfeeding. Mixed feeding is not advised. If the mother wants to stop breastfeeding, she can stop breastfeeding over one month after ensuring adequate nutrition from the complementary feeding and growth of the baby.[3,4] It is also important to ensure the right dose of nevirapine based on the weight of the infants as mentioned in **Table 2**.

Infant Born to Mother having Hepatitis B

The prevalence of hepatitis B infection in pregnant women may be between 0.8 and 1.1% in India.[5-11] In another study, the pooled

TABLE 2: Nevirapine (NVP) prophylaxis.[3,4]

Birth weight	NVP daily dose (in mg)	NVP daily dose (in mL)
<2,000 g	2 mg/kg OD	0.2 mL/kg OD
2,000–2,500 g	10 mg OD	1 mL OD
>2,500 g	15 mg OD	1.5 mL OD

prevalence of hepatitis B surface antigen (HBsAg) was reported to be 1,6% [95% confidence interval (CI), 1.4-1.8] among pregnant women.[11] The transmission of hepatitis B infection from mother to child can occur during antenatal, natal, and breastfeeding. The risk of infectivity is higher when the infant is born to a mother who is serologically positive for both HBsAg and hepatitis B e antigen (HBeAg) in the absence of postexposure immune prophylaxis and the risk of chronic hepatitis B infection may increase in infants to 70-90% by the age of 6 months.[7]

Recommendations

Breastfeeding can safely be practiced under preventive measures: Hepatitis B vaccine and immunoglobulins within 12 hours of delivery. If there is a delay in getting vaccination breastfeeding should not be withheld. If there is sore/cracked nipple stop breastfeeding temporarily for a few days or until the problem is corrected and use pasteurized donor's milk to feed the babies.[1-3,7]

Infant Born to Mother having Hepatitis C

The risk of transmission of hepatitis C through breastfeeding is negligible.[12,13]

Recommendations

Breastfeeding can safely be given to the babies immediately after delivery. If there is a sore/cracked nipple stop breastfeeding temporarily for a few days or till the problem is corrected and, in such a situation, pasteurized donor's milk can be given.

Mother with COVID-19 and Breastfeeding

The risk of transmission of COVID-19 through breastfeeding is not known.[14-20]

Recommendations

The most babies born to COVID-19-positive mothers remain mildly symptomatic or asymptomatic. Immediate skin-to-skin contact between mother and baby and early initiation of breastfeeding under respiratory and hand hygiene has a positive impact on breastfeeding and survival of infants.

Mother with H1N1

No evidence to suggest the risk of transmission of H1N1 through breastfeeding.[21,22]

Recommendations

Breastfeeding can safely be practiced with the appropriate hand and respiratory hygiene.

Mothers with HSV Infection and Breastfeeding

The risk of transmission of HSV through breastfeeding is negligible.[23-25]

Recommendations

Breastfeeding can safely be given with appropriate hygiene. If lesions are on the nipple or breast; withhold breastfeeding on that side till lesions are healed and continue breastfeeding on the other side of the breast under proper preventive measures like covering the site of the lesion. It is important to maintain milk flow on the lesion side by regular expression of breast milk and that should be discarded.

Mother with Varicella Zoster Virus Infection and Breastfeeding

The primary mode of transmission of varicella zoster virus (VZV) is airborne and through contact with vesicular lesions.[26,27]

Recommendations

Breastfeeding is advisable for varicella exposed as well as infected newborns in view of the breast milk antibodies that may be protective. Though varicella deoxyribonucleic acid (DNA) is found in the mother's milk by polymerase chain reaction (PCR) testing, transmission is uncertain. *Considering the benefit versus risk, breastfeeding is safely given with appropriate hygiene in mothers with no active lesions over the breast.* If the mother gets varicella infection >5 days before delivery, continue breastfeeding without separating baby and mother. If the mother gets varicella infection within 5 days before or within 2 days after delivery, start expressed breast milk feeding and separate mother and baby until the lesions are healed and then start breastfeeding thereafter. If the mother gets varicella after 2 days of delivery, starts expressed breast milk feeding and separate the mother and baby until the lesions are healed and start breastfeeding thereafter.

Mothers with Cytomegalovirus Infection (CMV) and Breastfeeding

Cytomegalovirus infection may be transmitted placentally; via aspiration of secretions in the birth canal, or by exposure to infected secretions such as breast milk, saliva, or blood products. The prevalence of congenital CMV infection is reported to be 0.23–0.64% and 1.3–2.3% in very low birth weight infants. Postnatal CMV infection is generally asymptomatic in full-term babies whereas babies born before 30 weeks of pregnancy and/or weighing <1,500 g may have a higher chance of getting sick from CMV through breast milk.[28-33]

Recommendations

There are no recommendations against breastfeeding by mothers who are CMV-seropositive. However, infants born <30 weeks of gestational age and <1,500g who acquire CMV from breast milk may be at risk of developing a late-onset sepsis-like syndrome. The potential benefits of human milk versus the risk of CMV transmission should be considered when deciding between the breastfeeding of very premature babies by mothers known to be CMV-seropositive. Freezing and pasteurization of breast milk can decrease the risk of transmission; however, freezing does not eliminate the risk of transmission.

Mother with Tuberculosis and Breastfeeding

The risk of transmission of TB through breastfeeding is negligible.[34,35]

Recommendations

Breastfeeding is safe and should be continued with good respiratory hygiene. The modern antitubercular drugs are so efficacious that maternal separation is not recommended unless she is sick, nonadherent to therapy, or has drug resistance to TB. The infant should be put on Isoniazid (INH) (10 mg/kg) prophylaxis therapy for 6 months along with vitamin B6. All infants born to mothers with TB should be given Bacillus Calmette-Guérin (BCG) vaccination at birth even if they are on preventive INH prophylaxis therapy.

It is also important to evaluate for TB in the baby before stopping the INH prophylaxis therapy. If the baby turns out to be positive for TB, switch over to the standard antituberculosis treatment (ATT) regimen as per the new National Tuberculosis Elimination Programme (NTEP) pediatric guideline 2022.

KEY MESSAGES

- Breastfeeding is the cornerstone for the growth, development, and survival of infants and children.
- Breastfeeding is safe for most maternal infections with appropriate preventive measures.
- Breastfeeding can safely be given in infants born to mothers with HBsAg under the cover of postexposure immune prophylaxis.
- In mothers living with HIV, a balanced decision should be taken after weighing the risk over the benefits.
- Breastfeeding can safely be given to infants born to mothers with TB under good respiratory hygiene.
- Maternal separation is not recommended unless the mother is sick, nonadherent to therapy, or has drug-resistant TB (DRTB).
- All infants born to mothers with TB should receive preventive INH prophylaxis therapy for 6 months along with vitamin B6.
- All infants born to mothers with TB should be vaccinated for BCG even if the infant is on INH prophylaxis therapy.

REFERENCES

1. Aryeetey R, Dykes F. Global implications of the new WHO and UNICEF implementation guidance on the revised Baby-Friendly Hospital Initiative. Matern Child Nutr. 2018;14(3):e12637.
2. World Health Organization. Guideline: Updates on HIV and Infant Feeding. Geneva: World Health Organization; 2016.
3. National AIDS Control Organization, World Health Organization, United Nations Children's Fund. Guideline: Updates on HIV and Infant Feeding: The Duration of Breastfeeding, and Support from Health Services to Improve Feeding Practices among Mothers Living with HIV. Geneva: World Health Organization; 2021.
4. NACO. National Guidelines for HIV Care and Treatment. New Delhi: NACO, Ministry of Health and Family Welfare, Government of India; 2021.
5. Chen X, Chen J, Wen J, Xu C, Zhang S, Zhou YH, et al. Breastfeeding is not a risk factor for mother-to-child transmission of hepatitis B virus. PloS One. 2013;8(1):e55303.
6. Chatterjee S, Ravishankar K, Chatterjee R, Narang A, Kinikar. Hepatitis B prevalence during pregnancy. Indian Pediatr. 2009; 46:1005-8.
7. Singh R, Chaudhary M, Shrivastava K, Agarwal BV, Mitra S. Seroprevalence of Hepatitis B Infection among Antenatal Women in a Tertiary Care Center in Eastern UP and Assessment of the Associated High-risk Factors. J South Asian Fed Obstet Gynaecol. 2022;13(6):378-81.
8. Dwivedi M, Misra SP, Misra V, Pandey A, Pant S, Singh R, et al. Seroprevalence of hepatitis B infection during pregnancy and risk of perinatal transmission. Indian J Gastroenterol. 2011;30:66-71.
9. Sibia P, Mohi MK, Kumar A. Seroprevalence of hepatitis B infection among pregnant women in one of the institutes of Northern India. J Clin Diagnos Res. 2016;10(8):QC08.
10. Nguyen MH, Keeffe EB. Are Hepatitis B e Antigen (HBeAg)-Positive Chronic Hepatitis B and HBeAg-Negative Chronic Hepatitis B Distinct Diseases? Clin Infect Dis. 2008;47(10):1312-4.
11. Pandey S, Lohani P, Roy R, Bhar D, Ranjan A, Kumar P, et al. Prevalence and knowledge of hepatitis B infection in pregnant women in a primary health center of Patna district, Bihar. J Family Med Prim Care. 2021;10(10):3675-81.
12. Giri S, Agrawal D, Afzalpurkar S, Kasturi S, Gopan A, Sundaram S, et al. Prevalence

of hepatitis B virus and hepatitis C virus infection in patients with inflammatory bowel disease: a systematic review and meta-analysis. Intest Res. 2023;21(3):392-405.
13. Mast EE. Mother-to-infant hepatitis C virus transmission and breastfeeding. Protecting Infants through Human Milk: Adv Exp Med Biol. 2004;554:211-6.
14. Zhu H, Wang L, Fang C, Peng S, Zhang L, Chang G, et al. Clinical analysis of 10 neonates born to mothers with 2019-nCoV pneumonia. Transl Pediatr. 2020;9(1):51-60.
15. Liu X, Chen H, An M, Yang W, Wen Y, Cai Z, et al. Recommendations for breastfeeding during Coronavirus Disease 2019 (COVID-19) pandemic. Int Breastfeed J. 2022;17(1):28.
16. Lubbe W, Botha E, Niela-Vilen H, Reimers P. Breastfeeding during the COVID-19 pandemic–a literature review for clinical practice. Int Breastfeed J. 2020;15(1):1-9.
17. World Health Organization. Breastfeeding and COVID-19. Geneva: World Health Organization; 2020.
18. Singh V, Parakh A. What is new in the management of childhood tuberculosis in 2020? Indian Pediatr. 2020;57:1172-6.
19. Sullivan SE, Thompson LA. Best practices for COVID-19–positive or exposed mothers—Breastfeeding and pumping milk. JAMA Pediatr. 2020;174(12):1228-9.
20. Yang N, Che S, Zhang J, Wang X, Tang Y, Wang J, et al. Breastfeeding of infants born to mothers with COVID-19: a rapid review. Ann Transl Med. 2020;8(10):618.
21. Satpathy HK, Lindsay M, Kawwass JF. Novel H1N1 virus infection and pregnancy. Postgraduate Medicine. 2009;121(6):106-12.
22. Rasmussen SA, Kissin DM, Yeung LF, MacFarlane K, Chu SY, Turcios-Ruiz RM, et al. Preparing for influenza after 2009 H1N1: special considerations for pregnant women and newborns. Am J Obstet Gynecol. 2011;204(6):S13-20.
23. Lamounier JA, Moulin ZS, Xavier CC. Recommendations for breastfeeding during maternal infections. J Pediatr (Rio J). 2004;80:S181-8.
24. Lawrence RM, Lawrence RA. Given the benefits of breastfeeding, what contraindications exist? Pediatr Clin North Am. 2001;48(1):235-51.
25. Gantt S, Orem J, Krantz EM, Morrow RA, Selke S, Huang ML, et al. Prospective characterization of the risk factors for transmission and symptoms of primary human herpesvirus infections among Ugandan infants. J Infect Dis. 2016;214(1):36-44.
26. American Academy of Pediatrics. Red Book: 2021-2024 Report of the Committee on Infectious Diseases. Itasca, IL: American Academy of Pediatrics; 2021. pp. 831-43.
27. Weimer KE, Singh T, Permar SR. Viral infections. In: Eichenwald EC, Hansen AR, Martin CR, Stark AR. Cloherty and Stark's Manual of Neonatal Care, 9th edition. Philadelphia: Wolters Kluwer; 2023. pp. 660.
28. Pass RF, Anderson B. Mother-to-child transmission of cytomegalovirus and prevention of congenital infection. J Pediatric Infect Dis Soc. 2014;3(Suppl 1):S2-6.
29. Forsgren M. Cytomegalovirus in breast milk: reassessment of pasteurization and freeze-thawing. Pediatr Res. 2004;56(4):526-8.
30. Resch B. How to Provide Breast Milk for the Preterm Infant and Avoid Symptomatic Cytomegalovirus Infection with Possible Long-Term Sequelae. Life (Basel). 2022;12(4):504.
31. Bardanzellu F, Fanos V, Reali A. Human breast milk-acquired cytomegalovirus infection: certainties, doubts, and perspectives. Curr Pediatr Rev. 2019;15(1):30-41.
32. Park HW, Cho MH, Bae SH, Lee R, Kim KS. Incidence of postnatal CMV infection among breastfed preterm infants: a systematic review and meta-analysis. J Korean Med Sci. 2021;36(12): e84.
33. Bryant P, Morley C, Garland S, Curtis N. Cytomegalovirus transmission from breast milk in premature babies: does it matter? Arch Dis Child Fetal Neonatal Ed. 2002;87(2):F75-7.
34. Loto OM, Awowole I. Tuberculosis in pregnancy: a review. J Pregnancy. 2012; 2012:379271.
35. National Tuberculosis Elimination Programme. Paediatric TB Management Guideline 2022. New Delhi: Ministry of Health and Family Welfare, Government of India; 2022.

CHAPTER 31

Breastfeeding and Metabolic Disorders

Prathik Bandiya, Mahesh Kamate

"When in doubt, Nutrition is first"

INTRODUCTION

Inborn errors of metabolism (IEM) are a diverse group of metabolic disorders that can present from the neonatal period to childhood. Most of these conditions mimic sepsis in the neonatal period. A high index of suspicion should be kept for the diagnosis of these conditions. In this chapter, the basic principles of feeding in commonly encountered inborn errors of metabolism are described.

The biochemical processes that occur to maintain normal cellular function are commonly termed "metabolism". An error or interference in any of these pathways leads to either excessive accumulation of the substrate or deficiency of the end product leading to end-organ dysfunction.[1] This group of disorders is called inborn errors of metabolism.

The incidence of common IEMs varies depending on the geographical distribution, ethnicity, and degree of testing. Conditions such as galactosemia and phenylketonuria (PKU) are extremely rare, especially in our population with an incidence of 1:41027 and 1:20513, respectively.[2] The incidence of other conditions such as organic acidurias, aminoacidopathies, and fatty acid oxidation (FAO) disorder is approximately 1:100000.[1]

GENERAL PRINCIPLES OF FEEDING/DIETARY MANAGEMENT

The following are the few general principles in the management of any IEM:
- Withhold feeds upon initial suspicion until the specific diagnosis is established.
- Replacement of specific metabolite/nutrient when there is a block in the metabolic pathway.
- Use of specific vitamins for enzyme induction in some IEMs
- Early initiation of a special diet and lifelong restriction of the certain substrate if needed.

In the following sections, feeding in common IEMs, especially during the neonatal period and infancy, is described.

FEEDING IN AMINO ACID DISORDERS

The basic principle of feeding in any aminoacidopathy is to avoid the accumulation of toxic metabolite by limiting or complete the stoppage of feeds.

Phenylketonuria

Phenylketonuria is the first IEM for which dietary treatment was available. The etiology of brain damage is due to excessive accumulation of phenylalanine in the blood which can lead to various neurological (seizures, tremors), behavioral (hyperactivity, self-injury), and psychological (depression, anxiety, agoraphobia) manifestations. The accumulation of phenylalanine is due to the absence of the enzyme *phenylalanine hydroxylase* or co-factor tetrahydrobiopterin (BH4). The absence of this enzyme also results in phenylalanine not getting converted to tyrosine; hence, it becomes a conditionally essential amino acid and needs to be supplemented.

Management

The cornerstone in the management of PKU is limiting the intake of phenylalanine, the offending amino acid. The restriction should be lifelong, and hence it is aptly called a "diet for life". Most centers target a phenylalanine concentration of ≥360 µmol/L as an indication of dietary management, and the goal of dietary treatment is to maintain phenylalanine concentrations between 120 and 360 µmol/L so that it provides adequate phenylalanine for growth and development and also prevents toxicity.

Stepwise Management of Phenylketonuria

Step 1: The first step is to remove the phenylalanine from the diet to quickly reduce the phenylalanine concentration. This period is called "washout period" and it depends on the initial blood concentration of phenylalanine. This is followed by the calculation of phenylalanine needs depending on the blood phenylalanine concentrations. The amount of phenylalanine to be prescribed after the washout period is mentioned in **Table 1**.

TABLE 1: Phenylalanine to be prescribed after the washout period depending on initial blood concentration.[3]

Blood phenylalanine levels (µmol/L)	Phenylalanine is to be prescribed after the washout period (mg/kg)
<600	70
600–1,200	55
1,200–1,800	45
1,800–2,400	35

TABLE 2: Recommended phenylalanine and tyrosine intake for a patient with phenylketonuria (PKU).[3]

Age (months)	Phenylalanine (mg/kg)	Tyrosine (mg/kg)
0–3	25–70	300–350
3–6	20–45	300–350
6–9	15–35	250–300
9–12	10–35	250–300

Step 2: Mature breast milk contains approximately 45 mg of phenylalanine and 53 mg of tyrosine per 100 mL of milk. Calculate the volume of breast milk that will provide the phenylalanine needs of the baby **(Table 2)**.

Step 3: Then calculate the protein requirement for the infant for that age and then subtract the protein provided by the calculated volume of breast milk from the total protein needs of the baby.

Step 4: Then supplement the remaining amount of protein from the phenylalanine-free formula. The final calculated volume of milk which includes both breast milk and special formula now contains a sufficient amount of protein. The calories provided by this volume of milk are also noted. If there is any deficit in calories, then additional calories need to be supplemented from a nonprotein source.

TABLE 3: Additional supplementation and therapies in phenylketonuria (PKU).

Supplements	Therapies
Tyrosine	To be supplemented in all cases as tyrosine is an essential amino acid in PKU
• Tetrahydrobiopterin (BH$_4$) • Sapropterin dihydrochloride (a synthetic form of BH$_4$)	This is the co-factor for the enzyme phenylalanine hydroxylase and is beneficial
Large neutral amino acids (LNAAs)	• LNAAs competitively inhibit phenylalanine for transport across the blood–brain barrier • Used mainly in adults and contraindicated in infants and young children.

In difficult situations, additional therapies can be tried **(Table 3)**.

Galactosemia

Classical galactosemia is a rare disorder of galactose metabolism characterized by a deficiency of the enzyme *galactose-1-phosphate uridylyltransferase* (GALT) which usually presents in the neonatal period. The other forms of galactosemia are due to deficiency of the enzyme galactokinase and galactose-4-epimerase. These enzyme deficiencies result in the accumulation of metabolites such as galactose, galactose-1-phosphate, galactitol, and galactonate and also lead to a deficiency of UDP-galactose and UDP-glucose.

It is one of the important causes of acute liver failure in a neonate. These neonates are also prone to gram-negative sepsis, especially *Escherichia coli*, and are at an increased risk of neurological complications, developmental delay, and speech issues despite lifelong treatment.

Principles of Dietary Management

- Restriction of galactose intake
- Supplementation of calcium and Vitamin D (long term).

The main dietary management of galactosemia is to restrict galactose from the diet. In neonates and infants, the main source of galactose is lactose, which is a combination of glucose and galactose. Hence, all the sources of lactose and galactose, including breast milk and dairy products, should be avoided. This is one of the rare scenarios where breast milk is absolutely contraindicated.

There are many commercial lactose-free formulas available in our country that can be used during the neonatal period. Another option is to use soy formula/milk or casein hydrolysate or elemental formula which is also devoid of galactose. The treatment should be initiated if there is a strong clinical suspicion even if the laboratory results are pending.

In soy formula, the protein source is soy protein isolate which may contain very small quantities of galactose and can be used. The elemental formula contains mainly L amino acids and contains no detectable galactose. In any preterm neonate with suspected galactosemia, elemental formula is recommended over soy formula.

During infancy, most standard guidelines recommend a galactose-free diet and also permit very small quantities of galactose from nonmilk sources, especially from caseinates and mature cheeses, as it is very difficult to completely eliminate galactose from the diet.[4]

The clinical monitoring of any neonate with galactosemia is based on the measurement of galactose-1-phosphate in blood along with clinical monitoring and serial anthropometry. These children are also prone to osteopenia and vitamin D deficiency and should be periodically monitored with vitamin D levels and DEXA scans.

Tyrosinemia

Feeding in tyrosinemia is similar to PKU, where the offending amino acid, tyrosine, needs to be restricted. As in any metabolic disorder, the main goal is to support normal growth by protein anabolism and prevention of catabolism and complications.

The principle in dietary management is to avoid a natural protein source that contains tyrosine and use a special formula that is tyrosine free to provide adequate protein, energy, and calories. These neonates also need to be treated with nitisinone (NTBC) for adequate metabolic control.

The calculation of diet is similar to that of PKU as mentioned previously.

Glutaric Acidemia Type 1

Glutaric acidemia type 1 (GA-1) is a disorder affecting the metabolism of tryptophan, lysine, and hydroxylysine due to a deficiency of enzyme *glutaryl-CoA dehydrogenase* which results in the accumulation of toxic metabolites such as 3-hydroxyglutaric acid and glutaric acid. These neonates mainly present with macrocephaly along with dystonia after any intercurrent illness. It is considered one of the cerebral palsy mimics.

Feeding/Dietary Principles

The main principle in the management of these neonates is to *restrict lysine and tryptophan* in the diet and supplement L-carnitine, riboflavin, and pantothenic acid.

The approximate protein and lysine intake in these neonates should be determined based on age, clinical status, and laboratory values. **Table 4** shows age-appropriate values.

Depending on the age, calculate the amount of breast milk needed to fulfil the lysine requirement for the baby and also the protein provided by the calculated volume of the breast milk. The rest of the protein requirement should be met by the special formula for GA-1. If there is any deficit in calories, then a protein-free medical food must be added. The required amount of water should be added taking into consideration the fluid requirement of the baby **(Table 1)**.

Urea Cycle Disorders[5,6]

Urea cycle disorders (UCD) are a group of disorders caused due to defects in any of the enzymes involved in the urea cycle pathway. The main feature of these disorders is an accumulation of ammonia due to a defect in one of the pathways involved in the clearance of ammonia. The accumulation of ammonia, glutamine, and other toxic metabolites results in various clinical manifestations such as poor feeding, lethargy, vomiting, irritability, coma, and death.

Neonates with severe forms of the disease usually present with metabolic crisis and encephalopathy. Infants and children can present with vomiting, failure to gain weight, hepatic dysfunction, convulsions, and developmental delay.

TABLE 4: Age-appropriate requirement of lysine and tryptophan in glutaric acidemia type 1 (GA-1).

Age (months)	Protein (g/kg)	Lysine (mg/kg)	Tryptophan (mg/kg)
0–6	2.75–3.5	65–100	10–20
6–12	2.5–3.25	55–90	10–12

Management

Clinical management includes management of acute crises and chronic nutrition management.

In an acute crisis, the main goal is to reduce the ammonia to normal levels either by hemodialysis (preferred) or by peritoneal dialysis. Intravenous (IV) 10% dextrose infusion along with electrolytes should be started to provide sufficient calories and to prevent endogenous protein catabolism. Protein restriction should be for a maximum of 24 hours.

Nitrogen scavengers: These drugs allow the excretion of nitrogen via alternate pathways. The commonly used medications are sodium benzoate and sodium phenyl acetate. Both drugs can be used during the time of acute crisis and can be continued during the maintenance phase. They are available in both IV and oral forms. IV formulation is not readily available in our country.

Replacement of urea cycle intermediates: Arginine (contraindicated in arginase deficiency) and citrulline need to be replaced depending on the type of UCD. They are available as an oral preparation.

Enteral feeds should be started as soon as possible. Initially, these need to be protein-free and dietary protein should be gradually reintroduced depending on ammonia levels.

Dietary Management

The main principles in the dietary management of urea cycle defect are to restrict dietary protein intake, prevention of catabolism by the provision of sufficient energy, use of nitrogen scavenging drugs, and specific amino acid supplementation **(Fig. 1)**.

As in any IEM, the first step is to calculate the total protein intake and the amount of protein that needs to be supplemented as essential amino acids (synthetic protein). These essential amino acids are not produced by the body and need to be supplemented.

From 1 month to infancy, the total protein intake will range from 1.2 to 2.2 g/kg/day and the essential amino acid requirement is 0.6–1.1 g/kg/day. The guidelines recommended by the World Health Organization (WHO) can be safely used to calculate the protein and energy requirement **(Table 5)**.

The total protein requirement should be met as approximately 50% from essential amino acids and the other 50% from the

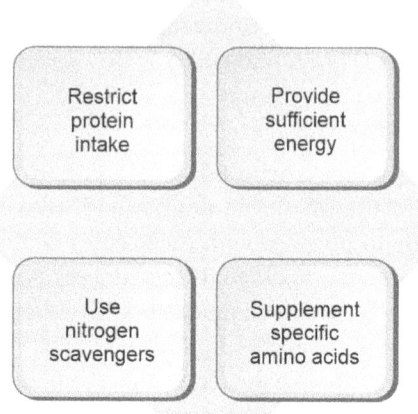

Fig. 1: Principles of dietary management.

TABLE 5: Protein and energy requirement till 1 year of age.

Age group (months)	Protein (g/kg/day)	Energy (kcal/kg)
1	1.77	80–81.2
2	1.50	
3	1.36	
4	1.24	
6	1.14	
12	1.14	82

Source: WHO Technical Report Series 2007.

whole protein. Few others recommend at least 30% of essential amino acids among the total protein requirement. Whatever the ratio, it is of paramount importance to supplement essential amino acids in the diet.

Once the protein requirement is calculated, the next step is to calculate the volume of breast milk that needs to be given for the calculated amount of whole protein.

After the calculation of protein requirement from breast milk and special formula, one has to make sure that adequate calories are being provided by the total volume. If not, then additional energy should be provided by a protein-free source, for example, medium-chain triglyceride (MCT) oil, commercial protein-free formulas. A metabolic specialist should be consulted to add additional citrulline or arginine. Serial monitoring of ammonia levels should be done for proper titration of protein intake.

Breastfeeding in Urea Cycle Disorders

Breastfeeding can be given in UCD, and many authors have described successful breastfeeding in these cases. The amount of protein and volume of breastfeeding given to a neonate vary during each feed and also during the day. The amount of protein given to a neonate can be limited by giving the prescribed amount of protein-free formula before breastfeeds followed by breastfeeding.[7,8]

FEEDING IN ORGANIC ACIDEMIAS

Organic acidemias are characterized by the disordered metabolism of propiogenic amino acids such as valine, isoleucine, threonine and methionine, and odd-chain fatty acids. The common disorders in this group are propionic acidemia and methylmalonic acidemia.

Principles of Feeding in Organic Acidemias

- Restrict offending amino acids (propiogenic amino acids and odd-chain fatty acids).
- Provide high-energy and moderate-protein diet.
- Provide sufficient energy to prevent catabolism.

The total protein intake should include both intact protein and special amino acid formula. The amount of protein required is based on the weight of the child, the severity of the disease, nutritional status, and the laboratory values of amino acids. In severe organic acidemias, nearly 50% of the protein requirement should be met by amino acid formula. These special amino acid formulae are devoid of the propiogenic amino acids and serve as an initial formula to be started after the metabolic crisis. This supplement should contain appropriate amounts of carbohydrates, fats, minerals, and vitamins. Breast milk is then gradually introduced depending on the severity of the condition. The WHO guidelines on protein intake provide a rough estimate of protein intake for these children **(Table 5)**.

Once the total protein intake is determined, at least 50% of the total protein need must be met by breast milk or standard infant formula (if breast milk is not available). This protein is called intact protein. Then calculate the amount of offending amino acids from this intact protein source (from breast milk). The approximate daily requirement of these amino acids is mentioned in **Table 6**.

The rest of the remaining protein requirement needs to be provided by special amino acid formulae. These special amino acid formulae are devoid of these precursor amino acids. Once the protein requirement is calculated from breast milk (intact protein) and

TABLE 6: Requirement of propiogenic amino acids in organic acidemias.[9]

Nutrient	Age	
	0–6 months	6 months to 1 year
Isoleucine (mg)	110–60	90–40
Methionine (mg)	50–20	40–15
Threonine (mg)	125–50	75–20
Valine (mg)	105–60	80–40
Protein (g)	2.5	2.5
Energy (kJ)	100–125% of RDA for age	

(RDA: recommended dietary allowance)

special formula, check if the required calories are met by the calculated amount. If not, then add protein-free medical food. These formulae contain only carbohydrates, fat, and micronutrients.

BREASTFEEDING IN METHYLMALONIC ACIDEMIA/ PROPIONIC ACIDEMIA (MMA/PA)

Breast milk and feeding can be given safely in nonclassical forms of the disease where the risk of metabolic crisis is very low. In these conditions, the advantage of breast milk is its low protein content, reduction in gut propionate, and protection from infections. Whatever the proportion of breast milk and special formula, the amount given should be titrated according to growth, metabolic tolerance, and severity of the condition.

FEEDING IN MAPLE SYRUP URINE DISEASE

Maple syrup urine disease (MSUD) is an IEM caused due to deficiency of enzyme *branched-chain keto acid dehydrogenase* that is involved in the metabolism of keto acids, namely leucine, isoleucine, and valine. The resulting enzyme deficiency results in the accumulation of these keto acids which result in various clinical manifestations such as lethargy, vomiting, irritability, weight loss, tone abnormalities, seizures, coma, and death. There are several variants of MSUD, and the presentation of each varies depending on the severity of the deficiency.

Most of these clinical manifestations are caused due to accumulation of leucine and 2-oxo-isocaproic acid.

Principles of Feeding

- Restriction of branched-chain amino acids, mainly leucine
- Supplementation of thiamine (in thiamine-responsive forms).

Acute Nutritional Management

The following steps need to be followed for acute reduction of branched-chain amino acids:

- *Special formula:* Start special formula which is devoid of branched-chain amino acids.
- *Promote anabolism:* By providing sufficient calories
- *Supplementation of valine and isoleucine:* This is done to prevent deficiency of these amino acids, and this will also ensure rapid reduction in the blood levels of leucine. The blood levels will not fall if valine and isoleucine are not supplemented.

Nutritional Management in a Stable Case of Maple Syrup Urine Disease

Once the metabolic crisis is over and the neonate is started on a special diet, subsequent adjustments in feeds are based on the blood concentrations of branched-chain amino acids. Based on blood levels of leucine, the initial goals are set. The amount of leucine that needs to be supplemented is also determined based on the clinical status

TABLE 7: Requirements of Branched-chain amino acids in maple syrup urine disease (MSUD).[3]

Dietary components	Acute period	Asymptomatic case
Energy	120–140	100–120
Protein	3–4	2–3.5
Leucine	0	40–100
Valine	80–120	30–95
Isoleucine	80–120	30–95

TABLE 8: Target blood levels of branched-chain amino acids in maple syrup urine disease (MSUD).[3,10,11]

	mg/dL	µmol/L	Normal values
Leucine	1.3–3.9	100–300	50–215
Valine	2.3–4.6	200–400	85–200
Isoleucine	1.3–3.9	100–300	25–90

of the individual. **Table 7** gives a rough guide of energy, protein, and branched-chain amino acids requirement in both acute and asymptomatic cases.

The amount of breast milk that provides the desired amount of leucine is calculated. The energy and protein in that volume of breast milk are also noted. The total protein requirement is also calculated. Now, the protein provided by breast milk is deducted from the total protein requirement. The remaining protein requirement is met by the branched-chain amino acid formula.

Valine and isoleucine content in the calculated amount of breast milk is noted and if there is any deficit in amount, then an additional amount is added as per the requirement of the baby.

Note: While calculating the diet for MSUD, only the leucine content is taken into account. This is because the valine and isoleucine content in the food is about half of the leucine content. If the diet is calculated only based on leucine, then the infant will not get any additional valine and isoleucine. Monitoring of these cases is done by maintaining the target blood levels as mentioned in **Table 8**.

Breastfeeding in Maple Syrup Urine Disease

There are very few reports which describe successful breastfeeding in milder forms of MSUD.[12] However, exclusive breastfeeding is not recommended as it can precipitate a metabolic crisis. Most of the time, it is a combination of breastfeeding with special amino acid formula, where these special formulae are given before breastfeeds.

FATTY ACID OXIDATION DEFECTS

Fatty acid oxidation defects are the group of disorders characterized by a defect in the metabolism of fatty acids. Fatty acids are used as fuel during periods of fasting, reduced calorie intake due to any reason, or in periods of increased calorie expenditure like sepsis. The main tissues which are affected are the brain, skeletal muscle, heart, and liver. These disorders can be due to defects in enzymes that metabolize long-chain, medium-chain, and short-chain fatty acids or due to defects in carnitine metabolism. Common clinical features include hypoglycemia, vomiting, seizures, encephalopathy, cardiac dysfunction, and sudden infant death. Symptomatology varies depending on the type of metabolic defect, age, and associated co-morbidities.[13,14]

Principles of Feeding in Fatty Acid Oxidation Defects

Dietary management depends on the type of FAO defect.

Long-chain Fatty Acid Oxidation Defect (LCFAOD)

- Restriction of long-chain fatty acid intake
- Supplementation of MCT, carbohydrate-rich food, and carnitine
- Avoidance of fasting.

Medium-chain Fatty Acid Oxidation Defect

- Restriction of medium-chain triglycerides
- Supplementation of carnitine (if low or during illness)
- Avoidance of fasting.

Neonates with fatty acid oxidation defects, especially LCFAOD, who present acutely, should be provided with a quick energy source, usually in the form of intravenous dextrose. Once stabilized, they can be started on feeds.

In any neonate diagnosed on new born screening or in any asymptomatic neonate who is accepting breast feeds well with no end-organ involvement [normal liver function test (LFT), electrocardiogram (ECG), and creatine phosphokinase (CPK)], no additional treatment is required and close monitoring for clinical signs should be considered. These neonates can be safely breastfed as per standard WHO recommendations.

In neonates and infants who have severe forms of LCFAOD, the total long-chain fatty acid intake should be 8–10% of the energy needs. MCT should also be supplemented to 10–30% of the total energy intake. The usual dose of MCT in infancy is 2–3 g/kg/day.

During the neonatal period and early infancy, this condition may not manifest, since the neonates are frequently fed during this period. Fasting up to 6–8 hours in early infancy and up to 12 hours at the end of the first year can be easily tolerated. Hence, breastfeeding can be continued as per schedule. After 6 months of age, in very severe cases uncooked corn starch (1 g/kg/day) may be introduced during night-time to provide a steady supply of glucose. These patients also require supplementation with docosahexaenoic acid (DHA) in a dose of 50 mg/day.

Neonates and infants with medium-chain acyl-CoA dehydrogenase deficiency (MCAD) can be breast fed and do not require any special diet. However, these patients should avoid medium-chain triglycerides.

GLYCOGEN STORAGE DISEASES

Glycogen storage diseases (GSD) are a group of disorders due to deficiencies of various enzymes involved in the glycogen pathway. They may present with various clinical manifestations, the most common of which is fasting hypoglycemia. The clinical features depend on the type of enzyme affected and the organ affected. One of the most common disorders which presents in the neonatal period and infancy is GSD type 1, also called Von Gierke disease.

Feeding in Glycogen Storage Disease Type 1[14,15]

This condition is due to a defect in the enzyme glucose-6-phosphatase which presents in hypoglycemia, especially during fasting. It can present during the neonatal period but more often presents at 3–4 months of age.

Principles of Management

- *What to avoid:* Galactose (and lactose), fructose (and sucrose), excessive fat
- *Supplement:* Carbohydrates (glucose, glucose polymers, uncooked cornstarch <2 years of age)

The neonates affected with this condition should be fed once in 2–3 hours to avoid hypoglycemia. The type of feed includes special formulae that do not contain sucrose, lactose, or fructose. Glucose or uncooked starch can also be given via nasogastric (NG) feeding.

A soy-based formula can also be used. Sometimes, this may not be tolerated and special formula needs to be used. The glucose requirements in these infants are between 8 and 10 mg/kg/min. Fasting hypoglycemia should be avoided by providing bolus feeds during night-time.

Cornstarch can be given at a dose of 1.6 g/kg every 4 hours for children <2 years of age which acts as a source of glucose that is released slowly. MCTs can also be supplemented in these neonates and infants to improve growth.

Breastfeeding

Breast milk contains lactose; hence, it should be used cautiously in this condition. Nevertheless, breastfeeding can be continued as long as the metabolic and clinical goals are met. Clinicians usually need to keep a higher target of laboratory parameters when breastfeeding is given.

KEY MESSAGES

- Feeding in IEM needs to be individualized based on the nature of the condition and metabolic defect.
- Breastfeeding can be continued in milder varieties of IEMs with adequate follow-up.
- Proper attention to growth and other nutritional deficiencies should be taken into account while managing these cases.

Educational Websites for Doctors and Dieticians

www.gmdi.org
www.imd-nutrition-management.com
www.metabolic.ie
www.nutricialearningcenter.com

REFERENCES

1. Kamboj M. Clinical approach to the diagnoses of inborn errors of metabolism. Pediatr Clin North Am. 2008;55(5):1113-2.
2. Kommalur A, Devadas S, Kariyappa M, Sabapathy S, Benakappa A, Gagandeep V, et al. Newborn screening for five conditions in a tertiary care government hospital in Bengaluru, South India: Three years experience. J Trop Pediatr. 2020;66(3):284-9.
3. Bernstein LE, Rohr F, Helm JR (Eds). Nutrition Management of Inherited Metabolic Diseases: Lessons from Metabolic University, 1st edition. New York: Springer; 2015.
4. Welling L, Bernstein LE, Berry GT, Burlina AB, Eyskens F, Gautschi M, et al. Galactosemia Network (GalNet). International clinical guideline for the management of classical galactosemia: diagnosis, treatment, and follow-up. J Inherit Metab Dis. 2017; 40(2):171-6.
5. Häberle J, Burlina A, Chakrapani A, Dixon M, Karall D, Lindner M, et al. Suggested guidelines for the diagnosis and management of urea cycle disorders: First revision. J Inherit Metab Dis. 2019;42(6):1192-130.
6. Häberle J, Boddaert N, Burlina A, Chakrapani A, Dixon M, Huemer M, et al. Suggested guidelines for the diagnosis and management of urea cycle disorders. Orphanet J Rare Dis. 2012;7:32.
7. MacDonald A, Depondt E, Evans S, Daly A, Hendriksz C, Chakrapani AA, et al. Breastfeeding in IMD. J Inherit Metab Dis. 2006;29(2-3):299-303.
8. Huner G, Baykal T, Demir F, Demirkol M. Breastfeeding experience in inborn errors of metabolism other than phenylketonuria. J Inherit Metab Dis. 2005;28(4):457-65.
9. Yannicelli S. Nutrition therapy of organic acidaemias with amino acid-based formulas: emphasis on methylmalonic and propionic acidaemia. J Inherit Metab Dis. 2006;29(2-3):281-7.
10. Frazier DM, Allgeier C, Homer C, Marriage BJ, Ogata B, Rohr F, et al. Nutrition management guideline for maple syrup urine disease: an

evidence- and consensus-based approach. Mol Genet Metab. 2014;112(3):210-7.

11. Morton DH, Strauss KA, Robinson DL, Puffenberger EG, Kelley RI. Diagnosis and treatment of maple syrup disease: a study of 36 patients. Pediatrics. 2002;109(6):999-1008.

12. Pichler K, Michel M, Zlamy M, Scholl-Buergi S, Ralser E, Jörg-Streller M, et al. Breast milk feeding in infants with inherited metabolic disorders other than phenylketonuria: a 10-year single-center experience. J Perinat Med. 2017;45(3):375-82.

13. Stanley C, Bennett M. Defects in metabolism of lipids. In: Kliegman R, St Geme J, Blum N, Shah S, Tasker R, Wilson K (Eds). Nelson Textbook of Pediatrics, 21st edition. Philadelphia: Elsevier; 2019. pp. 739-77 (Chapter 104).

14. Spiekerkoetter U, Lindner M, Santer R, Grotzke M, Baumgartner MR, Boehles H, et al. Treatment recommendations in long-chain fatty acid oxidation defects: consensus from a workshop. J Inherit Metab Dis. 2009;32(4):498-505.

15. Rake JP, Visser G, Labrune P, Leonard JV, Ullrich K, Smit GP. European Study on Glycogen Storage Disease Type I (ESGSD I). Guidelines for the management of glycogen storage disease type I - European Study on Glycogen Storage Disease Type I (ESGSD I). Eur J Pediatr. 2002;161(Suppl 1):S112-9.

CHAPTER 32

Breastfeeding during Emergency

G Guruprasad, Chaitali Raghoji, Durgappa H

"Breastfeeding is lifeline"

INTRODUCTION

Both calamity and disaster refer to events that cause damage, destruction, and loss. The most acceptable definition for natural calamities was given by the United Nations International Strategy for Disaster Reduction, also being recognized by the World Health Organization (WHO), is that "A sudden disruption of the functioning of a community or a society involving widespread human, material, economic, or environmental losses and impacts, which exceeds the ability of the affected community or society to cope using its own resources".

According to World Disaster Report 2016, on an average 600 natural or man-made disaster occur every year in the world. More than 1,420 million people were affected and more than 700,000 of people died worldwide from disaster. The vulnerability of India to disaster is higher as more than half of the land is prone to earthquakes; more than one-tenth of land is prone to floods and river erosions; more than three-fourths of the coastline is prone to cyclones or tsunami; and more than two-thirds of the agricultural land is prone to droughts. Natural disasters like floods, typhoons, tsunamis, and earthquakes displace millions of families and destroy a country's infrastructure and livelihood of survivors.

In these emergency situations, young children are more likely to become ill and die from malnutrition and diseases. Breastfeeding is the safest, often the best reliable choice for feeding infants and small children. Protecting, supporting, and promoting breastfeeding in disaster areas will help to ensure optimal nutrition to infant and young children.

Natural disasters are on rise worldwide often jeopardizing the human life. It is challenging to restore the life toward normalcy, especially in resource-limited countries.

Women and children are most vulnerable group during disasters. They often face difficulties in getting basic needs of life; safe shelters, food, and water. In addition, they also have insecure feeling, uncertainty of life, anxiety, fear, stress, poor access to health, and communication.[1]

They also find hurdles to breastfeed their babies due to lack of privacy, overcrowding, support, and assistance, often forcing them to start infant formula supplied at the disaster site by the donors. It is difficult to prepare safe formula during disaster, resulting in increased risk of contaminations and infections, which will have negative impacts on breastfeeding and health of babies. Hence, there is a need to put stringent rule in place during emergency to prohibit infant formula supply and encourage breastfeeding, which is safe, well-conditioned, clean, and available all time and needs no preparation.[1]

The disaster management committee should ensure all the basic needs of life, safety, and security to women and child. The healthcare professionals should specially be directed to pay an attention toward mother and baby on one-to-one basis and empower and enable the mothers to breastfeed their babies comfortably and safely by being supportive to them around the clock.[1]

PRESENTATIONS OF PAST SURVEY REPORTS

A survey from tsunami-affected villages in Pondicherry by Adhisivam B et al. found that according to 67% of mothers, breastfeeding was affected after Tsunami, and 4% felt that usage of milk powder has increased. 42% of women felt that breastfeeding once stopped cannot be restarted. In the post-tsunami period, it was found that almost 30% of mothers did not exclusively breastfeed for 6 months. Bottle-feeding incidence has increased. 58% of young children received bottle-feeding, and 51% of infants were fed with formula.[2]

In another study conducted at Chennai to know the awareness among public, volunteers and NGOs about IMS Act, bottles and infant foods showed that 88% of were unaware of the IMS act, 10% were partially aware and rest had some/full knowledge. In pre- and post-tsunami survey on breastfeeding, the incidence of breastfeeding was 72%, which was decreased to 52% after tsunami. Use of milk powder was around 16%, which increased to around 45% after tsunami period. The incidence of use of animal milk, cereals, and others usage also increased post-tsunami period. During emergencies, even in the previous healthy populations, the rates of infant mortality can increase up to 70 times higher than average. Child morbidity and crude mortality rates can increase by 20% in 2 weeks due to diarrhea and malnutrition. Lancet demonstrated that optimal breastfeeding and complementary feeding could reduce child mortality in children under 5 more than any other preventive measure by up to 26%.[2]

NATURAL DISASTERS AND ITS IMPACTS ON CHILD AND INFANT HEALTH

The following are the few health hazards:
- *Communicable disease:* Most commonly seen outbreaks are due to fecal contamination of food and water. Vector-borne disease transmission (dengue and malaria) increases, especially following floods and heavy rain. Zoonotic disease transmission is increased due to displacement of wild animals near human settlements.
- *Food and nutrition:* Disruption of food stock and public distribution system during a disaster are major cause of food shortage and hunger, leading to *malnutrition in children*. Child mortality rates can increase significantly.
- *Water and sanitation:* Damage to the water distribution and sewage disposal results in shortage of drinking water and problems of excreta or waste disposal, thus leading to spread of gastrointestinal infections (such as rotavirus diarrhea, *Salmonellosis, Escherichia coli*, and

typhoid) and blood-borne viruses (hepatitis A/C).
- *Mental health:* Problems were largely seen in industrialized or the urban areas of developing countries. Posttraumatic stress disorder (PTSD) is the most common manifestation.[1]

OPERATIONAL GUIDELINES ON INFANT AND YOUNG CHILD FEEDING IN EMERGENCIES (OG-IFE)

The world health assembly on infant and young child feeding (IYCF) requested all member states to develop tools for training, monitoring, advocacy, and preparedness for the implementation of OG-IFE.[3,4]

The three basic core principles of recommendations are:[1,5]

Principle 1: Exclusive Breastfeeding

Infants born into populations affected during disaster or an emergency, *the cleanest, safest food for an infant is human milk* and should exclusively breastfed till 6 months of age.

- Breast milk provides ideal nutrition for young infant, readily available without dependence on feeding supplies. It enhances the immune system, protects against diseases, especially diarrhea and respiratory infections, helps to maintain right temperature, and prevents from hypothermia in young infant. Hormone released during breastfeeding helps relieve maternal stress and anxiety in mothers.[1,5]

Barriers to Breastfeeding during a Disaster

- Lack of lactation support and psychological support, whether it is a new mother or a mother who has just weaned a baby.
- Being away from home—displaced having to being separated from family and other people who usually support the mother make the mothers emotionally weak and increase their stress levels **(Flowchart 1)**.

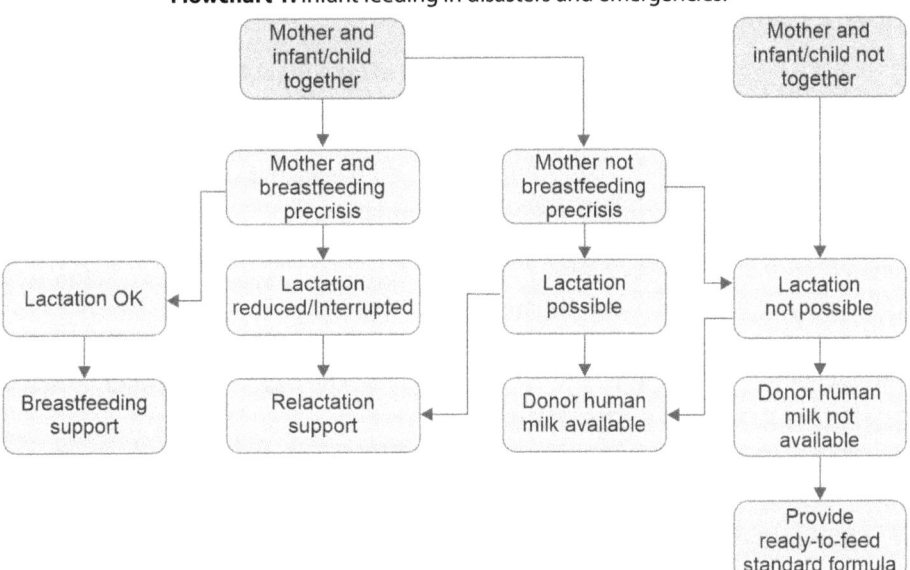

Flowchart 1: Infant feeding in disasters and emergencies.[6]

Principle 2: Breast-milk Substitutes

- The quantity, distribution, and use of breast-milk substitutes at the emergency site should be strictly restricted. In situation where mother's own milk is not available, the best option is donor human milk. While pasteurized donor milk from a regulated milk bank is preferred, it is often not available during disaster. If formula is given, recommend ready to feed standard formula.
- To those who have to be fed on breast-milk substitutes, nutritionally adequate breast-milk substitute should be made available and fed by cup or spoon only.
- The use of infant-feeding bottles and artificial teats during emergencies should be strictly discouraged.

Disadvantages of Formula use during Disaster or Calamities

It may not be available. It may become contaminated if prepared with unclean water or stored in nonsterilized containers. Errors in preparation may occur.[1,5]

Principle 3: Complementary Feeding

Children need hygienically prepared and easy to digest and eat foods. The traditional foods that caregivers would normally feed to older infants and young children may not be available during the time of emergencies and the foods that are available may be unfamiliar. Complementary food should be easy to chew, digest, safe, appealing to child and balanced.

MINIMUM RESOURCES REQUIRED FOR SAFE-FEEDING PRACTICES DURING DISASTERS

- Create safe havens for pregnant and breastfeeding mothers
- Fuel
- Clean water for washing utensils and preparing food
- Protect food from rodents, animals, and insects
- Time for frequent food preparation, feeding, and cleaning up
- Utensils for cooking and storing
- Containers for:
  - Transporting food and water to shelters
  - Storing water at shelters
  - Protecting storage of uncooked foods
  - Protecting storage of cooked food.[3]

INFANT AND YOUNG CHILD FEEDING-EMERGENCY (IYCF-E) TOOL KIT[4]

Save the children IYCF-E tool kits have been designed to promote best practice and rapid implementation of IYCF in emergencies. Tool kit aims to meet the needs of emergency nutrition program managers, coordinators, and advisors who are responsible for program design, implementation, and management of IYCF-E programs in emergency contexts.

The core tool kit contains a folder "Overview of IYCF-E Tool kit", each folder contains the following subfolders:

- Determine the need
- Program planning
- Caseload and supply needs
- Staff
- Orientation and training
- Proposal development, monitoring, and reporting
- Policy
- Coordination and communications.

FEEDING PRACTICES DURING PANDEMICS LIKE COVID-19

Currently world is going through coronavirus disease (COVID) pandemic wherein nearly

200 countries are affected and is expected to continue for another 18–24 months.

National Neonatology Forum (NNF India) along with Federation of Obstetric and Gynaecological Societies of India (FOGSI) and Indian Academy of Paediatrics (IAP) with WHO has provided following recommendations for IYCF when COVID-19 disease is suspected or confirmed in the mother.[7,8]

- Neonates born to mothers with suspected or confirmed COVID-19 infection, if both the neonate and mother are stable, rooming-in is practiced. Exclusive breastfeeding must be promoted. Mothers should practice respiratory hygiene and wear a triple layered mask while feeding.
- If the mother is sick and is unable to breastfeed the neonate her expressed breast milk should be given to the neonate with a clean cup and or spoon. Expression of breast milk has to be done after thorough handwashing and wearing a mask.
- Circumstances where mother is unable to breastfeed directly or either express her breast milk, the best option in this condition is to use donor human milk or formula feeds, provided appropriate precautions are taken to avoid promotion of breast-milk substitutes and use of feeding bottles by the health facility and the healthcare providers.
- Kangaroo Mother Care (KMC) should be practiced in stable low birth neonates who are eligible, irrespective of mothers COVID status.
- During disasters mothers should be provided breastfeeding counseling, basic psychosocial support, and feeding support to manage breastfeeding difficulties.
- Mothers who are breastfeeding should practice respiratory hygiene and follow respiratory etiquettes during feeding, and washing hands before touching the baby, and routinely cleaning and disinfecting surfaces should be followed.

Breastfeeding should be initiated within 1 hour of birth. Exclusive breastfeeding should continue for 6 months with timely introduction of adequate, safe, and properly fed complementary foods at age 6 months, while continuing breastfeeding up to 2 years of age or beyond.[9]

Breastfeeding Promotion Network of India (BPNI) suggests adaptation of the decision tree in this document by replacing "infant formula milk to the baby until the mother recovers" with "suitable breast-milk substitute including locally available, unmodified, boiled animal milk to the baby".[10]

TEN FEEDING PRINCIPLES OF WHO DURING DISASTERS[1]

1. The infants born into populations affected by emergencies should normally be exclusively breastfed from birth to 6 months of age.
2. The aim should be to create and sustain an environment that encourages frequent breastfeeding for children up to 2 years and beyond.
3. Quantity, distribution, and use of breast-milk substitutes or formula feeds during emergency situation should be strictly controlled.
4. To sustain growth, development, and health, infants from 6 months onward and older children need hygienically prepared and early to eat and digest foods.
5. Caregivers need secure uninterrupted access to appropriate ingredients with which to prepare and feed nutrient-dense foods to older infants and young children.

6. Because the number of caregivers is often reducing during emergencies as stress levels increase, promoting caregivers coping capacity is an essential part of fostering good feeding practices for infants and young children.
7. The health and vigor of infants and children should be protected, so that they are able to suckle frequently and maintain their appetite for complementary foods.
8. Nutritional status should be continually monitored for early identification of malnourished children, so that their condition can be assessed and treated, and prevented from deteriorating further.
9. To minimize an emergency's negative impact on feeding practices, interventions should begin immediately. The focus should be on supporting caregivers and channeling scarce resources to meet the nutritional needs of the infant and young children in their charge.
10. Promoting optimal feeding for infants and young children in emergencies requires a flexible approach based on continual careful monitoring.

KEY MESSAGES

- Natural calamities are on rise worldwide and often they are unpredictable.
- Mothers and babies are most vulnerable group during natural calamities; hence, they need to be cared optimally.
- Mother–baby friendly tents are essential to ensure breastfeeding practices.
- It is quiet crucial to ensure safety and security to the mother and baby throughout.
- All the healthcare professionals need to undergo disaster management training with special reference to women and child.
- Involving NGOs and community volunteers to take part in the disaster management may deload the work on healthcare professionals.
- It is always crucial to be prepared well in advance to handle the emergencies effectively.

REFERENCES

1. The World Health Organization. (2004). Guiding Principles for Feeding Infants and young children during emergencies. [online] Available from: https://www.who.int/publications/i/item/9241546069 [Last accessed November, 2023].
2. Adhisivam B, Srinivasan S, Soudarssanane MB, Deepak AS, Nirmal KA. Feeding of infants and young children in tsunami affected villages in Pondicherry. Indian Pediatr. 2006;43(8):724-7.
3. Infant Feeding in Emergency Core Group. (2017) Infant and young child feeding in emergencies. Operational guidance for emergency relief staff and programme managers developed by the IFE Core Group, version 3. [online] Available from: https://www.unhcr.org/media/infant-and-young-child-feeding-emergencies-operational-guidance-emergency-relief-staff-and [Last accessed November, 2023].
4. Save the Children, The TOPS Program, USAID. IYCF-E TOOL KIT: Rapid start up for emergency Nutrition Personnel; 2015.
5. UNICEF and World Health Organization. (2015). Breastfeeding. [online] Available from: https://www.who.int/health-topics/breastfeeding#tab=tab_2 [Last accessed November, 2019].
6. American Academy of Pediatrics. Infant Feeding During a Disaster. [online] Available from: https://www.acf.hhs.gov/ohsepr/factsheet/infant-feeding-during-disasters [Last accessed November, 2023].

7. Breastfeeding Promotion Network of India (BPNI). (2020). COVID 19 and breastfeeding update. [online] Available from: https://www.bpni.org/webinar-on-covid-19-and-breastfeeding-june-19-2020/ [Last accessed November, 2023].
8. National Neonatology Forum, India; Federation of Obstetric & Gynaecological Societies of India; Indian Academy of Pediatrics. (2021). Perinatal–Neonatal Management of COVID 19/Summary of Recommendations, version 3.0. [online] Available from: https://www.fogsi.org/wp-content/uploads/gcpr/perinatal-neonatal-management-of-covid-19.pdf [Last accessed November, 2023].
9. Ministry of Women and Child Development, Government of India. (2006). National guidelines on infant and young child feeding. [online] Available from: https://wcd.nic.in/sites/default/files/nationalguidelines.pdf [Last accessed November, 2023].
10. Infant feeding in emergency situations. A report from national convention of BPNI, 2005. [online] Available from: https://www.bpni.org/report/infant-feeding-emergency-situation.pdf [Last accessed November, 2023].

CHAPTER 33

Nursing Strike

Shashidhar A, Durgappa H, Anish B Samaga

"Nursing strike is physiological response of infants to say something is not right".

INTRODUCTION

A baby who has been breastfeeding well, suddenly refuses to nurse is called nursing strike.[1] The nursing strikes can be upsetting for the mother and baby. These are almost always temporary and will resolve within 2–4 days. The exact incidence is not known; however, in one study it was reported that about 24% of infants will have it at some point of time. These mothers commonly respond by weaning prematurely. The reasons for refusal of feed could be in the mother, baby, and mother-infant dyad as mentioned in the **Table 1**.[2]

This behavior of infant is often associated with the onset of menstrual cycle, dietary change, soap, perfumes, deodorant, breast engorgement, oversupply of milk, low milk supply, maternal stress, maternal separation, return to job, pregnancy, and oral contraceptives. It is also associated with stuffy nose, earache, teething, oral thrush, colic, distractions, and bottle-feeding. It is also important to differentiate it from weaning which usually occurs gradually in contrast to nursing strike. In most cases, it is due to minor reasons and rarely may signify underlying serious problem like sepsis.

MANAGEMENT[5-13]

- The most important principle is to remain calm and cool; maintain milk flow by regular expression of breast milk; and feed the baby with help of cup or spoon not with the bottle.

TABLE 1: Causes for nursing strike.[2,3,4]

Maternal factors	Infant factors	Common factors related to mother-infant dyad
• Acute stress	• Nasal obstruction	• Change in environment
• Change of smell	• Teething	• Use of pacifiers
• Change of diet	• Gastroesophageal reflex	• Maternal separation
• Menstrual cycle	• Oral thrush	• Return to work
• Change in nursing pattern	• Otitis media	• Low milk supply
• Application of cream for cracked nipple	• Infantile colic	
• Breast congestion	• Distractions	
• Pregnancy	• Bottle-feeding	
• Local infections of breast		

- Do not force the baby to feed at the breast during strike as it may worsen the condition.
- Identify and address the underlying reasons for refusal to breastfeed.
- Cuddle the baby and increase the closeness by maintaining skin-to-skin contact which might help in getting reattachment.
- Try to breastfeed the baby in relatively dark and isolated room.
- Try feeding when baby falls asleep or just after awakening when he/she will not be remembering the discomfort.
- Avoid distractions during nursing the baby like TV sound.
- You can take warm shower bath along with baby that might help your baby to breastfeed.
- You can play light music which may help in soothing the baby.
- Take care of all the triggers immediately that might have caused discomfort for the baby like recent change in the smell.
- Try feeding the baby in different positions that might help if the baby is having earache.
- Instill the saline nasal drops so that it runs along the lateral wall of the nose that will relieve the nasal congestion effectively.
- In case of oral thrush, topical antifungal like nystatin or miconazole mouth paint can be applied over the oral thrush thrice a day for 1 week.
- You can offer teethers to comfort the baby in case of itchy gums due to teething.
- If refusal is due to infantile colic, parental counseling and prescription of placebo is beneficial.

KEY MESSAGES

- Nursing strike is a physiological response that the baby is trying to say something is not right.
- Parental counseling about the transient problem is important.
- Identifying the underlying reasons and addressing them promptly is important.
- Most nursing strikes are temporary and resolve by 2-4 days.
- Patience is the key to success.

REFERENCES

1. Schanler RJ, Krebs NF, Mass SB. 2 ed. USA: American Academy of Pediatrics; 2013. Breastfeeding handbook for physicians.
2. Nayyeri F, Raji F, Haghnazarian E, Shariat M, Dalili H. Frequency of "nursing strike" among 6-month-old infants, at east Tehran health center and contributing factors. J Family Reprod Health. 2015;9(3):137-40.
3. Jalali F, Kamiab Z, Khademalhosseini M, Daeizadeh F, Bazmandegan G. Nursing strikes among infants and its affecting factors in Rafsanjan city. J Med Life. 2021;14(1):56-60.
4. Hill PD, Hanson KS, Mefford AL. Mothers of low birthweight infants: breastfeeding patterns and problems. J Hum Lact. 1994;10(3):169-76.
5. Wight NE. Management of common breastfeeding issues. Pediatr Clin North Am. 2001;48(2):321-44.
6. Grueger B; Canadian Paediatric Society; Community Paediatrics Committee. Weaning from the breast. Paediatr Child Health. 2013;18(4):210-1.
7. Lawrence RA, Lawrence RM. Breastfeeding: A Guide for the Medical Professional, 9th edition. Amsterdam, Netherlands: Elsevier; 2021.
8. Huggins K. Nursing Mother's Companion: The Breastfeeding Book Mothers Trust, from Pregnancy Through Weaning, 8th edition. Boston: Harvard Common Press; 2022.
9. Dewey KG. Nutrition, growth, and complementary feeding of the breastfed infant. Pediatr Clin North Am. 2001;48(1):87-104.
10. Mohrbacher N, Stock J. The Breastfeeding Answer Book. Schaumburg, IL: La Leche League International; 1997.
11. Mohrbacher N. Breastfeeding Answers Made Simple. Texas: Hale Publishing; 2010.
12. Mohrbacher N. Breastfeeding Answers: A Guide for Helping Families, 2nd edition. Texas: Hale Publishing; 2020.
13. Winchell K. Nursing strike: misunderstood feelings. J Hum Lact. 1992;8(4):217-9.

34. Relactation and Induced Lactation

Shobha C Banapurmath, CR Banapurmath

"Breastfeeding is a beautiful thing, one of the most beautiful things that exist in nature. Think about how a woman can literally feed her baby with her body! In my eyes, this is a certain form of beauty, of divinity! To know that my body can not only form and bring another human being into the world, but that I can actually feed babies with my own milk from my own breasts—that puts me in a state of awe each time I think about it. It is an honour to be a woman."
—C JoyBell C

INTRODUCTION

Maternal instincts to give birth to a child, and then on to nurture it with her own milk is what keeps our civilization alive. Mothers all over the world go through various challenges during breastfeeding phase. Health workers have to be trained to support and help mothers to initiate, establish lactation, and relactation.

The concept of relactation has traveled a long way. Forty years ago, the health trainer used to suggest to the trainees not to waste time on the futile exercise of relactation, but to focus and give guidance in other areas of infant feeding. It was considered a time-consuming exercise. With passing time, as we have learned more about how breastfeeding works, it is now realized that if the mother is adequately motivated and she has a helpful support group, she can be successful with her attempts at relactation.

The first few weeks of postpartum has been identified as a critical time for establishing lactation or for early termination breastfeeding.[1] Relactation is much time-consuming and needs intensive and continuing support. Hence, every effort must be made to support the mother from the very beginning of her confinement, during delivery and later on for breastfeeding. When the mother receives appropriate guidance regarding how to initiate, establish, and sustain breastfeeding, relactation should rarely be necessary.

DEFINITIONS ASSOCIATED WITH RELACTATION

- *Establishing lactation:* When the lactation gap is <15 days, the process is called as establishing lactation.[1]
- *Relactation*: When the lactation gap is >15 days, the process is called relactation.[2]
- *Partial relactation:* Partial lactation is termed when the top-up supplements can be reduced by more than half.[3]
- *Complete relactation:* Complete relactation is termed when no top milk is supplemented.[3]

PHYSIOLOGICAL BASIS OF LACTATION AND RELACTATION

Production of breast milk depends on secretion of milk by the mammary cells of secretory alveoli and removal of milk by the infant. Prolactin and oxytocin hormones play a major role. Prolactin response can be induced by satisfactory suckling of an infant and the response is greater during night. Removal of the milk from the breast requires action of oxytocin hormone which is released in response to suckling. Oxytocin causes small muscles to contract which surround the secretory alveoli and its secretion can be affected by the mother's psychological state, hence support and encouragement are important ways of enhancing oxytocin response. The infant suckling at the breast is the most effective method and best way to stimulate the nipple and to remove milk provided that the infant is well attached and suckles effectively at its mother's breast. The more frequently and for longer duration the infant suckles, the more milk is produced. To remove milk effectively, an infant needs to be well attached to the breast.[4,5] The part of the breast beneath the areola, where the milk collects in lactiferous sinuses, must be well inside the infant's mouth.

On the other hand, among babies who are bottle-fed, the way they remove milk from the bottle is entirely different from the way a baby would remove milk from the breast. A bottle-fed baby feeds with a closed mouth, whereas, a breastfed baby has to open its mouth widely to take a good amount of areola into its mouth and form a teat which traverses way into its mouth. The baby gently removes milk by peristaltic action of its tongue. In fact the tongue cups around the breast during effective milk removal by the baby. In a bottle-fed baby such action does not happen. Hence, bottle-fed babies find it confusing when mother tries to breastfeed, and this is referred to as nipple confusion. The most common cause for breast refusal is bottle-feeding. A similar situation also arises when babies get used to pacifiers.

SCOPE FOR RELACTATION IN CLINICAL PRACTICE

We come across multiple situations where scope for relactation exists. During newborn period many sick and preterm neonates are unable to effectively breastfeed. Sometimes, they are referred from other hospitals wherein baby-friendly practices may be suboptimal. Some parents wrongly start feeding top milk very early in newborn period or early infancy. Many mothers feel they have insufficient milk for their baby and start supplementing with spoon or may offer bottle-feeding. The infant develops nipple confusion which can result in breast refusal. Many babies may have latching problems and mothers land up with various breastfeeding problems.

Many young infants present with diarrhea, dysentery, and respiratory infections when supplementary feeds are given. This by far is the most common situation in clinical practice for sick babies to land up with pediatricians. We also come across mothers, when they visit with baby for routine immunization, who have stopped breastfeeding their babies for various reasons. Hence, in every situation of health contact with baby, it becomes important to assess the feeding history at all levels, be it a frontline worker, primary healthcare worker, counselor, or a pediatrician.

At the community level, the accredited social health activists (ASHA) workers, auxiliary nurse midwives (AWWs) or Anganwadi workers (ANMs) must be trained to evaluate the feeding history in their outreach programs and mothers must be provided the help as early as possible to overcome their breastfeeding difficulties. Home visits by well-trained breastfeeding counselors were found highly effective in extending the duration of exclusive breastfeeding.[6,7] In the very unfortunate circumstances where mother is experiencing illness or is not alive, the relatives such as aunts and grandmothers/caretaker could be encouraged for adoptive nursing. Sometimes lactating relative can breastfeed the young infant along with her nursing infant. During natural disasters when breastfeeding gets disrupted, a scope for relactation arises.

The "three pillars" which affect the success of relactation are:
1. Factors related to the infant
2. Factors related to mother
3. Role of support group.

Factors Related to the Infant

Relactation succeeds easily if an infant is willing to suckle at the breast, however, many infants need to be helped to take the breast as they would have difficulties attaching to the breast. Infants are more willing to take the breast when they are younger. Older infants tend to be less willing, especially if they have become used to feeding bottle. Therefore, it becomes necessary to stop using bottles and pacifiers to overcome an infant's unwillingness to suckle. However, even among the infants who have been used to nipple or artificial teats, such infants can learn to suckle at the breast if mothers are given skilled help. Sick or sedated infants will refuse to suckle as well as infants born with congenital anomalies, like cleft palate, micrognathia, would have difficulty with latching. Premature babies with low birth weight are at higher risk of lactation failure, especially when they are separated from mother or bottle-fed. With the advent of improved neonatal care interventions like kangaroo mother care (KMC), early enteral feeding of newborns with mother's own milk helps in establishing earlier lactation. If the desire to suckle is strong in the infant, even grandmothers have produced milk when they put the infant to soothe them in absence of their mothers. Such reports are published from India and Africa.[8,9]

Factors Related to Mother

Many mothers are unable to establish breastfeeding due to premature baby or illness in the mother or baby. Many mothers start feeding but are unable to feed after few days or months due to feeling of not enough milk and resort to supplementation through bottle or palada and as she shifts to top feeds, her breast milk decreases. This reduced secretion of breast milk is also observed in mothers who stop feeding due to breast conditions either due to separation of mother from the baby or mother had to return back to workplace. Many drugs and contraceptives hinder lactation. In some cases mothers are not willing to breastfeed or they find it very tiresome. Few of the Indian studies report that infants were already ill and admitted to hospital and when relactation was suggested, they were easily motivated.[10,11] While motivating, better compliance was noted as mothers were convinced about favorable effect of relactation on mother-child bonding.[12]

Role of Support Group

By far this is the most important pillar among the three. It is very essential for the mother to have ample physical, mental, and emotional support. A friendly, supportive, and relaxed atmosphere would calm her mind. It is also important that no negative remarks are made by anyone around her. Traditionally in Indian communities, the parturient mother is very strongly supported by her mother. Mothers with higher education and preoccupation with other works on their minds may find this simple task of breastfeeding as very difficult. For mothers attempting relactation, the entire mother's support group consisting of healthcare professionals, counselors, and all family members including her husband, have to be actively involved to support the mother in all possible ways. This aspect is the defining step in achieving success for the mother. In spite of many challenges, relactation would be successful if the mother is given adequate support.

Trained nurses and counselors have a large role to play. An excellent counseling skill along with active listening and ability to provide practical help to the mothers is crucial. If mothers are admitted in a lactation management unit (LMU),[10] they can share their success as well as obstacles faced with others. Telephonic suggestions can also help in this regard if the mother wants outpatient services.[12]

TECHNIQUES AND PROCEDURES ADOPTED IN RELACTATION

Mothers are taught to achieve proper attachment of the baby to their breast. This is the most important step in success of relactation. Health worker's help is needed, when the baby is awake and responsive. Some babies refuse to suckle at the breast; such babies are cajoled to suckle with the help of *drip and drop method*[13] **(Figs. 1A and B)**.

Drip and drop method is very simple. A helper, usually a relative of the mother, sits comfortably in front of the mother and pours milk, drop by drop, on upper part of breast and the drops of milk come to the baby's mouth. The baby is stimulated to suckle. The process is carried out for longer periods until the baby's hunger is satisfied. Providing adequate physical rest to the mother, motivation, counseling, and appreciation of mother's effort along with family support are crucial

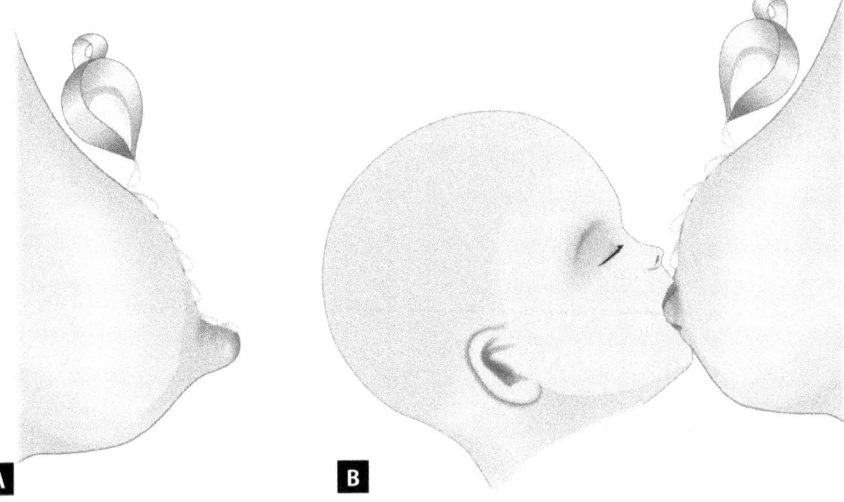

Figs. 1A and B: Drip and drop method. (A) Expressed breast milk is poured over the breast drop by drop using a spoon, allowing the milk to flow to the tip of the nipple; (B) Baby positioned with mouth wide open at the areola. Continue pouring and allow milk to drip into the baby's mouth. The baby learns to suck.

for the success of relactation. The advantage, however, is that the mother can soon learn to manage herself obviating the need for help from another person. **Figures 1A and B** shows the drip and drop method.

Lactaid or nursing supplementer is a commercially available container device as shown in **Fig. 2**, which is placed between the breasts of the mother. Milk is placed in the device. The infant receives milk through a flexible plastic tube connected to the container. The tip of the tube is held in place near the nipple by a small micropore adhesive plaster. As the infant suckles at the breast, he simultaneously draws the milk from the bag and at the same time, the breast receives suckling stimulation to enhance milk production. This method does not require another person to help the mother. The infant also does not get frustrated. However, nursing supplementers are expensive, not easily available and difficult to keep it clean.[12]

Relactation through Supplementary Suckling Technique

The supplementary suckling technique (SST) as shown in **Fig. 3** consists of cup of milk at one end, with a nasogastric feeding tube, through which the milk feed can pass along the nipple to the infant's mouth. The cup is placed not >10 cm below the level of the breast so that the milk does not flow too rapidly. One can adjust the flow of milk by elevating or depressing the level of the cup. When the infant sucks on the breast, along with the tip of the tube into its mouth, the milk from the cup gets sucked up through the tube by the baby. A caretaker initially can hold the cup until the mother herself can manage. In some cases, it may take 1–3 days' time for the baby and the mother to get used to the technique, however, gentle persuasion is needed. SST stimulates prolactin reflex which helps the breast to secrete more milk. The infant suckles and stimulates the breast at the same time the baby draws milk through the tube. The milk used for this technique may be either expressed mother's own milk or top milk.[14]

Kangaroo Mother Care

The KMC is where the mother is advised to hold the infant close to her, and sleep with the infant **(Fig. 4)**. Bedding-in is important in Indian scenario, as the maternal grandmother invariably takes up the responsibility of the

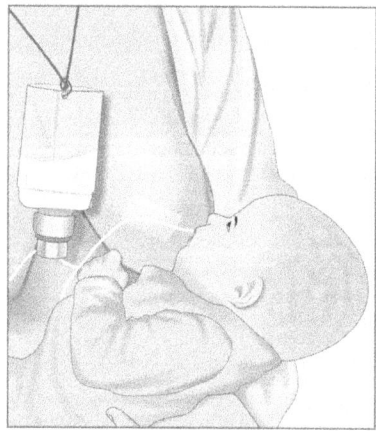

Fig. 2: Lactaid or nursing supplementer.

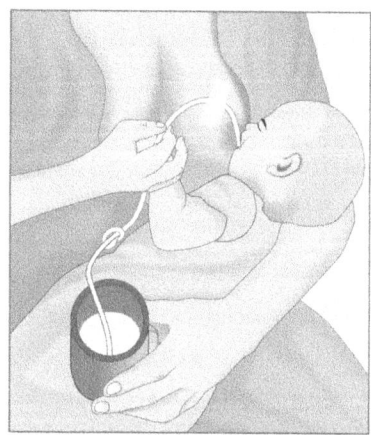

Fig. 3: Supplementary suckling technique (SST).

postpartum care. The maternal grandmother always wants her daughter to get good sleep and rest at night, hence she tries to keep the baby with her or a traditional swing "jhole"(hammock) is used to put the baby in it. This, however, should be avoided until lactation is well established. Skin-to-skin contact is part of the more extensive KMC and is useful for the wide range of breastfeeding problems, as it increases milk production. Many babies will spontaneously start breastfeeding with KMC. This intervention also helps the baby and mother because the baby enjoys the warmth and close proximity of its mother. The sense of smell also helps the baby for locating the nipple.[15]

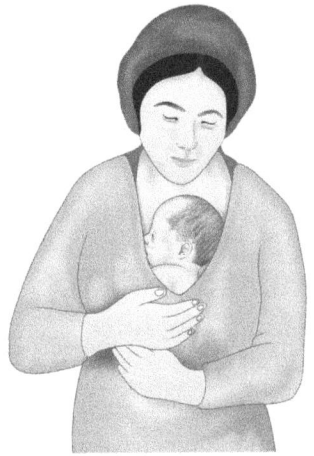

Fig. 4: Kangaroo mother care.

Hand Expression of Milk

Steps of How to Express Breast Milk by Hand (Fig. 5)

The mother should:
- Have a clean, dry, wide-necked container for the expressed breast milk
- Wash her hands thoroughly

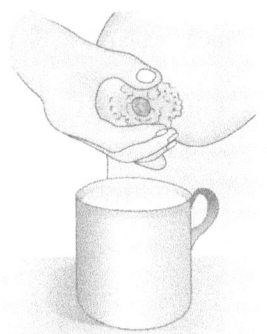
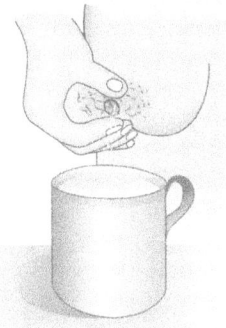
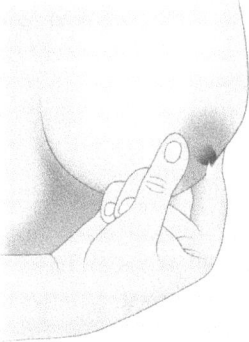

Fig. 5: Hand expression of milk.

- Sit or stand comfortably and hold the container under her nipple and areola
- Put her thumb on top of her breast and her first finger on the underside of her breast so that they are opposite each other about 4 cm from the tip of the nipple
- Compress and release her breast between her finger and thumb a few times. If milk does not appear, reposition her thumb and finger a little closer or further away from the nipple and compress and release a number of times as before.

This practice should not hurt, and if it is hurting, the technique is wrong.

At first, there may not be any milk secretion but after compressing a few times, milk starts to drip out. It may flow in streams if the oxytocin reflex is active. Mother is trained to compress and release all the way around her breast with her finger and thumb at the same distance from the nipple and express each breast until the milk drips slowly. Repeat expressing from each breast five to six times. Stop expressing when milk drips slowly from the start of compression, and does not flow.

Avoid rubbing or sliding her fingers along the skin.

Avoid squeezing or pinching the nipple itself.

Back Massage

Rubbing and massaging the upper back of the mother results in physical comfort and also stimulates release of oxytocin[16] **(Fig. 6)**. This can be repeated several times in the day. The traditional practice of hot water bath to lactating mothers also is associated with better secretion of oxytocin, since it acts in similar way of stimulating release of oxytocin.[16]

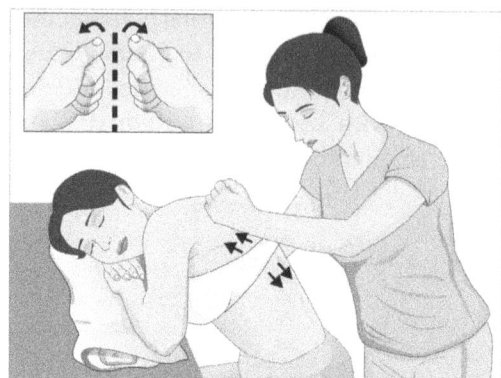

Fig. 6: Back massage to mother.

ACTUAL PROCESS AND PROGRESS TOWARD RELACTATION

Motivating the mother would be the first step of relactation. Mothers have to be shown the comfortable posture (seated or lying down) and techniques of how to get their baby "To attach" well onto the breast. While doing so, the mother first aims the baby's lower lip well below her inferior areola which is the defining step. If the attachment is not satisfactory, the mother is encouraged to let go and try again. After several attempts, once the baby learns to attach well to the breast, the next step would be to help the baby and mother to sustain the hold. For this to happen, "drop and drip" method is very useful to entice the baby to get a good attachment as well as to sustain the hold. In the initial stages, if the attachment is less satisfactory, mother is helped to procure good attachment by repeated attempts. If the baby is irritable, sleepy, or if the mother is exhausted, a break for a brief time will be a good alternative. Again the mother and the support team should try the process. This would go on for a day or two until a good attachment is procured by the baby and it suckles at the breast. The mother is encouraged to try several times till she becomes confident and relaxed. Within a few days, the baby is found suckling at the breast for longer periods of time. This is the time when the milk which is being dropped on the breast should be reduced in amount and also dropped infrequently. Care is taken not to allow the infant to get frustrated. When the milk supply is abruptly stopped, the infant becomes agitated and starts crying. If too much milk is poured, the baby becomes inactive or lazy. Hence, the person who drops the milk would do well to gauge the need of the baby and modulate the milk flow. Using this method, the interest of the baby at the breast can be sustained for longer periods. Effective suckling by the baby at the breast in turn will set the process of milk production by the breast. Initiation of relactation can be said to have been achieved when the infant is suckling at the breast spontaneously and milk can be expressed manually from the breast. Mothers may notice some changes in their breasts. They may feel that their breasts are feeling fuller and may leak some milk at times. Some mothers may feel tingling sensation at their nipples and squeezing sensation within their breasts. All mothers may not feel the fullness and tingling sensations despite being able to successfully nurse their infants. With passing time, infants will require less and less of supplemental top-up feeds as the mother's own milk supply steadily increases.

An exclusively breastfed growing baby will be passing clear colorless urine more than six times or more within 24 hours. This would indicate that the baby's fluid intake is adequate. Babies will be more active and interested in surroundings and sleep peacefully for longer periods. Gradually, the need for supplemental top-up feeds will go on decreasing. The stools also become much softer and semisolid, resembling that of the breastfed infant.

Among mothers who are relactating, it becomes essential to assess the growth and weight gain of the infant. Infant must be weighed periodically and it is better to weigh the infant on weekly basis. After the first 10 days of life among term born babies aged <6 months gain about 125 g of weight/week, or 500 g a month. Initially, the infant should be given full amounts of supplements, which could be 150 mL of full strength milk per kg/day. As the breast milk production increases, the supplements can be gradually reduced by about 15 mL/day. The other way for gradual reduction in the top-up supplements is: mothers are educated to observe urine output from 6 to 10 AM in the morning, and if the baby has passed dilute pale urine, once or twice in those 4 hours, she is advised to continue giving only breastfeeds for next 4 hours. By doing this, the mother gets motivated and also becomes confident with her own supply of breast milk. Similarly she must assess the infant's urine output for the whole day and vary the supplements of the top feeds accordingly. If the baby is not gaining weight at the end of a week, supplements should not be reduced. Sometimes, it is needed to even increase the supplements. There are several routines of giving supplements; a common pattern is to breastfeed early in the day or night and to give supplements later. Sometimes supplements have to be given for longer periods of time, depending on weight gain of the baby.

Studies on relactation vary according to the cultural practices of the area, region, or nation. In all settings, when mother is convinced about her own abilities, she is readily agreeable to continue her efforts. This is important for sustaining the ongoing breastfeeding.

For some nursing mothers, the mother-infant relationship is more important and milk production is less often a goal.[12] Mothers need to express positive feelings about nurturing the sick and preterm infants.[3] The most effective factor that increases and sustains breastfeeding is counseling and training the nursing mother for lactation.[17] In a study from Montana, participants reflected on the emotional aspects of the process. The common feelings expressed were rejection, anger, stress, and failure. However, not a single mother regretted her attempts. On the contrary, they felt stronger for having tried.[18]

Relactation was possible in most mothers in India as babies were admitted with life-threatening illnesses due to top feeding and bottle-feeding. After the babies recovered from serious illness, mothers expressed strong will to breastfeed.[2,10,11,19-21]

The role of galactogogues has been well researched in relactation. Motivation and training of the mothers has shown to increase the lactation performance, than giving metoclopramide or domperidone. Few of the studies[11,17] have conclusively shown that there is no statistical difference among the group receiving drugs enhancing prolactin like metoclopramide or domperidone.

RELACTATION AMONG MOTHERS OF OLDER INFANTS AND YOUNG CHILDREN

It is a common occurrence to come across mothers who have stopped breastfeeding their babies after having been feeding them successfully. The common reasons are illness in the mother or next pregnancy and abortion, feeling of not enough milk in the mother, or baby's refusal to breastfeed. If the lactation gap is less than a few weeks, an attempt at relactation will be easily successful.

Common presentation in such situations is that the infant is brought with diarrhea and dysentery. When enquired in depth, it leads to history of mother having recently stopped breastfeeding. Mothers when encouraged to reinitiate breastfeeding, they invariably have been able to relactate and on follow-up the babies have recovered satisfactorily.

INDUCED LACTATION

Induced lactation is the process of breastfeeding in a mother who has either never breastfed a baby or she had nursed years ago. Induced lactation is more challenging than relactation. It is important to have realistic expectations. Since nursing involves so much more than just transferring milk from breast to baby, it brings physical and emotional closeness. It is important to remember that prolactin and oxytocin, the hormones which govern lactation are pituitary and not ovarian hormones. They are produced in response to nipple stimulation. Many women have induced lactation with only mechanical stimulation. This consists of breast massage, nipple stimulation, and baby sucking at the breast. It is possible for some mothers to breastfeed without even having given birth to a baby. This is called as non-puerperal-induced lactation. There is documented evidence that such mothers have achieved exclusive breastfeeding.[22] There are many different factors that affect a women's ability to lactate like age of baby, previous breastfeeding experience, and willingness of the baby to take and suck at the breast.[4] Factors in the mother are also varied; her health, level of motivation, support from family, husband, and health professionals.[23]

For mothers who are planning adoptive nursing, it can be recommended to them to prepare for their baby's arrival, 6 months in advance; birth control pills containing estrogen and progesterone without the usual 1-week break at each month. This stimulates high levels of these hormones that are produced during pregnancy, and in turn they stimulate breast development. Two weeks before the baby's arrival, domperidone 10 mg three times a day has to be taken.[23] The dose is increased to 20 mg four times a day, later just 2 weeks before the birth of the baby and birth control pills are stopped. Domperidone is however continued.[24] Breast stimulation, nipple stimulation, and expression of breast milk manually or by pump must be continued. Initially milk output will be small but mothers must be encouraged to continue to do so. Once the baby is born, drop and drip method or nursing supplementer or SST must be used to entice the baby to attach well and to suckle at the breast to initiate lactation. Baby's growth must be monitored and depending on the mother's lactation and supplements must be reduced gradually. Care is being taken never to taper or stop top-up supplements suddenly, since there always will be a danger of hypoglycemia, hypernatremia, or failure to thrive. It is important to monitor the baby's weight gain, urine, and stool output. Domperidone is the drug of choice since it does not cross the blood–brain barrier and is much safer than other drugs.[25] European Medicines Agency (EMA) has issued guidelines in 2014 restricting the maximum dose and period for the use of domperidone,[26] as prolonged and larger doses of this drug has cardiac risk.[27] Mothers must receive adequate counseling which is done by active listening with respect and concern.[23] Mother's confidence levels must be raised but unrealistic expectations should be avoided. Technical information and success stories from other mothers must be shared. Mother-to-mother support groups who have induced lactation successfully must be formed.

INSHORT

Initiation of relactation and induced lactation are dependent on many factors like health status, financial and environmental status, working or nonworking mother, education of the mother, and more importantly her desire to breastfeed. Relactation is possible in most instances when the mother is adequately motivated and helped to get her baby well attached to her breast. Building the confidence of the mother and providing her good support along with follow-up help the mother to sustain her efforts. Most mothers are able to achieve exclusive breastfeeding as has been shown in several studies. Relactation is possible with good motivation and support to mothers. Studies have results showing that >85% mothers were able to relactate. Relactation is possible in outpatient practice as well. Relactation is simple, a no-cost technology, and can be taught easily to medical and paramedical workers.

Monitoring the feeding of newborns in neonatal intensive care unit (NICU), postnatal wards, and later in the community with the help of follow-up clinics, scouting to detect early breach in exclusive breastfeeding, and applying corrective measures instantly are crucial, since the younger the baby and the shorter the lactation gap, the easier it is to achieve relactation. Providing practical help and early intervention would also result in a strong and positive breastfeeding milieu for all breastfeeding mothers and obviate the need for relactation.

In older babies where mother has stopped breastfeeding, she can be easily motivated for relactation that prevents diarrhea, dysentery, and respiratory illnesses in their babies.

Induced lactation requires more intense efforts on the part of the mother, with her family support and the treating team.

Furthermore, there is a tremendous scope for induced lactation with the availability of newer modalities of treatment for women opting for surrogacy.

KEY MESSAGES

- Re-lactation is possible and satisfying to the mother, her family and the health care team.
- Motivating the mother and providing her with skilled help by an empathetic councilor is the cornerstone to help mothers to succeed with breastfeeding.
- Infants less than 2 months of age, babies having a lactation gap of less than a few weeks easily are able to latch well and succeed with improving breast milk transfer.
- Mothers experience emotional and psychological benefits with relactation.
- Induced lactation calls for more intense efforts from the mother, her family members and the treating team.

REFERENCES

1. Banapurmath S, Banapurmath CR, Kesaree N. Initiation of lactation and establishing relactation in outpatients. Indian Pediatr. 2003;40:343-7.
2. Banapurmath CR, Banapurmath SC, Kesaree N. Initiation of relactation. Indian Pediatr. 1993;31:1329-32.
3. Bose CL, D'Ercole AJ, Lester AG, Hunter RS, Barrett JR. Relactation by mothers of sick and premature infants. Pediatrics. 1981;67:565-9.
4. Woolridge MW. The 'anatomy' of infant suckling. Midwifery. 1986;2:164-71.
5. Woolridge MW. Aetiology of sore nipples. Midwifery. 1986;2:172-6.
6. Haider R, Ashworth A, Kabir I, Huttly SR. Effect of community-based peer counsellors on exclusive breastfeeding practices in Dhaka, Bangladesh: a randomised control trial [see comments]. Lancet. 2000;356:1643-7.
7. Lutter CK, Perez-Escamilla R, Segall A, Sanghvi T, Teruya K, Wickharn C. The effectiveness of a hospital-based program to promote exclusive breastfeeding among low-income women in Brazil. Am J Public Health. 1997;87:659-63.
8. Slome C. Nonpuerperal lactation in grandmothers. J Pediatr. 1956;9:550-2.
9. Banapurmath CR, Banapurmath S, Kesaree N. Successful induced non-puerperal lactation in surrogate mothers. Indian J Pediatr. 1993;60:639-43.
10. De NC, Pandit B, Mishra SK, Pappu K, Chaudhuri SK. Initiating the process of relactation: an Institute based study. Indian Pediatr. 2002;39:173-8.
11. Seema P, Patwari A K, Satyanarayana L. Relactation: an effective intervention to promote exclusive breastfeeding. J Trop Pediatr. 1997;43:213-6.
12. Auerbach KG, Avery JL. Relactation: a study of 366 cases. Pediatrics. 1980;65:233-5.
13. Kesaree N. Drop and drip method. Indian Pediatr. 1993;30:277-8.
14. Ministry of Health and Family Welfare. Supplementary suckling technique. Participant Manual: Facility Based Care of Severe Acute Malnutrition. Section 8.3. New Delhi: National Rural Health Mission, Ministry of Health and Family Welfare; 2011.
15. Hurst NM, Valentine CJ, Renfro L, Burns P, Ferlic L. Skin-to-skin holding in the neonatal intensive care unit influences maternal milk volume. J Perinatol. 1997;17:213-7.
16. Infant and Young Child Feeding. Model Chapter for Textbooks for Medical Students and Allied Health Professionals. Geneva: World Health Organization; 2009. pp. 32-5.
17. Sakha K, Behbahan AG. Training for perfect breastfeeding or metoclopramide: Which one can promote lactation in nursing mothers? Breastfeed Med. 2008;3:120-3.
18. Lommen A, Brown B, Hollist D. Experiential perceptions of relactation: A phenomeno-logical study. J Hum Lact. 2015;31:498-503.
19. Lakhkar BB, Shenoy VD, Bhaskaranand N. Relactation—Manipal experience. Indian Pediatr. 1999;36:700-3.

20. Mehta A, Rathi AK, Kushwaha KP, Singh A. Relactation in lactation failure and low milk supply. Sudan J Pediatr. 2018;18:39-47.
21. Tomar RS. Initiation of relactation: an Army hospital based study of 381 cases. Int J Contemp Pediatrics. 2016;3:635-8.
22. Szucs KA, Axline SE, Rosenman MB. Induced lactation and exclusive breast milk feeding of adopted premature twins. J Hum Lact. 2010;26:309-13.
23. Hormann E, Savage F. (1998). Relactation: Review of Experience and Recommendations for Practise. [online] Available from: https://www.ennonline.net/attachments/334/who-chs-cah-98-14-relactation-document.pdf [Last accessed November, 2023].
24. Kaufmann M. (2017). Relactation and induced lactation. [online] Available from: https://www.nct.org.uk/sites/default/files/related_documents/Kaufmann%20M%20Relactation%20and%20induced%20lactation.pdf [Last accessed November, 2023].
25. National Infant Feeding Network. The Use of Domperidone in Inadequate Lactation. 2014.
26. European Medicines agency. (2014). Domperidone-containing medicines. [online] Available from: https://www.ema.europa.eu/en/medicines/human/referrals/domperidone-containing-medicines [Last accessed November, 2023].
27. Newman J. Interpretation of Health Canada warning on domperidone. 2015.

SECTION 5

Promotion of Infant and Young Child Feeding Practices

35. **Global Networking and Promotion of Breastfeeding**
    Anita Nyamagoudar, Venkatasheshan, Mallesh Gowda, Bharathi Balachander

36. **Mothers Support Group and Breastfeeding**
    NS Mahanthashetti, Durgappa H, Roopa Bellad

37. **Infant Milk Substitute Act**
    Dhyanesh DK, Asha Doddamane Benakappa, Hari Dattatreya M

38. **Human Milk Banking**
    Adhisivam B, Roopa Bellad, Durgappa H

39. **Policy Making at the National Level for the Promotion of Breastfeeding**
    Shivananda R, Durgappa H

40. **Role of Research in Lactation: Present and Future**
    Sneha J Andrade, Jayashree Purkayastha, Leslie Lewis, Maria Pais

41. **Counseling in Breastfeeding**
    Anita Nyamagoudar, Udaykumar B, Durgappa H

CHAPTER 35

Global Networking and Promotion of Breastfeeding

Anita Nyamagoudar, Venkatasheshan, Mallesh Gowda, Bharathi Balachander

> "Mothers and babies form an inseparable biological and social unit; the health and nutrition of one group cannot be divorced from the health and nutrition of the other"
> —**World Health Organization**

INTRODUCTION

Although breastfeeding is a natural phenomenon, many mothers face challenges in exclusively feeding their babies. With professional help, mothers can successfully practice exclusive breastfeeding. To ensure professional help to mothers, many national and international initiatives have been taken up by governments and nongovernmental organizations (NGOs) across the world.

Initiation of breastfeeding within the first hour of life, exclusive breastfeeding till 6 months of age, and continued breastfeeding till 2 years of age along with complementary feeding are the three hallmarks of appropriate feeding practices. To ensure that every mother can sustain good feeding practices, many programs have been launched by various authorities across the globe and this chapter discusses the same.

MAGNITUDE OF THE PROBLEM

Worldwide, only 44% of infants are receiving breastfeeding within the first hour of birth. About 40% of infants are exclusively breastfed till 6 months of age.[1] Neonatal mortality rates were 33% higher among babies who initiated breastfeeding at 2–23 hours after birth, and >50% higher when initiated after day 1 as compared to babies who were breastfed within the first hour after birth.[2]

BABY-FRIENDLY HOSPITAL INITIATIVE

Introduction

In the year 1989, a joint statement was given by World Health Organization (WHO) and the United Nations Children's Fund (UNICEF). The statement listed Ten Steps to Successful Breastfeeding. These ten steps became part of the Baby-friendly Hospital Initiative (BFHI) which was published in the year 1991. BFHI is a global effort for protecting, promoting, and supporting breastfeeding across maternity and newborn service units.[3]

It is appealing to the public when a hospital is designated as "baby-friendly". However, data in 2017 showed that as little as 10% of the infants were born in facilities designated as "baby-friendly" then.[4]

The revision to the original version of BFHI was published in the year 2018. The topic of each of the ten steps is unchanged, but the wording of each one has been updated as per the evidence-based guidelines and global public health policy.[5]

The ten steps are subdivided into (**Box 1**):
- *Critical management procedures:* These are institutional procedures necessary to ensure that care is delivered consistently and ethically.
- *Key clinical practices:* These are standards for the individual care of mothers and infants.

Rationale for Each Step

Step 1: Facility Policies

Step 1a: Comply fully with the *International Code of Marketing of Breast-milk Substitutes* and relevant World Health Assembly resolutions.[6-8]

Rationale: Expectant mothers are influenced by attractive marketing strategies of infant milk substitutes. Healthcare workers may also be commercially influenced by infant milk substitutes affecting their professional activities and judgment.

Step 1b: Have a written infant feeding policy that is routinely communicated to staff and parents.

Rationale: It is a fact that policy drives practice. A written policy guarantees appropriate care to mother–infant pairs and also makes the staff accountable. It also helps to sustain the practices over time.

Step 1c: Establish ongoing monitoring and data management systems.

Rationale: Facilities need to record all the clinical practices related to breastfeeding inappropriate data management systems.

BOX 1: Ten Steps to Successful Breastfeeding (revised 2018).

Critical management procedures:
1. Firstly:
   a. Comply fully with the International Code of Marketing of Breast-milk Substitutes and relevant World Health Assembly resolutions
   b. Have a written infant feeding policy that is routinely communicated to staff and parents
   c. Establish ongoing monitoring and data management systems
2. Ensure that staff have sufficient knowledge, competence, and skills to support breastfeeding

Key clinical practices:
3. Discuss the importance and management of breastfeeding with pregnant women and their families
4. Facilitate immediate and uninterrupted skin-to-skin contact and support mothers to initiate breastfeeding as soon as possible after birth
5. Support mothers to initiate and maintain breastfeeding and manage common difficulties
6. Do not provide breastfed newborns any food or fluids other than breast milk, unless medically indicated
7. Enable mothers and their infants to remain together and to practice rooming-in 24 hours a day
8. Support mothers to recognize and respond to their infants' cues for feeding
9. Counsel mothers on the use and risks of feeding bottles, teats, and pacifiers
10. Coordinate discharge so that parents and their infants have timely access to ongoing support and care

Early initiation of breastfeeding and exclusive breastfeeding up to 6 months are considered *sentinel indicators*.

Step 2: Staff Competency

Ensure that staff members have sufficient knowledge, competence, and skills to support breastfeeding.

Rationale: A knowledgeable, skillful, and competent staff member can give timely help to the breastfeeding mother.

Step 3: Antenatal Information

Discuss the importance and management of breastfeeding with pregnant women and their families.

Rationale: A review of 18 qualitative studies[9] showed that not enough is discussed about breastfeeding during the antenatal period.

Step 4: Immediate Postnatal Care

Facilitate immediate and uninterrupted skin-to-skin contact and support mothers to initiate breastfeeding as soon as possible after birth.

Rationale: Immediate skin-to-skin contact propagates the rooting reflex, helps develop a healthy microbiome, and prevents hypothermia. Apart from increasing breast milk production, early initiation of breastfeeding has also been shown to prevent infant deaths.[10]

Step 5: Support with Breastfeeding

Support mothers to initiate and maintain breastfeeding and manage common difficulties.

Rationale: Both the new and experienced mothers face challenges while breastfeeding which are effectively reduced by appropriate postnatal counseling and by providing practical help.

Step 6: Supplementation

Do not provide breastfed newborns any food or fluids other than breast milk, unless medically indicated.

Rationale: Administration of any fluid or food to the newborn has harmful consequences like the risk of infection, lactation failure, cessation of breastfeeding within 6 weeks of life,[11] and altered intestinal microflora.[12]

Step 7: Rooming-in

Enable mothers and their infants to remain together and to practice rooming-in 24 hours a day.

Rationale: Rooming-in means that mother and baby stay together day and night. Rooming-in helps mothers to identify feeding cues in the baby and practice responsive feeding.

Step 8: Responsive Feeding

Support mothers to recognize and respond to their infants' cues for feeding.

Rationale: As part of a growing bond between the mother and the baby, the mother should be able to identify the baby's hunger and feeding cues, and the ready-to-feed state of the baby. It is also called demand feeding or baby-led feeding and does not restrict the duration or frequency of feeding. Time-based feeding is not recommended. Baby should be given as much and as many times a feed as it wants. Crying is a late cue and the baby will not position and attach well during periods of irritability and distress.

Step 9: Feeding Bottles, Teats, and Pacifiers

Counsel mothers on the use and risks of feeding bottles, teats, and pacifiers.

Rationale: Proper guidance is needed for the use or avoidance of feeding bottles, teats, or pacifiers. A word of caution has to be exercised about their use as there are concerns with hygiene, oral formation, and identification of feeding cues. Mothers need to be explained that the physiology of sucking from the breast is different from the physiology of sucking from any of the abovementioned materials.[13]

Step 10: Care at Discharge

Coordinate discharge so that parents and their infants have timely access to ongoing support and care.

Rationale: Since the postnatal period is dynamic for the mother as well as the baby, it is important to advise the mother regarding the likely challenges she may face after discharge and how best she can find solutions. It may be related to circumstances, for example, varying milk production, infant growth, colic, the mother's return to work, etc. Additional support must be ensured for the mother by referring her to a variety of resources that are available in the community. Active follow-up care by a healthcare worker along with print media and/or online information can help as point of contact in case of need.

Additional Practical Information about Baby-friendly Hospital Initiative[14,15]

- The Ten Steps to Successful Breastfeeding is also applicable to *preterm and sick babies* but needs to be adapted and individualized as per the baby's condition.
- There are *implementation guidelines* for each step of BFHI described by WHO.
- There are *global standards* for each step of BFHI. At last 80% of healthcare workers and mothers should be able to practice the guidelines appropriately.
- Maternity and newborn service units can apply through proper channels for recognition as a "baby-friendly" hospital.
- Step 4 includes "skin-to-skin contact" and uses the terms "immediate" and "as soon as possible". Skin-to-skin contact means placing the baby on the mother's chest or abdomen with no clothing separating them. The words "as soon as possible" suggest that an occasional delay may be permitted to assess for any critical medical issues in the mother and the baby. The global standards describe "up to 5 minutes" for skin-to-skin contact and "within 1 hour" for initiation of breastfeeding.
- Step 7 describes rooming-in. As per global standards, the mother and the baby should not be separated for >60 minutes per 24-hour period.
- BFHI implementation is voluntary at present for healthcare facilities. However, scaling up the program as mandatory coverage is the way forward for national implementation of the program.
- BFHI guidance says that the global standards for each step should exceed 80%. This may not be a realistic goal for many countries. Hence, such countries can have a multiyear action plan to achieve percentages >80%.

MOTHERS' ABSOLUTE AFFECTION[16]

"Mothers' Absolute Affection (MAA) Ek Sankalp" was launched in 2016 under National Health Mission (NHM) for the promotion of breastfeeding.

Goal: It was initiated to revitalize efforts toward promotion, protection, and support of breastfeeding practices through the health system to achieve higher breastfeeding rates.

Components of the Program

- *Awareness generation:* Building an enabling environment and demand generation through mass media (TV and radio) and mid-media (song, drama, theatre, folk, puppet shows, video vans, fairs, and exhibitions).
- *Community-level interventions:* Capacity building of community health workers—accredited social health activists (ASHAs),

Anganwadi workers (AWWs), and auxiliary nurse midwives (ANMs)—on breastfeeding and community dialogue by ASHAs through mothers' meetings; lactation support and interpersonal communication by skilled ANMs at subcenters.
- *Health facility strengthening:* Capacity building of ANMs/nurses, doctors on lactation support, and management at facilities and role of reinforcement on breastfeeding at all delivery points
- *Monitoring:* Monitoring and awards/recognition.

BREASTFEEDING PROMOTION NETWORK OF INDIA[17]

On December 3, 1991, the Breastfeeding Promotion Network of India (BPNI) was founded in Wardha, Maharashtra.

The BPNI has launched the "Stanpan Suraksha" app, the first of its kind app, for supporting and promoting breastfeeding and reporting infant milk substitutes. Any person can photograph inappropriate infant food promotion and send it to BPNI. The database has been created citywise and information are available regarding trained breastfeeding counselors. Mothers can enroll themselves as breastfeeding counselors through this app **(Fig. 1)**.

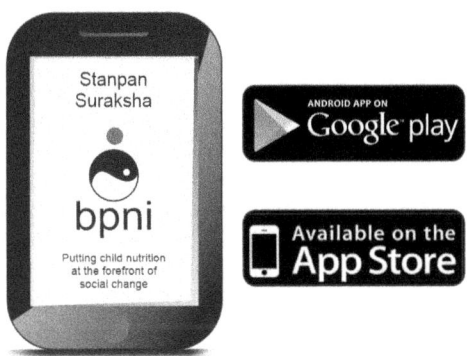

Fig. 1: Stanpan Suraksha app.

INTERNATIONAL BABY FOOD ACTION NETWORK[18]

International Baby Food Action Network (IBFAN) was founded in the year 1978 consisting of 273 public interest groups in 168 countries. IBFAN monitors compliance with the International Code of Breast-Milk Substitutes.

The BPNI AND IBFAN South Asia jointly worked for World Breastfeeding Trends Initiative (WBTi) to assess the progress of implementation of *global standards for infant and young child feeding* at a national level.

WORLD ALLIANCE FOR BREASTFEEDING ACTION[19]

Global networking for breastfeeding promotion was launched in 1991 based on the Innocenti Declaration for the promotion, protection, and support of breastfeeding. World Alliance for Breastfeeding Action (WABA) works to integrate breastfeeding with each of the Sustainable Development Goals (SDGs).

The WABA offers breastfeeding advocacy and practice course and technical support to access the knowledge and expertise of experts within the field. WABA supports and promotes activities like the celebration of World Breastfeeding Week (August 1–7 every year), the promotion of a warm chain for breastfeeding, and the "Empowering Parents" campaign.

GLOBAL BREASTFEEDING COLLECTIVE[20]

Initiated by WHO and UNICEF, Global Breastfeeding Collective brings together people responsible for implementation and donors from government, philanthropists, international organizations, and civil society.

Global Breastfeeding Collective calls for:
- Raising funds for breastfeeding promotional activities
- Enforcement of strong legal measures against infant milk substitutes
- To enable working mothers by paid family leave and workplace breastfeeding measures
- Implementation of Ten Steps to Successful Breastfeeding
- Improve access to skilled breastfeeding counseling
- Strengthen links between health facilities and communities
- Strengthen monitoring systems of breastfeeding promotional projects and policies.

QUALITY IMPROVEMENT INITIATIVE

Overall, quality improvement initiatives are required for the effective implementation and sustaining of breastfeeding promotional activities. Each step of BFHI can be implemented effectively by applying quality improvement initiatives.

The core methodology of quality improvement initiative is PDSA (Plan, Do, Study, Act) cycle **(Fig. 2)**.

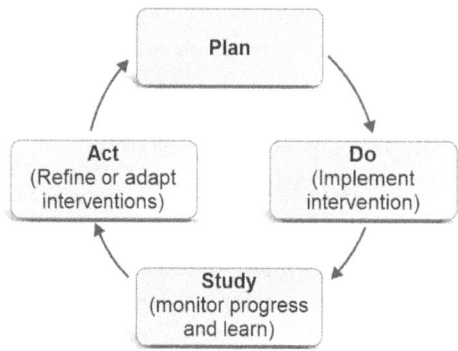

Fig. 2: PDSA (Plan, Do, Study, Act) cycle of quality improvement initiative.

KEY MESSAGES

- Breastfeeding promotional activities are vital for neonatal and infant survival.
- The goal is to protect, promote, and support appropriate breastfeeding practices.
- Ten Steps to Successful Breastfeeding are a vital part of the BFHI (revised in 2018).
- There is a rationale for the implementation of each step of BFHI and global standards have been set to achieve at least 80% of the expected standards.
- At the national level, MAA and Stanpan Suraksha app are efforts at community outreach for support of breastfeeding.
- Quality improvement initiatives are essential for the integration of feeding policies into clinical practice.

REFERENCES

1. United Nations Children's Fund. (2023). UNICEF data: Monitoring the situation of children and women. Infant and young child feeding. [online] Available from: [http://data.unicef.org/topic/nutrition/infant-and-young-child-feeding/ [Last accessed November, 2023].
2. Smith ER, Hurt L, Chowdhury R, Sinha B, Fawzi W, Edmond KM, et al. Delayed breastfeeding initiation and infant survival: a systematic review and meta-analysis. PLoS One. 2017;12(7):e0180722.
3. World Health Organization. (1989). Protecting, promoting and supporting breast-feeding: The special role of maternity services. A joint WHO/UNICEF statement. [online] Available from: http://apps.who.int/iris/bitstream/10665/39679/1/9241561300.pdf [Last accessed November, 2023].
4. World Health Organization. (2017). National Implementation of the Baby-friendly Hospital Initiative. [online] Available from: http://apps.who.int/iris/bitstream/10665/255197/1/9789241512381-eng.pdf?ua=1 [Last accessed November, 2023].
5. World Health Organization. (2017). Guideline: protecting, promoting, and supporting

breastfeeding in facilities providing maternity and newborn services. [online] Available from: https://iris.who.int/bitstream/handle/10665/259386/9789241550086-eng.pdf?sequence=1 [Last accessed November, 2023].
6. World Health Organization. (1981). International Code of Marketing of Breast-milk Substitutes. [online] Available from: https://iris.who.int/bitstream/handle/10665/40382/9241541601.pdf?sequence=1 [Last accessed November, 2023].
7. World Health Organization. (2017). The International Code of Marketing of Breast-Milk Substitutes. Frequently Asked Questions—2017 update. [online] Available from: https://iris.who.int/bitstream/handle/10665/254911/WHO-NMH-NHD-17.1-eng.pdf?sequence=1 [Last accessed November, 2023]. Geneva: World Health Organization; 2017.
8. World Health Organization. Code and Subsequent Resolutions. [online] Available from: https://www.who.int/teams/nutrition-and-food-safety/food-and-nutrition-actions-in-health-systems/code-and-subsequent-resolutions [Last accessed November, 2023].
9. Pérez-Escamilla R, Martinez JL, Segura-Pérez S. Impact of the Baby-friendly Hospital Initiative on breastfeeding and child health outcomes: a systematic review. Matern Child Nutr. 2016;12(3):402-17.
10. NEOVITA Study Group. Timing of initiation, patterns of breastfeeding, and infant survival: prospective analysis of pooled data from three randomised trials. Lancet Glob Health. 2016;4(4):e266-75.
11. DiGirolamo AM, Grummer-Strawn LM, Fein SB. Effect of maternity-care practices on breastfeeding. Pediatrics. 2008;122(Suppl 2):S43-9.
12. Guaraldi F, Salvatori G. Effect of breast and formula feeding on gut microbiota shaping in newborns. Front Cell Infect Microbiol. 2012;2:94.
13. Bu'Lock F, Woolridge MW, Baum JD. Development of co-ordination of sucking, swallowing and breathing: ultrasound study of term and preterm infants. Dev Med Child Neurol. 1990;32:669-78.
14. World Health Organization. (2018). Implementation guidance: Protecting, promoting and supporting breastfeeding in facilities providing maternity and newborn services: the Revised Baby-friendly Hospital Initiative. [online] Available from: https://www.unicef.org/media/95191/file/Baby-friendly-hospital-initiative-implementation-guidance-2018.pdf [Last accessed November, 2023].
15. World Health Organization, United Nations Children's Fund. (2020). Protecting, promoting and supporting breastfeeding in facilities providing maternity and newborn services: the revised Baby-friendly Hospital Initiative 2018 implementation guidance. Frequently asked questions. [online] Available from: https://iris.who.int/bitstream/handle/10665/330824/9789240001459-eng.pdf?sequence=1&isAllowed=y [Last accessed November, 2023].
16. Ministry of Health and Family Welfare, Government of India. (2016). MAA (Mothers' Absolute Affection). Program for Promotion of Breastfeeding. Operational guidelines, 2016. [online] Available from: https://nhm.gov.in/MAA/Operational_Guidelines.pdf [Last accessed November, 2023].
17. Breastfeeding Promotion Network of India. [online] Available from www.bpni.org [Last accessed November, 2023].
18. International Baby Food Action Network. [online] Available from www.ibfan.org [Last accessed November, 2023].
19. World Alliance for Breastfeeding Action. [online] Available from waba.org.my [Last accessed November, 2023].
20. Global Breastfeeding Collective. [online] Available from: www.globalbreastfeedingcollective.org [Last accessed November, 2023].

CHAPTER 36

Mothers Support Group and Breastfeeding

NS Mahanthashetti, Durgappa H, Roopa Bellad

"Many women are surprised by the passion they come to feel about breastfeeding. If you meet another breastfeeding mother, anywhere in the world, you feel a connection no matter how different her culture is, and no matter how long ago you or she breastfed your babies. Not many of us felt this passionately about breastfeeding until we did it ourselves, and many of us remember it as one of the best things we did in our lives. The experience is just that powerful".

INTRODUCTION

Breastfeeding though said to be "natural" for an Indian mother, is many a times daunting and demanding to some others. Rightful support needs to be provided to these mothers as it can lead to breastfeeding problems and many times even to lactation failure. This threat has resulted in global and national support for achieving the World Health Organization (WHO) guidelines mainly to encourage early initiation, the practice of exclusive breastfeeding up to 6 months of age by all mothers, and to continue breastfeeding until 2 years of age.[1] Though, the incidence of breastfeeding is on the increase after many years of decline, we are far from achieving the proposed levels outlined in Healthy People 2010 objectives of a 75% breastfeeding initiation rate at hospital discharge, with 50% of infants still breastfeeding at 6 months and 25% breastfeeding at 12 months.[2] Even the latest rates of early initiation of breastfeeding and exclusive breastfeeding (EBF) are far from encouraging being 25.9-78.8% and 28.3-79.4% (EBF-NFHS-5).[3] Breastfeeding is not influenced by the mother's decision alone but by many factors, such as sociocultural, community, and family norms. Hence, to follow the WHO guidelines for appropriate breastfeeding practices, the mother requires support, especially professional help, and support from the community and family. Providing skilled help and support from the family, community, and healthcare providers helps in successful breastfeeding.[4] A large national survey found that healthcare provider encouragement has a positive influence on breastfeeding initiation across all strata as it resulted in mothers initiating breastfeeding four times more.

CRITICAL STAGES BREASTFEEDING MOTHERS REQUIRING SUPPORT

At birth—early initiation "within the first hour of birth" is the best start for successful breastfeeding. This is possible only if the healthcare personnel provide the right support required for the first breastfeeding. The key elements required to achieve this are enumerated here.

Prepare the Mother in the Antenatal Period

This is the most important factor for the successful initiation of breastfeeding. A woman should know that for successful breastfeeding, the right start is a must. She should in fact be well prepared to feed her baby within 1 hour of birth. She should be educated about this guideline in the antenatal period itself, not once but repeatedly during each visit to the health center, so much so that she should demand to breastfeed her baby immediately after delivery. Support should be provided by the healthcare provider or Accredited Social Health Activist (ASHA) worker (who should be present during delivery) or a family member in case the labor room has a high workload. Because healthcare providers can and do influence their patient's decisions about the choice of infant feeding, it is important to train healthcare providers, to provide comprehensive and strategic plans to protect, support, and recommend breastfeeding. This plan should be initiated right from the initial patient contact and throughout the antenatal period. Then, a collaborative approach with the hospital system would ensure successful breastfeeding in mothers. It is a well-known fact that early initiation of breastfeeding results in exclusive breastfeeding for 6 months of age.

A recent Cochrane review analysis which evaluated 34 randomized controlled trials in 29,385 women, found that mothers who were encouraged by healthcare providers to breastfeed were less likely to stop breastfeeding at 4 months after the birth and more likely to breastfeed exclusively in the first 3 months after the birth.

Critical Phase

The first breastfeed-support is required to ensure proper latching and proper positioning of the baby during breastfeeding. All healthcare providers should be aware of the checklist for proper positioning and latching and this should be implemented in every healthcare setting. Early initiation of breastfeeding (EIBF), though known to be protective of the newborn, the prevalence is low, i.e., 41.8%—NFHS-5 data which is well below the expected 90%.[5] The data also showed that less than four antenatal care (ANC) visits and caesarian deliveries were associated with delayed EIBF. Higher maternal education and delivery in health facilities promoted EIBF. First, breastfeeding should always be observed and any rectification should be suggested at the earliest. "A task well begun is half done" is very true for successful breastfeeding. Early initiation is particularly important as it has been shown to decrease neonatal mortality.[6-8] Early initiation may also facilitate the subsequent practice of EBF, as was demonstrated in Indonesia, where early initiation was associated with a 3.66 times higher likelihood of EBF.[9] Support is especially required for primigravida mothers, very young mothers, sick mothers, mothers who have undergone caesarian section deliveries and mothers with low birth weight (LBW), and preterm or sick babies.

Ongoing Support to Mothers to Practice Exclusive Breastfeeding

Practicing successful EBF for 6 months is a challenge to every mother. As per the Baby-Friendly Hospital Initiative (BFHI) guidelines, it is important to discuss the management of breastfeeding not only with pregnant women but with their families too. Once a mother is away from the hospital support, the mother is on her own to decide and manage her newborn and this includes breastfeeding issues. Hence the mother with breastfeeding problems looks up to her family members.

Especially her mother, aunt, and mother-in-law, and sometimes to her neighbors for help. If the family members are not adequately trained, many times the support and the advice given are not appropriate or even wrong. Hence, healthcare providers must train the family members about the support required for optimal breastfeeding practices.

Various support groups for breastfeeding have been developed globally. Some interventions that can be easily practiced are enumerated here.

Postnatal Mother's Meetings

Mother's meetings are routinely practiced during the ANC checkups. This can be continued till 1 year after the birth of the baby. Advice regarding optimal breastfeeding, problems of breastfeeding, and ensuring optimal complimentary feeding should be given priority apart from discussing, immunization, mother's postpartum issues, birth spacing, etc.

Lactation Counselors and Clinics

Lactation clinics need to be established in every community and well-trained lactation counselors should be available to every mother to provide support to breastfeeding mothers. The government or nongovernmental organizations (NGOs) should take up this responsibility.

Establishment of Peer Counselors to Support Breastfeeding Mothers

Community-based peer counseling has been suggested to be a promotion strategy for breastfeeding with support extending beyond the hospital. The vast majority of published EBF peer counseling trials have found a positive impact of peer counseling on EBF. Community support by peer counselors can be mothers who have successfully breastfed their babies and can take the responsibility of providing support to breastfeeding mothers. Breastfeeding peer support was initially developed in the 1950s in America through the formation of the La Leche League.[10] Since then, breastfeeding peer support services have mushroomed with the help of international and national organizations and also at community levels. A recent Cochrane review of interventions to increase the duration of breastfeeding reported that skilled support, peer or professional, actively offered to lactating women can increase breastfeeding duration rates.[11] Breastfeeding peer support can be offered in person (at home, hospital, or community locations, such as via breastfeeding groups), via telephone or short message service (SMS), or via social media, e.g., Facebook groups. While the primary need for breastfeeding peer support is to help women sustain self-feeding methods, it is also known to identify and address cultural barriers.[11] Training of peer counselors and support from the government or NGOs is essential. Randomized controlled trials were conducted in Belgaum, Karnataka, India, and Dhaka, Bangladesh showed that peer counselor support to breastfeeding mothers promoted early initiation of breastfeeding and exclusive breastfeeding significantly.[12,13] Findings from these studies indicate that trained community-based peer counselors, within the context of a baby-friendly hospital, is a good strategy to promote EBF.

Using Technology as Support Tools for Breastfeeding

Teleconsultation, telephonic helplines, and the use of technology such as breastfeeding apps and videos will go a long way in providing support and helping breastfeeding mothers. A study conducted in Belagavi, India on the integration of mHealthApp with community-based peer counselors to educate women promoted EBF at 6 months of age.[14]

Vulnerable mothers: Literature has shown that mothers who stopped exclusive breastfeeding early were more likely to be single, less educated, and have no friends or family who breastfed. Such mothers should be identified early by healthcare providers and provide more support and guidance for breastfeeding or connect them with support groups in the community to ensure adequate breastfeeding.[15]

Breastfeeding Support for Indian Mothers: This is a Facebook peer-to-peer support group for breastfeeding mothers, their partners, and family members, founded in 2013, with >1,35,000 members helping mothers 24 × 7 for no monetary benefits.[16]

Working mothers: Today majority of the mothers need to work to support the family. About 70% of the employed mothers of infants younger than 3 years have full-time jobs and around one-third of these mothers return to their jobs within the first 3 months postpartum.[15] Therefore, it is important to understand workplace-related barriers and facilitators influencing the initiation and continuation of breastfeeding. The World Bank estimates that female labor force participation has increased from 23% in 1990 to 33% in 2017 (The Global Economy, 2018).[17] Recent data from India state that 20% of our women are employed (as per World News https://www.reuters.com) in organized sectors and the maternity leave is extended to 6 months by the government. But in unorganized sectors, the mother needs to get back to work much earlier. Secondly, no special efforts, have been made by the health services to reach employed women despite the large numbers employed in industries and other factories where long working hours, inadequate access to health information, and time and space for breastfeeding/expressing breast milk (BM) makes breastfeeding lactation, particularly challenging.[18] Lack of adequate maternity protection and inadequate breastfeeding support can hinder breastfeeding. This is supported by surveys that have shown breastfeeding prevalence to be as low as 10% among readymade garment workers [United Nations Children's Fund (UNICEF), 2019]. These mothers do need support such as education of family members and providing creche at the workplace, which will help our mothers practice optimal breastfeeding. The "Maternity Benefits Act" demands that an employer should provide nursing breaks to mothers to feed their babies, and should provide clean, private facilities to express and store milk at work. Mothers should be informed about their legal entitlements and reasons why continued breastfeeding is important so that they can plan to breastfeed and at the same time be aware of obstacles that they may face on return to work.[18]

Support for Mothers with Preterm and Low Birth Weight Babies

Breastfeeding in LBW babies can be challenging. These mothers require continuous support from healthcare providers as breastfeeding a preterm or LBW infant is a complex process. Mothers encounter numerous barriers and challenges to successful breastfeeding that are not experienced by mothers of full-term, healthy infants[18]. Providing support to these mothers is labor-intensive and time-consuming and requires continuous education, supervision, and support.[18] Optimal measures such as practicing Kangaroo Mother Care, expression of breast milk and spoon or paladai feeding, having a human milk bank for donor milk, and trained nurses and faculty to provide support to the mothers will ensure optimal and successful breastfeeding in these babies who require breast milk more than any other babies. Another intervention can be provided help from peer counselors working in collaboration with the infant's healthcare team to ensure that mothers and families receive the help they need for the optimal practice of breastfeeding in these vulnerable babies[18.]

NATIONAL PROGRAMS TO SUPPORT MOTHERS

The government is struggling hard to increase the rates of EBF in India from the existing 59.3–70% which is the WHO and UNICEF target for 2030.[19] The steps taken are as follows:
- Establishment of Breastfeeding Promotion Network of India (BPNI) to promote breastfeeding and recognize baby-friendly hospitals.
- Mother's Absolute Affection Program (MAA)[20]—established in August 2016 by the Government of India. The main objectives of this program are as follows:
  - To build a breastfeeding environment by creating awareness among pregnant and lactating mothers, families, and the community to promote optimal breastfeeding.
  - Reinforce lactation support services by training government hospital nurses, Auxiliary nurse midwives (ANMs), and ASHA workers to provide the right information and counseling support to breastfeeding mothers.
  - Community services of ASHA workers to be enhanced to provide support to breastfeeding mothers by conducting mother's meetings and referring mothers who require more support.
  - Providing incentives and recognition to health facilities that show high rates of breastfeeding and also implementation of processes for lactation management.
- Development and implementation of Indian National Guidelines on Infant and Young Child Feeding by the Ministry of Women and Child Development Food and Nutrition Board, Government of India.
- *Amendment of Maternity Benefits Act for working mothers:* This act was passed in Rajya Sabha in 2016 and implemented in 2017. Under this act, every establishment having >50 employees should have a crèche facility within a 500-m distance or in the common facility, which mothers could visit four times a day. Secondly, paid nursing breaks should be provided to nursing mothers till their baby reaches 15 months of age (Maternity Benefits Act 1961, amended in 2017 April 2, 2021).
- *Accreditation of human milk bank:* Establishment of Lactation Management Centres in Public Health facilities by National Health Mission (NHM) Guidelines have been developed by NHM to establish human milk banks at healthcare facilities in government centers so that every babies especially preterm, LBW babies and sick babies receive human milk.

KEY MESSAGES

- The mother support group is one of the most cost-effective strategies for the promotion of breastfeeding in the community.
- They form a bridge between community and healthcare professionals.

REFERENCES

1. World Health Organization. (2021). Infant and young child feeding. [online] Available from: https://www.who.int/news-room/fact-sheets/detail/infant-and-young-child-feeding [Last accessed November, 2023].
2. Anderson AK, Damio G, Young S, Chapman DJ, Pérez-Escamilla R. A randomized trial assessing the efficacy of

peer counseling on exclusive breastfeeding in a predominantly latina low-income community. Arch Pediatr Adolesc Med. 2005;159(9):836-41.
3. Sheila AC, Vir SC. The 5th National Family Health Survey – 5 of India: a sub-national analysis of child nutrition.
4. World Health Organization. (2018). Health Topics: Breastfeeding. [online] Available from: https://www.who.int/health-topics/breastfeeding#tab=tab_1 [Last accessed November, 2023].
5. International Institute for Population Sciences (IIPS) and ICF. (2021). National Family Health Survey (NFHS-5), 2019-21. [online] Available from: https://dhsprogram.com/pubs/pdf/FR375/FR375.pdf [Last accessed November, 2023].
6. Takahashi K, Ganchimeg T, Ota E, Vogel JP, Souza JP, Laopaiboon M, et al. Prevalence of early initiation of breastfeeding and determinants of delayed initiation of breastfeeding: Secondary analysis of the WHO Global Survey. Sci Rep. 2017;7:448688.
7. Smith ER, Hurt L, Chowdhury R, Sinha B, Fawzi W, Edmond KM; et al. Delayed breastfeeding initiation and infant survival: A systematic review and meta-analysis. PLoS One. 2017;12(7):e0180722.
8. Phukan D, Ranjan M, Dwivedi LK. Impact of timing of breastfeeding initiation on neonatal mortality in India. Int Breastfeed J. 2018;13:27.
9. Parashmanti BA, Hadi H, Gunawan IM. Timely initiation of breastfeeding is associated with the practice of exclusive breastfeeding in Indonesia. Asia Pac J Clin Nutr. 2016;25(Suppl 1):S52-6.
10. Thomson G, Balaam MC, Hymers K. Building social capital through breastfeeding peer support: insights from an evaluation of a voluntary breastfeeding peer support service in North-West England. Int Breastfeed J. 2015;10:15.
11. Renfrew MJ, McCormick FM, Wade A, Quinn B, Dowswell T. Support for healthy breastfeeding mothers with healthy term babies. Cochrane Database Syst Rev. 2012;16(5):CD001141.
12. Durgappa A, Raghavendra B, Parimala, Satish D, Hegade S, Shetti MNS. Effect of peer counseling on breastfeeding practices in the rural community: Randomized control trial. Int J Health Sci Res. 2012;8(8):8-19.
13. Haider R, Ashworth A, Kabir I, Huttly SR. Effect of community-based peer counsellors on exclusive breastfeeding practices in Dhaka, Bangladesh: a randomised controlled trial [see comments]. Lancet. 2000;356(9242):1643-7.
14. Short VL, Bellad RM, Kelly PJ, Washio Y, Ma T, Chang K, et al. Feasibility, acceptability, and preliminary impact of an mHealth supported breastfeeding peer counselor intervention in rural India. Int J Gynecol Obstet. 2021;156(1):48-54.
15. Dagher RK, McGovern PM, Schold JD, Randall XJ. Determinants of breastfeeding initiation and cessation among employed mothers: a prospective cohort study. BMC Pregnancy and Childbirth. 2016;16(1):194.
16. Kumar M. (2021). India's female labour participation rate falls to 16.1% as pandemic hits jobs. [online] Available from: https://www.reuters.com/world/india/2021-08-03 [Last accessed November, 2023].
17. Haider R, Thorley V, Yourkavitch J. Breastfeeding practices after a counselling intervention for factory workers in Bangladesh. Matern Child Nutr. 2021;17(2): e13113.
18. Rossman R. Breastfeeding peer counselors in the United States: helping to build a culture and tradition of breastfeeding. J Midwifery Womens Health. 2007;52(6):631-7.
19. Griswold M, Palmquist A; Evidence Review Working Group of the Global Breastfeeding Collective. Breastfeeding and Family-Friendly Policies; An evidence brief. [online] Available from: https://www.unicef.org/sites/default/files/2019-07/UNICEF-Breastfeeding-Family-Friendly%20Policies-2019.pdf [Last accessed November, 2023].
20. Ministry of Health and Family Welfare (Government of India). (2016). Programme for Promotion of Breastfeeding. [online] Available from: http/nhm.gov.in/MAA/Operational Guidelines.pdf [Last accessed November, 2023].

CHAPTER 37

Infant Milk Substitute Act

Dhyanesh DK, Asha Doddamane Benakappa, Hari Dattatreya M

"Ignorantiajuris non excusat-Ignorance of law is not an excuse".[1]

INTRODUCTION

Case scenario 1: In a mother and child hospital, a mother of a term, healthy baby complained of inadequate milk secretion because of a sore nipple. The pediatrician prescribed formula milk without addressing the mother's issue. Is it a violation of the IMS (Infant Milk Substitutes) act?

Case scenario 2: In a maternity hospital, at the time of discharge, all the mothers were given infant formula milk as "TONIC" to their babies, as the formula milk company has promised a foreign tour to the doctor. Is it a violation of the IMS act?

In both cases, the answer is YES. "No person shall take part in the promotion of infant milk substitutes or infant foods". It is a clear violation of the IMS act and a punishable offense.

HISTORY OF IMS ACT

"Breastfeeding was the best, is the best, and will remain the best". As far as infant feeding is concerned, breastfeeding has been a part of our culture since ancient times, but with progressive transition, breastfeeding practices have gradually gone downhill.[2] Globally, it is estimated that 1.5 million babies die each year, because they are not adequately breastfed.[3] The International Code of Marketing of Breast Milk Substitutes was adopted by the World Health Assembly in 1981 to promote breastfeeding and to regulate the marketing of breast-milk substitutes and feeding bottles. In India, nearly one million children die each year because of improper feeding practices. The government of India recognized this code and adopted the Indian National Code for the protection and promotion of breastfeeding in December 1983. The international code is mainly regulatory. It regulates the promotion, sale, and marketing of teats, bottles, milk substitutes, and baby foods. The code insists that companies provide scientific unbiased and factual information about infant feeding. It does not prescribe any punishment to the offenders but gives power to the individual state government to frame their own specific rules to tackle the menace of artificial feeding. Based on the recommendation of "The WHA" (*World Health Assembly*), Indian government enacted the Infant Milk Substitute, Feeding Bottles, and Infant Foods (Regulation, Promotion, Supply, and Distribution) act 1992 (IMS act), which came into force on August

1st, 1993. It was further amended in 2003 to strengthen certain provisions and close any loopholes infant formula companies had found.[4]

OBJECTIVES OF THE IMS ACT

- To protect breastfeeding from commercial promotion and thus prevents malnutrition and deaths in infants and children.
- The IMS act regulates the marketing strategies of baby food manufacturers.[5]

IMPORTANT PROVISIONS OF THE IMS ACT[4]

Section 2(f) defines what is infant food: Infant food is any food (by whatever name called) being marketed or otherwise represented as a complement to the mother's milk to meet the growing nutrition needs of the infant after the age of 6 months and up to the age of 2 years.

Section 2(g) defines infant milk substitute: Infant milk substitute means any food being marketed or otherwise represented as a partial or total replacement for a mother's milk for an infant up to the age of 2 years.

Section 3: This is a very important section that deals with certain provisions about infant milk substitutes, feeding bottles, and infant foods.
- No person can advertise or take part in the publication of any advertisement for the distribution, sale, or supply of infant milk substitutes or feeding bottles, or infant foods.
- No person shall give an impression or create a belief in any manner that feeding of infant milk substitutes and infant foods are equivalent to or better than mother's milk.
- No person shall take part in the promotion of infant milk substitutes, feeding bottles, or infant foods.

Section 4: Deals with provisions about incentives for the use or sale of infant milk substitutes or feeding bottles or infant foods.
- No person can supply or distribute samples of infant milk substitutes or feeding bottles or infant foods or gifts of utensils or other articles.
- No person shall contact any pregnant woman or mother of an infant.
- No person shall offer the inducement of any other kind to promote the use or sale of infant milk substitutes or feeding bottles or infant foods.

Section 5 of the act states about the donation of infant products:
- No person shall donate or distribute infant milk substitutes or feeding bottles or infant foods to any person except to an orphanage.
- No person shall donate or distribute any informational or educational equipment or material relating to infant milk substitutes or feeding bottles or infant foods. But donation or distribution through the healthcare system under prescribed conditions and restrictions can be made.

Section 6: This mentions what information and labels should be there on containers of infant milk substitutes or infant foods. Every container thereof or any label affixed thereto indicates in a clear conspicuous and easily readable and understandable manner, the words "Important notice" in capital letters in such language as may be prescribed and indicating there under the following particulars in the same language.
- A statement "mother's milk is best for your baby" in capital letters.
- A statement that infant milk substitutes or infant food should be used only on the advice of a health worker as to the need for its use and the proper method of its use.

- A warning that infant milk substitutes or infant food are not the sole sources of nourishment for an infant.
- The instruction for its appropriate preparation and warning against the health hazards of its inappropriate preparation.
- No container shall have a picture of an infant or woman or both.
- No container shall have pictures or other graphic materials or phrases designed to increase the sale ability of infant milk substitutes or infant food.
- No container shall use on it the word "humanized" or "maternalized" or any other similar words.

Section 7: States that educational and other materials relating to the feeding of infants contain certain particulars, such as:
- The benefits and superiority of breastfeeding.
- The preparation for, and the continuance of breastfeeding.
- The harmful effects on breastfeeding due to the partial adoption of bottle-feeding.
- The difficulties in reverting to breastfeeding infants after a period of feeding by infant milk substitute.
- The financial and social implications of making use of infant milk substitutes and feeding bottles.
- The health hazards of improper use of infant milk substitutes and feeding bottles.

Section 8: Mentions the responsibility of the healthcare system.
- No person can use any healthcare system or the display of placards or posters relating to or for the distribution of materials to promote the use or sale of infant milk substitutes or feeding bottles or infant foods.
- No person who produces, supplies, distributes, or sells infant milk substitutes or feeding bottles or infant food can make any payment to any person working in the healthcare system to promote the use or sale of such substitutes or bottles or food.
- No person except a health worker can demonstrate feeding with infant milk substitutes or infant foods to the mother of an infant or any member of her family.
- No person except an institution or organization engaged in the healthcare system can distribute infant milk substitutes or feeding bottles to a mother who cannot resort to breastfeeding and who cannot afford to purchase infant milk substitutes or feeding bottles.

Section 9: This section of the IMS act is a very important section that deals with inducement to a health worker for promoting the use of infant milk substitutes.
- No person who produces, supplies, distributes, or sells infant milk substitutes or feeding bottles, or infant food shall offer or give directly or indirectly any financial inducements or gifts to a health worker or any member of his family to promote the use of such substitutes or bottles or foods.
- No producer, supplier, or distributor shall offer or give any contribution or pecuniary benefit to a health worker or any association of health workers, including funding of seminar meetings, conferences, educational courses, contests, fellowships, research work, or sponsorship.

Section 11: Mentions standards of infant milk substitute feeding bottles or infant foods and should be as for the standards specified under the Food Safety and Standards Act, 2006.

Section 13: Gives power to any food safety officer or authorized officer to seize infant milk substitutes or feeding bottles or infant food if the provisions of this act have been or are being contravened. And liable for confiscation as per Section 14.

PUNISHMENT FOR VIOLATING IMS ACT

Section 20 of the IMS act mentions *Punishment* and *Penalty*. If there is a violation of provisions of Sections 3, 4, 5, 7, 8, 9, 10 and rules made under Section 26 of the Act shall be punishable with *Imprisonment* up to 3 years or with *fine* up to 5,000 rupees or with *both*. When an offense under this act has been committed by a company shall be liable to be proceeded against and punished accordingly as per *Section 22*.

IMPLEMENTATION AND MONITORING OF THE IMS ACT

The monitoring of the IMS act is undertaken by four nongovernmental organizations (NGOs), food safety officials, and other government officials authorized by the government as specified in Section 21(1). The Breastfeeding Promotion Network of India (BPNI) has been widely involved and successful in monitoring the IMS act. It conducts events to create awareness of infant formula, develop monitoring tools, regularly monitors product labeling and promotional activities of the infant formula companies, timely report to the ministry of women and child development, and files cases if violations of the law.[6] Exclusive breastfeeding rates have increased from 36.8% in 2000 to 58.3% in 2005 to 64.9% in 2014 compared with the Global average of 38% due to promotional, educational, and training activities regarding infant and young child feeding and also due to enforcement of legislation such as IMS act.[7]

ACTIONS ARE TAKEN FOR VIOLATING IMS ACT

Breastfeeding Promotion Network of India has a surplus of reports and letters regarding the success of monitoring the IMS act. (1) In 2010, an annual conference for Parenteral Nutrition and Enteral Nutrition sponsored by Nestle Nutrition Institute was canceled by the organizer when they received letters from BPNI and the Ministry of Health and Family Welfare. (2) In 2012, the regional Food and Drug Administration raided Nestle factory, which was using inappropriate graphics. Nestle was fined after the event. (3) In February 2016, the Indian Journal of Pediatrics blocked the circulation of their February issue, which contained infant formula advertisement.[8,9]

LIMITATIONS OF THE IMS ACT

1. Rules and regulations regarding infant food advertisements have many let-out clauses as compared to that for infant milk substitutes and feeding bottles.
2. There are no strict rules to address the issue of sponsoring scientific sessions, inducements, and other gifts by infant food manufacturers.
3. However, there are restrictions for infant food companies and health workers, but the chemists have been spared from many provisions of the act. The chemists continue to advertise and promote baby food products through the shops.
4. There is an acute need for prohibition and monitoring, promotion, and sales of IMS products, especially in e-marketing.[10]

STRATEGIES FOR THE EFFECTIVE IMPLEMENTATION OF THE ACT

Even though the government has enacted and passed the act, things are not working out as they expected. To defeat the aim of the act, the manufacturers always look for loopholes in the law that are used by them for their benefit.

ROLE OF PARENTS

To make the act work, the parents have to play a very important role. The parents should know that exclusive breastfeeding till 6 months is a must for every child; it is the right of every child. After 6 months if the child is started on complementary feeds and accepting cereals, pulses, vegetables, fruits, etc. then *artificial food* is not at all essential. Every relative including the husband must help the mother in breastfeeding.[2,9]

ROLE OF NONGOVERNMENTAL ORGANIZATIONS

Various voluntary organizations like BPNI and the Association for Consumer Action on Safety and Health have already taken up the cause of fighting the menace of commercial foods by filing criminal cases against companies violating the IMS act. Because of this in 1996, Johnson and Johnson decided to stop marketing feeding bottles in India. These organizations also booked criminal prosecution against Nestle for violating the act. They are authorized by the Government of India.[11,12] These NGOs still need to be more vigilant for the effective implementation of the IMS act.

ROLE OF HEALTH WORKERS

The health workers along with relatives must counsel and motivate the mother and build her confidence in removing various misconceptions related to breastfeeding.[2,13] Health education regarding the advantages of breastfeeding and the disadvantages of commercial food must be imparted to the mother and her relatives. Human lactation management training workshops and the Baby Friendly Hospital Initiative movement help in such education. All of us who are working for the betterment of child health must take a pledge to protect support and promote breastfeeding.

ROLE OF PROFESSIONAL BODIES

Professional bodies should develop Joint Action Plan for promoting, supporting, and protecting breastfeeding and improving awareness about the IMS act. Professional bodies like Indian Academy of Pediatrics (IAP), Federation of Obstetric and Gynaecological Societies of India (FOGSI), Indian Medical Association (IMA), Human Milk Banking Association (HMBA), and others can provide training platforms. These bodies also provide an internal platform for anonymous reporting of violations of the IMS act by its members.[6]

KEY MESSAGES

- The IMS act was enacted to promote, protect, and support breastfeeding.
- Rational and judicious use of infant milk substitutes is not banned under the IMS act.
- The aim is to prevent indiscriminate, unscientific, and overuse of artificial milk.
- It is our moral responsibility to monitor the violations of the act and report them to the appropriate authorities.
- Proper and optimal nutrition in infancy is one of the major strategies to prevent malnutrition-related mortality and morbidity in our future generation.[6]
- Save IMS Act and Save the Child.

REFERENCES

1. Black's Law Dictionary, 11 edition. Thomson Reuters; 2019. p. 719.

2. Tiwari SK, Pushpa C. The IMS act 1992: need for more amendments and publicity (editorial). Indian Pediatr. 2003;42:743-46.
3. World Health Organization. (1993). Infant and young child nutrition. EB93/17. [online] Available from: https://iris.who.int/bitstream/handle/10665/171779/EB93_17_eng.pdf?sequence=1 [Last accessed November, 2023].
4. Bare Act. The Infant milk substitutes, Feeding Bottles, And Infant foods (Regulation of production, supply, and Distribution) act, 1992. New Delhi: Universal Law Publishing Co. Pvt. Ltd.; 2010.
5. Choudhury P. Protecting IMS Act: Balancing trade interest and child health (editorial). Indian Pediatr. 2005;211-13.
6. Kumta NB. Why the act? Indian Pediatr. 1995;783-85.
7. Wolters DD, Phan LTH. The cost of not breastfeeding. The global results from a new tool. Health Policy and Plan. 2019;34:407-17.
8. Tiwari S. IMS acts the way forward. J Indian Medicolegal Ethics Assoc. 2019;7:71-6.
9. Tiwari S, Bharadva, Mishra S. IMS act: appraisal and recommendations in improving breastfeeding. India J Medicolegal Ethics Assoc. 2020;8(1):8-12.
10. Srivatsav RN. A balanced view. Indian Pediatrics. 1995;32:1189-91.
11. BPNI. (2017). Protecting breastfeeding. [online] Available from: https://old.bpni.org/protecting-breastfeeding [Last accessed November, 2023].
12. Gupta, Singh CU, George J. Under attack an Indian law to protect breastfeeding. BPNI, New Delhi: D K Fine Arts Press. 1998. p. 1011.
13. WHO and UNICEF. (1989). Ten steps to successful breastfeeding in protecting, promoting, and supporting breastfeeding, the special role of Health Services a joint WHO-UNICEF statement. [online] Available from: https://www.who.int/teams/nutrition-and-food-safety/food-and-nutrition-actions-in-health-systems/ten-steps-to-successful-breastfeeding [Last accessed November, 2023].

CHAPTER 38

Human Milk Banking

Adhisivam B, Roopa Bellad, Durgappa H

"Human milk is like ice cream, penicillin, and the drug ecstasy all wrapped up in two pretty packages".

—Florence William

INTRODUCTION

According to the World Health Organization (WHO) all infants should be exclusively breastfed for the first 6 months. Due to some reason, if a mother is unable to feed her infant directly, mother's own milk (MOM) should be expressed and fed to the infant. If MOM is unavailable, the next best option would be to use pasteurized donor human milk (PDHM). A human milk bank (HMB) is a service established to recruit breast milk donors, collect donor milk, process, screen, store, and dispense PDHM to the eligible babies who are usually preterm. Though the first HMB of India was started in 1989 at Mumbai, the growth of HMBs has not been proportionate to the phenomenal increase in neonatal intensive care units (NICUs) and preterm deliveries. Nevertheless, there has been renewed interest in this area over the past few years and nearly 80 HMBs are operational in the country today. During pandemics and disasters, HMB has a major role to play.[1]

RATIONALE

In India 27 million babies are born every year of which 3.5 million are preterm and 7.5 million have low birth weight (LBW).[2,3] An estimated 47% of babies born in India are small for gestational age (SGA). All these neonates are vulnerable in terms of survival and cognitive development and usually have feeding problems due to their medical conditions. Often, direct breastfeeding is not possible for these babies. The next best alternative is expressed breast milk, preferably from the same biological mother. When expressed breast milk is not adequate or available, these newborns are usually fed with infant formula milk. However, feeding formula milk is associated with high risk of sepsis and necrotizing enterocolitis (NEC), thus significantly decreasing the chance of both newborn survival as well as quality of long-term development. PDHM can save these vulnerable infants from the adverse effects of formula milk. PDHM has several benefits similar to MOM.

ELIGIBILITY TO RECEIVE PASTEURIZED DONOR HUMAN MILK FROM A HUMAN MILK BANK[4]

Usually preterm babies and sick infants are given priority for receiving PDHM.

Some infants whose mothers have postpartum illnesses or those infants whose mothers have transient lactation failure also are provided with PDHM. It is also useful for conditions including post-gastrointestinal surgeries, short gut syndrome, and sepsis. If PDHM supply is sufficient, it may also be used for adopted or abandoned neonates.

ELIGIBILITY TO DONATE MILK FOR A HUMAN MILK BANK

Any healthy lactating mother can volunteer to donate breast milk for the HMB. The potential donors could be mothers whose babies are in the NICU, mothers in the postnatal wards, and Kangaroo Mother Care (KMC) wards, mothers of babies visiting well-baby follow-up clinics/immunization sessions, and lactating women among the staff of the hospital. There is no money involved either for donating or receiving milk in the HMB.

Mothers with one or more of the following conditions may not be eligible for donating breast milk.
- Mother acutely ill or hemodynamically unstable
- Mother with hepatitis B, human immunodeficiency virus (HIV), hepatitis C, human T-cell lymphotropic virus (HTLV), or syphilis
- History of high-risk behavior and likely to have sexually transmitted diseases
- Presence of local infection of the breasts, including fungal infections
- Drug abuse, alcoholism, or tobacco use in the mother.

EQUIPMENT NEEDED FOR A HUMAN MILK BANK

Pasteurizer/Shaker-Water Bath

Holder pasteurization (HoP) involves treating donor milk at 62.5°C for 30 minutes followed by cooling. A conventional pasteurizer is expensive and massive and often may not be appropriate for the quantity of milk collected in the HMB on a daily basis. A shaker water bath provided with microprocessor-controlled temperature regulator, electronic timer device, and shaker speed controller can act as a pasteurizer in resource-restricted settings.

Deep Freezers

To store donor milk at -20°C, deep freezers are required in the HMB. Digital display of temperature with inbuilt alarms can be useful and the deep freezers need not be opened frequently to check the temperature. It is preferable to store pre- and post-pasteurized donor milk separately.

Refrigerators

The refrigerators are needed to store donor human milk (DHM) before and after pooling for subsequent processing. DHM from the refrigerator should be thawed before pooling and also before dispatching. It would be nice to have two separate refrigerators designated for pre- and post-pasteurization.

Hot Air Oven/Autoclave

If a central sterilization facility is available in the hospital, it can be used for sterilizing the containers. In case it is not available, then a hot air oven or autoclave in HMB may be used.

Breast Milk Pumps

For milk banking, hospital-grade electric pumps are preferred as they yield better volume of expressed milk and are relatively painless and comfortable to use. However, milk can be expressed manually by hand or using manually operated pumps as preferred by the donating mother. The breast milk pump and their parts may be sterilized as per the instructions of the manufacturer.

Containers

Although plastic containers are widely used, for Indian setting, wide-mouthed stainless steel containers (200 mL capacity) provided with good tight fitting or screwed caps are equally good. These stainless steel containers are sturdy, easy to clean, and autoclave.

Generator/Uninterrupted Power Supply

As it is essential that the appropriate temperature should be maintained for storing DHM, provisions for uninterrupted power supply and backup in case of interruption should be available in the HMB.

Human Milk Analyzer

It is desirable to have a human milk analyzer, which can estimate calorie, protein, and fat of a milk sample using infrared spectroscopy. The results of milk analysis can help in targeted fortification.

PERSONNEL REQUIRED FOR HUMAN MILK BANK

A team of professionals is needed for establishing and maintaining the services of a HMB. The team may include pediatricians, neonatologists, nurses, lactation counselors, microbiologist, laboratory technician, and housekeeping staff. The team should focus on sustaining and improving donor pool and also work collectively on quality improvement strategies in the HMB.

COLLECTION OF BREAST MILK

After proper counseling, checking suitability for donation, getting written informed consent, history taking, physical examination, and sampling for laboratory tests, the donor is sent to the designated breast milk collection area in the HMB. Breast milk is collected by a trained staff with hygienic precautions, after the method of breast milk expression is chosen by the donor. Washing the breast with water before expression is as good as washing with disinfectant. The donor mother can express milk manually or using breast pumps. It is advisable to use a new container for each pumping. Expressed DHM should be collected in properly labeled sterile containers and stored in the refrigerator before pooling.

PROCESSING

Raw DHM from multiple donors is usually pooled before pasteurization to facilitate the process of processing and storage. Addition of fresh DHM to the frozen milk may result in defreezing with hydrolysis of triglycerides and hence should not be done. Fresh raw breast milk should be chilled before adding to frozen DHM. Pasteurization is carried out by Holder's method.

Microbiological screening of donor milk can be done before and after pasteurization. Pre-pasteurization screening can result in wastage of donor milk to the tune of about 30%, and hence, most centers in India practice only post-pasteurization testing. Even after pasteurization, the endotoxins of organisms may be still present in the milk in some cases, but they have not been found to have any clinical effect on the neonates. A bacterial count of 10^5 CFU/mL or more in raw breast milk can be considered as an indicator of poor quality of milk. No growth should be noted in post-pasteurization microbiology cultures. In case of post-pasteurization culture positivity, the whole batch should be discarded.

STORAGE

Pasteurized milk awaiting culture report should be kept in dedicated freezer taking precautions not to disburse it till the culture reports are available. Storage should be done in the same container that is used for pasteurization. It is advisable not to transfer processed milk in other containers as it can cause contamination. Culture negative PDHM should be kept at -20°C in tightly sealed container with clear mention of expiry date. The temperature and maximum storage time for DHM is mentioned in **Table 1**.

DISBURSAL

After receiving the physician's requisition from NICU and taking informed consent from the parents of the recipient neonate, PDHM should be disbursed. Preterm neonates should preferably be administered PDHM from preterm donors. It should be done on first-in-first-out basis from the storage. Transport of PDHM should be done under cold storage in the same pasteurized container till its use. Frozen PDHM should be thawed by either defrosting the milk rapidly in a water bath at a temperature not exceeding 37°C or under running lukewarm water taking precautions to prevent contamination. Milk should not be refrozen after being thawed as this increases the hydrolysis of the triglycerides in the milk. While bringing to room temperature, it should be gently agitated to make a homogenous mixture before use and should be used preferably within 3 hours **(Table 2)**.

LABELLING AND RECORD KEEPING

Human milk bank should have an operational objective of ensuring full traceability from individual donation to recipient and maintaining a record of all storage and processing conditions. Written standard operating procedures should be followed. Confidentiality of records should be maintained by the HMB. Record keeping at all levels should be meticulous for donor record file containing consent form, donor's and her child's data, screening reports, pasteurization batch files, and PDHM disbursal.

GENERAL GUIDELINES FOR STAFF OF HUMAN MILK BANK[1]

- Standard operating procedures for strict asepsis in the HMB should be adhered to.
- Strict hand hygiene should be ensured during all steps of handling DHM.
- While handling raw and pasteurized DHM, gloves should be used.
- Regular health screening should be done for all HMB staff.
- An ongoing training program for HMB staff should be in place.

HAZARD ANALYSIS CRITICAL CONTROL POINTS[5]

Hazard Analysis Critical Control Points (HACCP) planning is a critical step in ensuring the safety and quality of any food product, including donated and processed human milk. HACCP planning is useful and is possible for any HMB, regardless of size, resources, or location. The objective of

TABLE 1: Temperature and duration of human milk storage.

Location	Temperature	Duration
Fresh raw milk	Room temperature (<25°C)	Up to 6 hours
Refrigerator (unpasteurized milk)	4°C (+2 to +4°C)	24 hours
Freezers:		
Unpasteurized milk	-20°C	3 months
Pasteurized Milk		6 months

TABLE 2: Steps involved in processing human milk.

Sl no	Process	Place	Equipment	Personnel
1	Counseling potential donors	Postnatal wards/NICU/HMB	—	Lactation counselor Nurse Pediatrician
2	Screening the willing mothers	Postnatal wards/NICU/HMB	—	Nurse Pediatrician
3	Milk expression	Postnatal wards/NICU/HMB	Hospital-grade breast milk pumps	Lactation counselor Nurse
4	Pooling/storing	HMB	Refrigerators and deep freezers Containers	HMB nurse
5	Pasteurization	HMB	Pasteurizer/Shaker-water bath	HMB nurse
6	Post-pasteurization testing	Microbiology lab	Bacterial culture media	Microbiologist/laboratory technician
7	Storing	HMB	Deep freezers and refrigerators Containers	HMB nurse
8	Dispensing	HMB	Containers	HMB nurse

(HMB: human milk bank; NICU: neonatal intensive care unit)

HACCP is to identify and prevent, eliminate, or reduce to acceptable levels any biological, chemical, or physical hazard that would be likely to occur in a food production or distribution environment. Through HACCP, food safety is addressed at every phase of the process, including procurement, handling, distribution, processing, and consumption. HMB processes involve many steps where contamination can occur and also where alteration of nutritional or immunological properties may take place. HACCP provides a solution for balancing the priorities of safety and quality within each location's own needs and limitations.

SCALING UP HUMAN MILK BANKING IN INDIA[6]

The Government of India launched the "National Guidelines on Lactation Management Centers in Public Health Facilities" in July 2017. The vision of this initiative is to make breast milk universally available for all infants by establishing comprehensive lactation management centers (CLMC), lactation management units (LMUs), and lactation support units (LSUs) at the facility level.

CHALLENGES IN HUMAN MILK BANKING

Though starting a HMB is relatively easy, sustaining voluntary milk donation is an arduous task but essential. Educating and sensitizing donor mothers is the most crucial aspect of HMB. The purpose of counseling them is to promote breastfeeding and encourage milk donation for the HMB as a parallel effort. Dedicated lactation counselors for this purpose would be ideal. However, in resource-restricted settings innovative methods like peer group counseling may be equally effective with no added cost involved. Parallel promotion of exclusive breastfeeding and HMB can complement each other. Auditing and quality improvement strategies should also be inherent components of HMB.

As per National Guidelines on Lactation Management Centers in Public Health Facilities, donation should be done freely and voluntarily without any monetary benefits to the donor and with an understanding that the donated milk may be used to feed the baby of another mother admitted in the hospital free of any cost. However, there are ongoing efforts to commercialize donor milk. If mothers start selling their milk or companies indirectly do so, HMBs will run dry and infant formula use will increase. There is also a risk that DHM may be used for nonscientific indications, excluding the needy preterm neonates.

HUMAN MILK BANK IN THE CONTEXT OF COVID[7]

The coronavirus disease 2019 (COVID-19) pandemic is posing several challenges to HMB worldwide and has exposed the vulnerability in service provision and emergency preparedness. Currently, there is no evidence around severe acute respiratory syndrome-coronavirus 2 (SARS-CoV-2) transmissions from breastfeeding or human milk, and the virus is inactivated by heat treatment. If donor milk is provided during any separation linked to COVID-19, this should be for as short a time as possible as a bridge to receiving MOM. By reducing the amount of mother–infant separation time and supporting the use of MOM, the excess demand for donor milk will diminish, ensuring that the global supply can continue to be used for those who need donor milk most.

KEY MESSAGES

- If MOM is unavailable or insufficient, the next best option is to use PDHM.
- Parallel promotion of exclusive breastfeeding and human milk banking can complement each other.

REFERENCES

1. Bharadva K, Tiwari S, Mishra S, Mukhopadhyay K, Yadav B, Agarwal RK, et al. Human milk banking guidelines. Indian Pediatr. 2014;51:469-74.
2. Blencowe H, Cousens S, Oestergaard MZ, et al. National, regional, and worldwide estimates of preterm birth rates in the year 2010 with time trends since 1990 for selected countries: a systematic analysis and implications. Lancet. 2012;379:2162-72.
3. Vishnu Bhat B, Adhisivam B. Human Milk Banking and Challenges in Quality Control. Indian J Pediatr. 2018;85(4):255-6.
4. National Guidelines on Lactation Management Centers in Public Health Facilities. Ministry of Health and Family Welfare, Government of India: New Delhi; 2017.
5. PATH. Strengthening Human Milk Banking: A Resource Toolkit for Establishing and Integrating Human Milk Bank Programs—Establishing Quality Assurance: A Workshop for Developing a Hazard Analysis Critical Control Points Plan (Trainee Workbook). Version 2.0. Seattle, Washington, USA: PATH; 2019.
6. Nangia S, Chugh RS, Sabharwal V. Human milk banking: An Indian experience. Neoreviews. 2018;19:e201.
7. Shenker N; Virtual Collaborative Network of Human Milk Banks and Associations. Maintaining safety and service provision in human milk banking: a call to action in response to the COVID-19 pandemic. Lancet Child Adolesc Health. 2020;4(7):484-5.

Policy Making at the National Level for the Promotion of Breastfeeding

CHAPTER 39

Shivananda R, Durgappa H

> *"While breastfeeding may not seem the right choice for every parent, it is the best choice for every baby."*
>
> —Amy Spangler

INTRODUCTION

The world is losing millions of infants for not getting breastfed within 1 hour after birth and exclusive breastfeeding for 6 months. They do not reach their full growth potential, both physical and mental, and are subjected to many infectious diseases. Further, mothers do face the risk of breast cancer and malnutrition as a result of frequent pregnancies. Exclusive breastfeeding can save nearly 8,30,000 neonatal deaths every year. Globally, only 38% of infants are breastfed out of 135 million births every year.[1] The World Health Assembly (WHA) has set a target to increase the global exclusive breastfeeding rate from 38% in 2012 to 60% in 2025 and improve the health of the babies.[2] Currently, in India, only 55% of children are exclusively breastfed; to contribute to the global goal, India has to achieve a 65.7% rate of exclusive breastfeeding by 2025 as per the World Health Organization (WHO) tracking tool.

Many factors play a role in the despicable situation: Apathy of healthcare workers, societal factors like myths related to breastfeeding, cultural pressure, shortage of breastfeeding, lack of legislation or imperfectly implemented International Monetary Fund (IMF) Act, women's safety at workplace, obstacles to feeding in public places, maternity leave, and pressure from industries. Together, these barriers create a challenging environment for mothers, families, and the healthcare system to contribute to low rates.[3]

Policy makers at different levels from the international level to the community level play a crucial role in the successful promotion of breastfeeding. Global organizations can better support national organizations to monitor national activities, particularly regarding legislative violations, in implementing the promotion of breastfeeding. The breastfeeding rate is widely variable among the nations. Some countries are performing very well and some countries are not; however, the breastfeeding rate is stagnant and even declining in a few nations. Hence, political commitment plays a crucial and dominant role in this regard.

HOW TO ACHIEVE THE TARGETS OF BREASTFEEDING PROMOTION?

Breastfeeding promotion can be achieved by executable policies which involve the international, national, state, and institutional levels with effective implementation at the community level.

International Level

The WHO is encouraging its member countries to enact the IMF code into law, but with a varying success; the International Baby Food Action Network (IBFAN) continues to advocate for strengthening the code at both national and international levels. The WHO had success in encouraging most of its country members to enact the code into law, though with varying degrees of implementation of the International Code of Marketing of Breast-Milk Substitutes.[4]

Globally, 136 of 194 countries have some form of legal measures related to the International Code of Marketing of Breast-Milk Substitutes and subsequent resolutions adopted by the WHA, but only 44 countries have strengthened their regulations on marketing over the past 2 years. Legal restrictions are not covering the marketing of healthcare facilities. Only 79 countries prohibit the promotion of breast-milk substitutes and 51 countries have prohibited the distribution of free or low-cost supplies within the health care system.

National Level: Pivotal Role of Government

Breastfeeding-focused initiatives by the government facilitate and support policies. This could be achieved, by raising awareness, building the capacity of health workers from national to remote rural areas, and planning multifarious activities at all levels. The government must ensure that every mother has access to credible and complete information about breastfeeding and provide legal, infrastructural support to enable her to breastfeed wherever and as long as she wishes to.

In India, as per the National Family Health Survey 5 (NFHS-5) (2019–2021), only 41.8% of children under 3 years of age were breastfed within 1 hour of birth while only 54.9% of children were exclusively breastfed until 6 months. While this is a slight improvement over global statistics, it still means that nearly half of our children are not being breastfed according to WHO guidelines.

Breastfeeding is a natural and intimate act between a mother and a child and has become a complicated political issue involving several other stakeholders such as the family, society, government, and commercial firms, which are not acting under benign interest.

The infant food industry is underplaying the IMF Act; hence, the government has to implement this act strictly so that the food industry cannot subjugate. In the United Kingdom, the Baby Feeding Law Group [BFLG, a coalition of 23 nongovernmental organizations (NGOs) including UNICEF and UK IBFAN] aims to strengthen and report violations of the code. BFLG poses a website where code violations can be reported by the public resulting in the monitoring of reports by the relevant regulatory bodies.[4]

Human Milk Banking

India got its first human bank in 1989 in Lokamanya Tilak Municipal Medical College.[5] Milk banks play an important role in case a mother is unable to breastfeed due to either illness or ignorance and lack of an adequate support system.

Maternity Benefits

Women constitute only 27% of the Indian workforce with nearly 96% of them being employed in the informal sector. The challenge is in providing policy and infrastructure support for young working mothers to breastfeed while continuing to be part of the workforce. The Maternity Benefits (Amendment) Act, 2017, is applicable only to the formal sector as of now, by providing for a compulsory 26 weeks of paid maternity leave, an optional work-from-home facility, and a compulsory crèche facility with a minimum of 4 breaks per day for childcare.

Maternity Protection Legislation is beneficial to working mothers to continue breastfeeding to optimize breastfeeding practices but unfortunately, not all nations follow the same efficiently. Alive & Thrive (A&T), which has recently commenced activities in Indonesia and the Philippines, is advocating for an increase in paid maternity leave to 6 months.

The most challenge lies in the absence of infrastructural support to facilitate breastfeeding in public spaces. It is usually stigmatized in many parts of the country to breastfeed in public areas. No effort has been made to provide private nursing rooms in public spaces such as bus stops, malls, and railway stations. A mother is confined to a home to breastfeed her child.

The government of India launched the National Breastfeeding Promotion Program—MAA (mothers' absolute affection) to ensure that adequate awareness is generated among the masses, especially mothers, on the benefits of breastfeeding. The goal of the program is to enhance optimal breastfeeding practices, which include initiation of breastfeeding within an hour of birth, exclusive breastfeeding for the first 6 months, and continued breastfeeding for at least 2 years. The government will train nurses in government hospitals, accredited social health activists (ASHA), and auxiliary nurse midwives (ANM) to provide relevant information and counseling support to mothers for breastfeeding.[6]

UNICEF was the driving force behind the Baby-Friendly Hospital Initiative (BFHI) and the International Labor Organization (ILO). 10 steps to successful breastfeeding in maternity services were published by WHO and UNICEF in 1989. BFHI has made an impact in some countries in supporting breastfeeding activities. The 10 steps were reemphasized in the Innocenti Declaration on the protection, promotion, and support of breastfeeding, adopted in Florence, Italy, in 1990 and 2005.[4]

The BFHI guides the implementation, training, monitoring, assessment, and reassessment of the 10 steps to successful breastfeeding and the International Code of Marketing of Breast-Milk Substitutes, a set of recommendations to regulate the marketing of breast-milk substitutes.

Lactation Management Centers

The National Health Mission has taken the initiative to establish lactation management centers at secondary- and tertiary-level public health facilities to provide lactation support for breastfeeding mothers. This facility-based lactation management has the strategies to collect, process, store, and dispense the donor human milk with a provision of lactation support to the mothers.

Bangladesh and Indonesia have developed training for health workers at the community level and have been a part of the medical curriculum. Similarly, the UK has expanded BFI standards for universities to ensure evidence-based training for midwives and health visitors. Breastfeeding training must have consistency in the provision of information about breastfeeding and its alternatives by health professionals. Breastfeeding training can also help to support health workers and their professional associations to withstand the negative influence of Breast Milk Substitutes (BMS).

Role of Institutions

The head of the maternity institution has an important role in implementing the national policies on breastfeeding in coordination with state government and international agencies. It has the responsibility and commitment to training all cadres of health workers from paramedics such as nurses ANMs, and class 4 employees. Breastfeeding education materials are made available at the antenatal clinic, and all of them are to be appropriate and adequate in 15 points of BFHI. Maternity centers are the best places to help parents to understand the nitti-gritty of breastfeeding. The head of maternity centers must ensure that the messages of MAA, breastfeeding methods, and infant feeding issues reach the community by the means of exhibitions, street plays, role plays, flip charts, handouts, radio jingles, radio talks, and TV talks and involve opinion leaders and influencers to motivate breastfeeding.

Community Level

The Information, communication and education (ICE) material should be simple, brief, technically correct, understandable, pictorial, culturally appropriate, and field-tested, with minimal text which can be comprehensible by illiterate rural women. Any skilled birth attendant or nursing staff can provide this counseling and support with the necessary information. Ideally, it needs to start as part of antenatal service to educate and motivate mothers for exclusive breastfeeding and appropriate complementary feeding. Private practitioners also need to enhance and support this cause. Past studies confirm that counseling that works in breastfeeding is not of routine type but interpersonal, "one-to-one" or "group counseling" where attention can be paid to every client and problem/s identified and resolved. This calls for the skills and patience of the person.[7]

It is possible to promote optimal breastfeeding practices in low- to mid-socio-economic, rural, and high-socioeconomic urban settings. The messages should be promoted through different channels at multiple contacts. This strategy demands training to ensure consistency, repeated training, and higher coverage. Medically qualified physicians and private providers need to be engaged as they have a high degree of credibility and they must endorse messages given by higher bodies.

A specially trained cadre of lactation counselors is required, especially in the urban setting, if exclusive breastfeeding is to become universal; they need to be accessible to a new mother whenever she has breastfeeding problems. Lactation consultants should be available for the resolution of difficult breastfeeding problems.

■ KEY MESSAGE

Policy making at national level for improving IYCF will go a long way for the optimal health of children.

■ REFERENCES

1. Victora C, Bahl R, Barros A, Franca GVA, Horton S, Krasevec J, et al. Breastfeeding in the 21st Century: Epidemiology, Mechanisms and Lifelong Effect. Lancet. 2016; 387(10017):475-90.

2. World Health Organization. Breastfeeding in the Western Pacific. [online] Available from: https://www.who.int/westernpacific/health-topics/breastfeeding [Last accessed November, 2023].
3. World Health Organization. Global breastfeeding scorecard, 2017: Tracking progress for breastfeeding policies and programmes. [online] Available from: https://www.who.int/publications/m/item/global-breastfeeding-scorecard-2017-tracking-progress-for-breastfeeding-policies-and-programmes [Last accessed November, 2023].
4. National Family Health Survey (NFHS-5). International Institute for Population Sciences (IIPS) and ICF, 2019–21: India, Volume I. Mumbai: IIPS; 2021.
5. Tyebally Fang M, Chatzixiros E, Grummer-Strawn L, Engmann C, Israel-Ballard K, Mansen K, et al. Developing global guidance on human milk banking. Bull World Health Organ. 2021;99(12):892-900.
6. Ritika Rocque. MAA (Mother Absolute Affection) Programme. Int. J. Nur. Edu. and Research. 2020;8(1):117-120.
7. WHO Infant and Young Child Feeding: Model Chapter for Textbooks for Medical Students and Allied Health Professionals. Geneva: World Health Organization; 2009.

CHAPTER 40

Role of Research in Lactation: Present and Future

Sneha J Andrade, Jayashree Purkayastha, Leslie Lewis, Maria Pais

"Mother's milk, time-tested for millions of years, is the best nutrient for babies because it is nature's perfect food".
—Robert S Mendelsohn

INTRODUCTION

Breastfeeding does more than provide nutrition to support an infant's growth and development; it also benefits maternal health and offers an opportunity for the pair to bond. The American Academy of Pediatrics (AAP) recommends that infants be fed their mother's breast milk exclusively until they are at least 6 months sold.

Although breastfeeding is considered the "gold standard", not all women breastfeed their infants. The UNICEF's State of the World's Children Report 2011 reports that of the 136.7 million babies born worldwide each year, only 32.6% are breastfed exclusively for the first 6 months.

Many studies related to infant feeding, including breastfeeding and breast milk, are being conducted worldwide. Research in the field of lactation encompasses varied topics ranging from the benefits of breastfeeding and breast milk, the physiology of lactation, the sociocultural determinants of infant feeding, and the impact of government policies and laws on breastfeeding.

RESEARCH ON THE BENEFITS OF BREASTFEEDING

Numerous studies have consistently demonstrated that breastfeeding benefits not only the infant–mother dyad but also the community and even the environment.

Benefits to the Infant and Mother

The Promotion of Breastfeeding Intervention Trial (PROBIT) is an ongoing study enrolling 17,046 healthy mothers and infants that continues to examine the effects of breastfeeding promotion on rates of breastfeeding and the benefits of exclusive breastfeeding on child health. It has been found that prolonged and exclusive breastfeeding improves children's cognitive development.[1] However, PROBIT demonstrated that there were no long-term effects of breastfeeding on child behavior and maternal adjustment.[2]

Studies have also shown that exclusive breast milk feeding lowers the risk of death and necrotizing enterocolitis (NEC) in extremely low-birth-weight infants.[3] As childhood obesity has become an important public health problem worldwide, researchers are trying to explore the role of lactation and human milk components such as adiponectin on weight gain during infancy and childhood.[4] Lactoferrin, found in breastmilk, is thought to be protective of infants primarily due to its anti-inflammatory, anti-infective, and immune-regulatory properties, which have been widely documented in in vitro and animal models. However, further research is necessary to demonstrate the protective effects in children definitively.[5] In mothers, breastfeeding reduces the likelihood of postpartum hemorrhage and depression, morbidity, and mortality from several diseases later in life.[6]

Benefits to the Community

Evidence shows that breastfeeding has much human capital and future economic benefits for children, mothers, and countries. Moderate increases in breastfeeding rates have been shown to substantially impact healthcare costs in the first year of life.[7] A Cost of Not Breastfeeding Tool developed by researchers in Canada is a user-friendly online tool that summarizes the economic consequences of not breastfeeding and exposure to breastmilk substitutes in various countries. The tool computes regional and global estimates based on two user inputs [the discount rate and gross domestic product (GDP) growth rate]. This tool helps illustrate the significant costs of not breastfeeding and the potential economic benefits that could be generated by government investments in scaling up breastfeeding promotion and support strategies.[8]

Benefits to the Environment

A carbon footprint is the number of greenhouse gases (mainly carbon dioxide) released into the atmosphere by a particular human activity. Studies indicate that breastfeeding has a consistently lower carbon footprint than using breastmilk substitutes.[9] Production of infant milk substitutes affects the environment in various other ways, such as pollution, contamination of water and soil, use of nonrenewable resources such as land, water, fossil fuels, and biodiversity loss. Breastfeeding provides food security with a positive ecological impact.[10]

RESEARCH ON THE PHYSIOLOGY OF LACTATION

Women's breast health is a major area of research as good breast health and mammary gland development and function are essential to ensure optimal milk production and comfort during breastfeeding. These factors often determine how long a woman chooses to breastfeed and the quality of breastmilk she produces, which directly influences infant health.

Role of Adipophilin

Milk lipids, mainly triglycerides, provide a majority of the calories, essential fatty acids, and bioactive lipids necessary for a newborn's growth and development. These calorific demands are met by the ability of mammary glands of most species to produce and secrete large amounts of lipid during lactation. Studies in mice have shown that the formation and secretion of milk lipids are initiated during the second half of gestation when the mammary gland differentiates into a secretory organ, and this process is regulated by the protein adipophilin.[11]

Role of Estrogen Receptor

Estrogen receptor (ER) has been shown to play a central role in mammary gland development. Mammary glands of mice where ER was knocked out showed only a primary ductal structure that could not invade the mammary fat pad, illustrating that the ER is required for normal ductal elongation. Repressor of ER activity (REA) was initially identified as a coregulator that repressed the activity of estrogen. Research has shown that the repressor of ER activity is a protein required for mammary gland development during puberty, maturation during pregnancy, and function during lactation. Changes in the levels of REA may also be linked to breast tumorigenesis.[12]

Role of Zinc transporter

Approximately 1-3 mg of zinc (Zn) is transferred from the mammary gland into milk each day to provide optimal Zn for the developing infant. Studies have demonstrated that a mutation in the gene that encodes for Zn transporter ZnT2 decreases milk Zn concentration by 75% in lactating women. Suboptimal Zn transfer to the developing infant during lactation results in serious adverse effects such as growth retardation, compromised cognitive development, and higher morbidity and mortality.[13]

Maternal Depression and Breastmilk Content

Perinatal depression is a common mental health condition observed during pregnancy and lactation. It has been demonstrated that depression during pregnancy alters breast milk content, including fatty acids, which are crucial for infant health and development. However, additional large longitudinal studies are required to trace the course of depressive symptoms and fatty acid status of breastmilk over longer periods.[14]

RESEARCH ON THE DETERMINANTS OF BREASTFEEDING

Research on infant feeding not only is not limited to the benefits and biology of breastfeeding, but also includes studies of factors that affect breastfeeding practices, methods, and duration. Breastfeeding duration may also be affected by partner or family support or how well an infant is suckling.

MATERNAL HEALTH AND LACTATION

Studies have shown that women with high prepregnant body mass index (BMI) have reduced lactation duration which is probably due to a lack of comfort or confidence with one's body. Further research into the interplay between weight status, body image, and breastfeeding outcomes may reveal behavioral targets amenable to modification and intervention that may subsequently improve breastfeeding outcomes for overweight women and their infants.[15] The role of breastfeeding in infants born to mothers with human immunodeficiency virus (HIV) infection has been debated. Studies have shown that in developing countries, the benefits of breastfeeding outweigh the risks of HIV transmission, especially with the use of antiretroviral drugs in both the mother and the infant.

Family Support and Breastfeeding

Support from partner and family members can play an important role in a mother's decision to begin, continue, or stop breastfeeding postnatally. Several studies have been done to determine the effect of specific types of partner support on breastfeeding initiation, exclusivity, and duration. Partner support in the form of verbal encouragement, the sensitivity of the partner to the nursing mother's needs, assistance to prevent and manage breastfeeding difficulties, and helping with household chores led to improved breastfeeding behavior. To increase the impact of breastfeeding policies and interventions among new mothers, breastfeeding programs should consider the involvement of partners.[16] The older generation, especially the infant's grandmothers, plays a pivotal role in the different aspects of pregnancy and child-rearing decision-making within the family. This is even more evident in low- and middle-income countries like India where older women are often seen as owners of traditional knowledge. It has been demonstrated that grandmothers can improve exclusive breastfeeding rates and they should be included in programs that seek to influence breastfeeding.[17]

RESEARCH ON THE ROLE OF EDUCATION AND BREASTFEEDING PRACTICES

Breastfeeding education is feasible and must not be overlooked. Health education can be provided at multiple levels such as schools, health care providers, antenatal and postnatal mothers, and even the community at large.

Prenatal and Postpartum Education

Evidence-based, prenatal breastfeeding education is one of the World Health Organization's 10 steps to support breastfeeding. Exclusive breastfeeding of the neonate during the hospital stay is a public health goal and it is associated with prolonged duration of breastfeeding.[18] Mothers' knowledge about infant health benefits was found to be directly related to the intention to exclusively breastfeed. Improving maternal knowledge of exclusive breastfeeding recommendations might encourage mothers to breastfeed their infants for the recommended 6-month duration. Combined prenatal and postpartum lactation counseling interventions, across the continuum of care, are effective in reinforcing breastfeeding intention and duration.[19] Further research is required on what educational medium may be the most effective in increasing breastfeeding knowledge.[20]

School Education

Advocating positive beliefs about breastfeeding in adolescents is an important antecedent of future breastfeeding. Studies have shown that education of primary and secondary school children may be an effective way to increase breastfeeding knowledge, foster positive attitudes, build a culture where breastfeeding is the norm, and, finally, increase future intentions to breastfeed. More research on the impact of school-based health education programs on breastfeeding is needed.[21]

Education of Pediatric Residents

To increase breastfeeding rates, health care providers must provide appropriate support and counseling for breastfeeding mothers and infants. Evidence-based knowledge is the critical first step in ensuring that residents are satisfactorily prepared for this role. Resident education regarding lactation is a key component that is lacking in many current residency training programs. Research demonstrated that a mandatory 2-week lactation rotation program for pediatric residents increased their knowledge and perceived confidence related to breastfeeding. Other groups of medical and nursing students could also benefit from such lactation rotations.[22]

RESEARCH ON GOVERNMENT POLICIES AND LAWS RELATED TO BREASTFEEDING

Public health services can play a central role in creating a supportive breastfeeding environment. Public health professionals need to explore ways to improve legal support for all mothers wishing to breastfeed. Researchers can identify the laws that have the most impact and assist policymakers in converting them into policy.

Breastfeeding and Government Policies

Women are more likely to breastfeed in nations with a strong breastfeeding-friendly environment where breastfeeding is protected, promoted, and supported. Most countries, however, have not graded breastfeeding as a high political priority and have failed to invest politically and financially to support mothers to breastfeed. There is a need for evidence-based frameworks that can guide and empower countries to prioritize breastfeeding on the national agenda and help them invest in scaling up programs embedded in breastfeeding-friendly environments.[23] Many hurdles to breastfeeding exist at the societal rather than individual level. Studies have identified the following areas which require investment including health services, health promotion at the population level, support of maternal legal rights, protection of maternal health, and reducing the reach of the infant milk substitute industry. Even though individual support is important, breastfeeding must be considered a public health concern. Focusing only on solving individual issues may not lead to the cultural changes that are needed to normalize breastfeeding.[24]

Breastfeeding and the Law

Returning to work and embarrassment about breastfeeding, especially in public, remain challenges for many mothers. Studies have demonstrated that for women to successfully breastfeed outside of the home environment, whether at work or in public, additional support is needed. In India, the Maternity Benefits Act requires employers to provide nursing breaks of prescribed duration for new mothers to express breast milk for the nursing child. These nursing breaks are fully paid and are available until a child reaches the age of 15 months. Such laws that support breastfeeding may increase breastfeeding rates.[25]

KEY MESSAGES

- Though it is recommended that every child be exclusively breastfed for the first 6 months of life, breastfeeding rates worldwide are not optimal.
- To improve breastfeeding rates, we need to extensively study varied topics ranging from the benefits of breastfeeding and breast milk, the physiology of lactation, the sociocultural determinants of infant feeding, and the impact of government policies and laws on breastfeeding.
- The responsibility of giving infants "the best start in life" through exclusive breastfeeding lies with the family, health care professionals, society, and government.

REFERENCES

1. Kramer MS, Aboud F, Mironova E, Vanilovich I, Platt RW, Matush L, et al. Breastfeeding and child cognitive development: new evidence from a large randomized trial. Arch Gen Psychiatry. 2008;65(5):578-84.
2. Kramer MS, Fombonne E, Igumnov S, Vanilovich I, Matush L, Mironova E, et al. Effects of prolonged and exclusive breastfeeding on child behavior and

maternal adjustment : Evidence From a large, randomized trial. Pediatrics. 2008;121(3): e435-40.
3. Manuscript A. NIH Public Access. 2010; 29(1):57-62.
4. Woo JG, Guerrero ML, Guo F, Martin LJ, Davidson BS, Ortega H, et al. The second year of life. J Pediatr Gastroenterol Nutr. 2012;54(4):532-9.
5. Ochoa TJ, Pezo A, Cruz K, Chea-woo E, Cleary TG. Clinical studies of lactoferrin in children. Biochem Cell Biol. 2012;467:457-67.
6. Martines J. Breastfeeding and maternal health outcomes: a systematic review and meta-analysis. Acta Paediatr. 2015;104(467): 96-113.
7. Stuebe AM, Jegier BJ, Schwarz EB, Green BD, Reinhold AG, Colaizy TT, et al. An online calculator to estimate the impact of changes in breastfeeding rates on population health and costs. Breastfeed Med. 2017;12(10):645-58.
8. Walters DD, Phan LTH, Mathisen R. The cost of not breastfeeding: global results from a new tool. Health Policy Plan. 2019;34(6): 407-17.
9. Karlsson JO, Garnett T, Rollins NC, Röös E. The carbon footprint of breastmilk substitutes in comparison with breastfeeding. J Clean Prod. 2019;222:436-45.
10. Zadkovic S, Hons BA, Lombardo N, Hons BA. Breastfeeding and Climate Change: Overlapping Vulnerabilities and Integrating Responses. J Hum Lact. 2020;37(2):323-30.
11. Russell TD, Schaack J, Orlicky DJ, Palmer C, Chang BH, Chan L, et al. Adipophilin regulates maturation of cytoplasmic lipid droplets and alveolae in differentiating mammary glands. J Cell Sci. 2011;124(Pt 19): 3247-53.
12. Park S, Zhao Y, Yoon S, Xu J, Liao L, Lydon J, et al. Repressor of Estrogen Receptor Activity (REA) Is Essential for Mammary Gland Morphogenesis and Functional Activities: Studies in Conditional Knockout. Endocrinology. 2015;152:4336-49.
13. Mccormick NH, Kelleher SL. ZnT4 provides zinc to zinc-dependent proteins in the trans-Golgi network critical for cell function and Zn export in mammary epithelial cells. Am J Physiol Cell Physiol. 2012;303(3):C291-7.
14. Keim SA, Daniels JL, Siega-riz AM, Dole N, Herring AH, Scheidt PC. Depressive Symptoms during Pregnancy and the Concentration of Fatty Acids in Breast Milk. J Hum Lact. 2012;28(2):189-95.
15. Hauff LE, Demerath EW. O Body image concerns and reduced breastfeeding duration in primiparous overweight and obese women. Am J Hum Biol. 2012;349:339-49.
16. Ogbo FA, Eastwood J, Page A, Arora A, Mckenzie A, Jalaludin B, et al. Prevalence and determinants of cessation of exclusive breastfeeding in the early postnatal period in Sydney, Australia. Int Breastfeed J. 2017;12:16.
17. Negin J, Coffman J, Vizintin P, Raynes-green C. The influence of grandmothers on breastfeeding rates: a systematic review. BMC Pregnancy Childbirth. 2016;16:91.
18. Kellams AL, Gurka KK, Hornsby PP, Drake E, Riffon M, Gellerson D, et al. The impact of a prenatal education video on rates of breastfeeding initiation and exclusivity during the newborn hospital stay in a low-income population. J Human Lact. 2015;2016;32(1):152-9.
19. Andaya E, Bonuck K, Barnett J, Lischewski-Joel J. Perceptions of primary care-based breastfeeding promotion interventions: Qualitative analysis of randomized controlled trial participant interviews. Breastfeed Med. 2012;7(6): 417-22..
20. Wallenberg JT, Jhongbe T, Rosario S, Masho SW. Knowledge of Breastfeeding Recommendations and Breastfeeding duration: A Survival Analysis on Infant Feeding Practices II. Breastfeed Med. 2017;12:156-62.
21. Glaser DB, Roberts KJ, Grosskopf NA, Basch CH. An evaluation of the effectiveness of school-based breastfeeding education. J Hum Lact. 2016,32(1).46-52.
22. Albert JB, Heinrichs-Breen J, Belmonte FW. Development and evaluation of a lactation rotation for a pediatric residency program. J Hum Lact. 2017;33(4):748-56.
23. Buccini S, Fiedler AJH, Doucet K, Pérez R, Gubert MB. Development and pretesting of "Becoming Breastfeeding Friendly": Empowering governments for global scaling up of breastfeeding programs. Matern Child Nutr. 2019;15(1):e12659.
24. Brown A. Breastfeeding as a public health responsibility: a review of the evidence. JHND. 2017;(10):759-70.
25. Manuscript A. NIH Public Access. 2014;1-16.

CHAPTER 41

Counseling in Breastfeeding

Anita Nyamagoudar, Udaykumar B, Durgappa H

"Breastfeeding is the right of every mother and baby"
—**World Health Organization**

INTRODUCTION

Breastfeeding counseling plays a pivotal role in the promotion of breastfeeding for infants and young children. Pregnant women, breastfeeding mothers, and caregivers need to be counseled on the benefits of breastfeeding and the harms associated with infant milk substitutes.[1]

DEFINITION

Breastfeeding counseling is a "conversation where someone with adequate training listens and responds to a mother's feelings and thoughts related to breastfeeding while respecting her situations and wishes".[2]

IMPORTANCE OF BREASTFEEDING COUNSELING

Breastfeeding counseling provides an opportunity to learn about the adequacy of breast milk secretion, sustenance of breastfeeding, breastfeeding difficulties in the mother, and breastfeeding status in working mothers.

WHO CAN PROVIDE COUNSELING

Healthcare professionals, community health workers, and voluntary peer support groups willing to help mothers and babies can provide counseling.

The World Health Organization (WHO) has framed guidelines for counseling in breastfeeding mothers to provide uniform and evidence-based recommendations across the globe. The following text summarizes the WHO guidelines adapted for counseling in breastfeeding.[3]

RECOMMENDATIONS[4]

Breastfeeding counseling should be provided:
- To all pregnant women and mothers with young children
- In both the antenatal period and postnatally and up to 24 months or longer
- At least six times and additionally as needed
- Through face-to-face counseling and may, in addition, be provided through telephone or other remote modes of counseling context-specific recommendation
- As a continuum of care, by appropriately trained healthcare professionals and community-based lay and peer breastfeeding counselors.
- Breastfeeding counselling should anticipate and address important challenges and contexts for breastfeeding, in addition to establishing skills, competencies, and confidence among mothers.

BEST PRACTICE STATEMENT (WHO)[1-4]

Protection, promotion, and support of breastfeeding, in accordance with international guidance, are essential in emergencies. Breastfeeding counseling should be an integral part of emergency preparedness plans for infant and young child feeding and both initial and sustained responses.

TIMING OF BREASTFEEDING COUNSELING

- During pregnancy
- Soon after birth and the postpartum period
- Enable caregivers to access appropriate help as needed.

FREQUENCY OF BREASTFEEDING COUNSELING[5]

A minimum of six breastfeeding counseling contacts as follows:
1. Before birth (antenatal period)
2. During and immediately after birth (perinatal period up to the first 2-3 days after birth)
3. 1-2 weeks after birth (neonatal period)
4. First 3-4 months (early infancy)
5. 6 months (at the start of complementary feeding)
6. After 6 months (late infancy and early childhood), with additional contacts as necessary.

The counseling during breastfeeding is divided into **(Fig. 1)**:
- Listening and learning skills
- Confidence and support skills

Listening and Learning Skills[3,5]

- Use helpful nonverbal communication
- Ask open questions

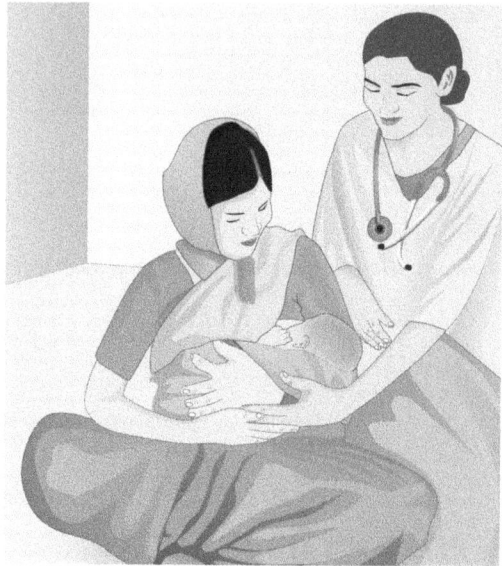

Fig. 1: Breastfeeding counseling.

- Use responses and gestures that show interest
- Reflect on what the mother says
- Empathize and show that you understand how she feels
- Avoid words that sound judging.

Helpful Nonverbal Communication[3,5]

- Keep your head level
- Pay attention
- Remove barriers
- Take time
- Touch appropriately.

Confidence and Support Skills[3,5]

- Accept what a mother thinks and feels
- Recognize and praise what a mother and baby are doing right
- Give practical help
- Give a little relevant information
- Use simple language
- Make one or two suggestions, not commands.

In addition to the abovementioned skills, additional history and examination may be needed based on the situation. A few examples are cited further.

How to Help with a Baby who Cries a Lot[6]

- *Look for a cause:*
  - Listen and learn:
    - Help mother to talk about feelings (guilt or anger)
    - Empathize
  - Take a history:
    - Learn about baby's feeding and behavior
    - Learn about mother's diet, coffee, smoking, drugs
    - Pressures from family and others
  - Assess a breastfeeding position at the breast and length of the feed
  - Examine baby's illness or pain (treat or refer as appropriate):
    - Check growth.

How to Help a Mother who Thinks that she Does not Have Enough Breastmilk

- *Understand her situation:*
  - *Listen and learn:* To understand why she lacks confidence, empathize
  - *Take a history:* To learn about pressures from other people
  - *Assess breastfeeding:* To check the baby's attachment to the breast
  - *Examine the mother:* Breast size may cause a lack of confidence.

How to Help a Mother Whose Baby is not Getting Enough Milk[6]

- *Look for a cause:*
  - *Steps to take:* What you may learn about
    - *Listen and learn:* Psychological factors and how a mother feels
    - *Take a history:* Of breastfeeding factors, contraceptive pills, and diuretics
    - *Assess a breastfeeding:* Baby's position at the breast—bonding or rejection
    - *Examine the baby's:* Illness or abnormality and growth
    - *Examine the mother's:* Nutrition and health.

WHAT MAKES GOOD COMMUNICATION?[7,8]

- Clarity
- Providing adequate time to listen
- Integrity
- Being nonjudgmental
- Allowing the mother to make her choice
- Be available for follow-up.

In a nutshell, *praise, inform, and suggest*—praise the mother for what she is doing right, give relevant information to solve the difficulty that a mother may be facing, and suggest steps for improvement if required. This should enable successful breastfeeding among all the postnatal mothers.

KEY MESSAGES

- Breastfeeding counseling is the most effective way to enhance breastfeeding practices.
- Timely skilled counseling and support are crucial in the sustenance of breastfeeding.
- Listening and learning, nonverbal communication, and confidence building are important steps in improving breastfeeding practices.
- Recognizing and praising the mother for what she is doing right is a key factor in building her confidence.
- Empathizing with her and her support group goes a long way in establishing a good rapport.

REFERENCES

1. United Nations Children's Fund (UNICEF), World Health Organization, Implementation Guidance on Counselling Women to Improve Breastfeeding Practices. New York: United Nations Children's Fund; 2021.
2. World Health Organization. Guideline: counselling of women to improve breastfeeding practices. Geneva: World Health Organization; 2018.
3. World Health Organization, UNICEF. Infant and young child feeding counselling: an integrated course: trainer's guide, 2nd edition. Geneva: World Health Organization; 2021.
4. World Health Organization CDD Programme, UNICEF. Breastfeeding counselling: A training course. Participants' manual. Part one. Sessions 1-9.
5. McFadden A, Siebert L, Marshall JL, Gavine A, Girard LC, Symon A, et al. Counselling interventions to enable women to initiate and continue breastfeeding: a systematic review and meta-analysis. Int Breastfeed J. 2019;14(1):1-9.
6. World Health Organization. Implementation guidance: protecting, promoting, and supporting breastfeeding in facilities providing maternity and newborn services: the revised Baby-Friendly Hospital Initiative 2018. Geneva: World Health Organization; 2018.
7. Gupta A, Dadhich JP, Suri S. How can global rates of exclusive breastfeeding for the first 6 months be enhanced? ICAN: Infant Child Adolesc Nutr. 2013;5(3):133-40.
8. WIC Works Resource System. Infant Nutrition and Feeding Guide: A Guide for Use in the WIC and CSFP Programs. Alexandria, VA: US Department of Agriculture, Food and Nutrition Service; 2008.

Index

Page numbers followed by *b* refer to box, *f* refer to figure, and *t* refer to table

A

Accredited Social Health Activists 227, 244, 249, 268
Acetaminophen 108
Acetylcholine, synthesis of 25
Acid-binding protein 35
Acidemia, propionic 212
Acini, number of 12
Acquired immunodeficiency syndrome 163
Adipokines 26
Adipophilin, role of 272
Air swallowing, excessive 196
Alcoholism 261
Allergic disorders 44, 180
Alveolar structure 19*f*
Alzheimer's disease 67
American Academy of Pediatrics 271
Amino acid
  disorders 206
  essential 210
  large neutral 208
  propiogenic 211
Amphetamines 175
Amylase 24
Analgesics 136
  ibuprofen 138
Anemia 196
  macrocytic 67
  maternal 65
Anethum graveolens 109
Anganwadi workers 227
Anorexia nervosa 185
Antenatal
  care 249
  counseling 133
  period 249
Antibiotics 138
Antibodies 22
Anticancer drugs 108
Antimicrobial agents 22
Antioxidant 24, 26
Antipsychotics, first-generation 186
Antiretroviral drugs 200
Anuria 167
Anxiety 16, 33, 149
Appetite, loss of 159
Arachidonic acid 24, 58
Areola 18
Arginase deficiency 210
Arginine 210
Artificial feeding
  methods 178
  risks of 176*f*
Asparagus racemosus 109
Asthma, risk of 180
Atenolol 108
Atopic dermatitis, risk of 180
Attention-deficit hyperactivity disorder 49
Autoclave 261
Autocrine control 15
Autoimmune disorders 45
Auxiliary nurse midwives 227, 245

B

Baby's sleep pattern 142
Baby Feeding Law Group 267
Baby-Friendly Hospital Initiative 4, 8, 76, 133, 241, 244, 268
Bacillus Calmette-Guérin vaccination 203
Bacterial cell wall 24
Bacteroidetes 120
Barium 24
Basal metabolic rate 28, 70
Behavior
  problems 178
  therapy 185
Bifidobacterium 37, 38
  breve 28
Binge-eating 185
  disorder 187
Biopsy, excisional 151
Biotin 30
Birth weight 202
  extremely low 92, 93
  low 92, 165, 249
  very low 49, 93, 155, 174
Bitot spots 67
Blind-ended tubes 12
Blood
  borne viruses 219
  concentration 207*t*
  flow, relation of 15
  phenylalanine levels 207
  vessels 18
Body mass index 28, 36, 37*f*, 273
Bottle-feeding 133, 178, 179, 182, 224
  baby, positions for 182
  effects of 179
  historical aspect of 178
  preparation of 181
  prevalence of 178
  problems of 180*t*
  reasons for 178
  storage of 181
Botulinum toxicity 54
Branched-chain amino acids
  requirements of 213*t*
  target blood levels of 213*t*
Breast 13, 16, 127
  abscess 135, 138
  anatomical problems of 127
  anatomy of 11
  asymmetry 127
  changes 14
  congestion 224
  developmental stages of 13*t*
  engorgement 135, 136
  examination, prenatal 151
  functional unit of 12
  gross anatomy 16
  hypoplastic 151
  irradiation 151
  local infections of 224, 261
  location 11
  massage 95
    gentle 136
  nulliparous 12
  overdevelopment of 127
  parenchyma 16
  physiology of 11
  pump 128
  shells 128
  support 85
  surgery 151
  tissue 15
  underdevelopment of 127
Breast development 235
  anomalies 127
  intrauterine environment for 12

Index

Breast milk 14, 19, 22-24, 30, 33-36, 37f, 43, 57, 106, 152, 154, 174, 201, 279
  amount of 213
  and genetics 33
  carbohydrates components of 24
  cholesterol content of 38
  collection of 262
  component 38, 38t
  composition of 22, 34, 57, 57
  content 58, 273
  dietary fat of 57
  donors 260
  epigenetic effects of 35
  fatty acid 58
  jaundice, persistent 175
  multinutrient fortification of 95
  nourishes 106
  nutrients 60
  production of 227
  pumps 261
  quality of 57, 58
  quantity of 22
  removal
    frequency of 22
    inefficient 137
  secretion 22, 148f, 149
    adequacy of 87
    amount of 22
  substitutes 175, 220
    disadvantages of 175
    influence of 269
    promotion of 221
    risks of 172, 175
    use of 174
  types of 103
Breastfeeding 3, 6, 7, 34, 36, 42-44, 46, 77, 85, 98, 101, 106, 108, 131, 133, 138, 143, 147, 152, 154, 155, 174, 175, 200, 201t, 202, 203, 206, 212, 213, 215, 217, 236, 241, 242b, 243, 248, 250, 267, 271, 273, 275, 277, 279
  ad libitum 152
  and law 275
  and maternal
    infections 200
    medications 106
  and metabolic disorders 206
  and neurodevelopment 44
  and neuropsychiatric disorders 44
  and working mother 98
  barriers of 100b, 106, 131, 219
  benefits of 42, 46t, 47t, 271
  biology of 273
  breaks 101
  cessation of 135
  correct techniques of 151
  counseling 277, 278f
    frequency of 278
    importance of 277
    timing of 278
  delayed initiation of 53, 54b
  determinants of 273
  difficulties 4, 135, 178
  direct 93
  duration of 22
  during emergency 217
  education 152
  exclusive 98, 101, 219, 241, 249, 266
  failure 196
  harmful practices for 152
  in cradle position 88f
  in hospitalized children 161
  in side lying down position 88f
  in special circumstances 193
  in working mothers, guidance for 102
  incorrect technique of 135, 135b
  infrequent 15
  initiation of 53, 54, 241
  lack of knowledge of 149
  observation aid 90
  outcome measures 101t
  overcome barriers of 133
  peer support 250
  policies 101
  positions, modifications of 139
  practices 3, 45, 99f, 132, 155l, 254, 274
    advantages of 100
    impacts on 196
  process 195
  promotion 4, 9, 217, 266, 271
    network 4, 8, 221, 245, 252, 257, 267
  rate 266
  room 9
  sensitization programs 5
  strategies, modification of 139
  support 151, 245, 249, 251, 278
    groups for 250
    tools for 250
  technique of 85
  total duration of 87
Bulimia nervosa 186

C

Cadmium 24
Caffeine 108
Calcitriol 68
Calcium 23, 25, 26, 59
  absorption of 23
  supplementation of 208
Cancer 33, 36
  endometrial 45
Candida albicans 38
Carbimazole 175
Carbohydrates 24, 26
Cardiac dysfunction 43, 213
Cardiovascular diseases 33
Carnitine, supplementation of 214
Carotenes 26
Casein 24
Caveolin-1 35
Cavity, oral 93
Cefadroxil 138
Cefazolin 138
Cefuroxime 138
Cells 28
Cephalexin 138
Cerebral edema 169
Cerebral venous thrombosis 169
Cerium 24
Chemokines 27
Chest wall 95
Chloride 25, 26
Cholesterol 24, 38
Choline 25, 26, 60
Chromium 24
Citalopram 108
Citrulline 210
Cleft lip 137, 195, 196, 196b
  management of 196
  prevalence of 195
  severity of 195
Cleft palate 137, 195, 196, 196b, 197
  management of 196
  surgical repair of 198
Cloxacillin 138
Cnicus benedictus 109
Cobalt 24
Cocaine 175
Cognitive behavioral therapy 185, 187, 188
Cold compresses 136
Colostrum 22, 27, 27t, 154, 166
  secretion 15
Commensal bacteria 37
Communicable disease 218
Communication, nonverbal 278
Community
  Health workers, capacity building of 244
  level interventions 244
Complementary feeding 112, 112f, 113, 114, 220
  frequency of 115t

Comprehensive lactation
    management centers 264
Constipation, functional 119, 121
Continuous positive airway pressure
    81, 93
Conventional pasteurizer 261
Cooper's ligament 17, 17f
Copper 24, 26, 59
Coproporphyrinogen 65
Cornerstone 119
Coronavirus disease-2019
    COVID-19 200-202, 265
Cow's milk 173
    protein 173
        intolerance 175
Cradle 88
Craniofacial anomalies 195, 196
Creatine phosphokinase 214
Cretinism, presentation of 66
Cross cradle 88
Cup feeding 198
Cyclic vomiting syndrome 117-119
    episodes of 119
Cytokine 37, 44
    inhibitors 27
    varieties of 25
Cytomegalovirus 23, 200, 201
    infection 203
Cytoplasmic lipid droplets 14
Cytosol 65
Cytotoxic chemotherapy 175

D

Dancer hand position 197, 197f
Death, risk of 271
Decision-making arm 172
Deep pectoral fascia 16
Dehydration
    hypernatremic 165
    mild 167
    moderate 167
    severe 167
Dementia 67
Dendritic arborization 34
Deoxyribonucleic acid 25, 33, 45,
    67, 201
Depression 272, 273
    maternal 273
    postpartum 76
Depressive disorders 33
Diabetes mellitus 33, 49, 149
Diagnostic and statistical manual
    for mental disorders-V
        diagnostic criteria
            185-189
Diarrhea 54, 158, 200
    functional 117, 118, 121

Diarrheal diseases 43, 162
Diazepam 108
Dietary management 210, 213
    principles of 206, 208, 209, 210f
Dietary protein 58
Digestive system 22
Disaster Management Committee
    218
Docosahexaenoic acid 24, 36
    supplementation of 57
Donate milk 260, 261
Drip and drop method 229f
Drugs 108-110
    abuse 261
    pharmacokinetics of 107
Duct, branching of 12f
Dysbiosis 39
Dyschezia 121
    infant 117, 118

E

Eating disorders 184, 185, 189
    types of 184
Ectoderm 11
Efavirenz 200
Electronic timer device 261
Embarrassment 275
Embryology 11
Emotional molecules 33
Emtricitabine 200
Encephalopathy 213
Energy 58, 114t, 161, 210, 212
Entamoeba histolytica 38
Enterococcus 38, 137
Enzyme 44
    branched-chain keto acid
        dehydrogenase,
        deficiency of 212
    galactose-1-phosphate
        uridylyltransferase 208
    phenylalanine hydroxylase 207
Epidermal growth factor 28
Epigastrium 79
Epithelial cells 15
Erythrocytes 65
Escherichia coli 23, 120, 137, 208,
    218
Estrogen 12
    receptor 272
    role of 272
    window 12
European Medicines Agency 235
Eustachian tube 179
Exosomes 26, 34
Express breast milk 95, 96, 229f, 231
Extracellular volume, contraction
    of 165

F

Face, embryonic components
    of 195
Faciomaxillary surgery 196
Failure to thrive 196
Fats 26
Fatty acid 24, 37, 273
    essential 57
    metabolism of 213
    oxidation defects 213
    saturated 58
Fatty liver disease, nonalcoholic
    34, 38
Federation of Obstetric and
    Gynecological Societies
    of India 221, 258
Feeding 75, 158, 206
    atmosphere 75f
    behavior, normal 142
    bottles 9, 243, 254
    breast milk substitutes,
        long-term risks of 176
    cluster 143
    devices 196
    difficulty, elements of 197
    disorders 184, 185
        types of 184
    in disasters and emergencies
        219
    in low birthweight infants 92
    in preterm infants 92
    in small vulnerable newborn
        babies 92
    management, general principles
        of 206
    method of 114
    neophobia 190
    positions, modifications of
        196, 199
    practices 161
        and beliefs 159
        during COVID-19 220
        principles of 209, 211-213
        quantity of 161
        responsive 143, 243
        type of 161
Fetal nervous system 58, 60
Fluoxetine 108
Foeniculum vulgare 109
Folate 26, 30, 59, 60, 64, 67
    deficiency 67
    functions of 67
Follicle stimulating hormone 14
Food 113
    ingredients, principle of
        selection of 113
    neophobia 189
        incidence of 190

Football method 196, 197f
Foremilk 23
Formula milk 173t
Fungal infections 261
Fussiness 120

G

Galactagogues 109, 109t, 151
Galactocele 139
Galactophores 11
Galactopoiesis 15
Galactosemia 206, 208
    classical 174
Galega officinalis 109
Gastric content, habitual
        regurgitation of 119
Gastroenteritis 175
Gastroesophageal reflux 178
    disease 117, 224
        management for 118
Gastrointestinal disorders,
        functional 117, 122
Gastrointestinal infections 179
Gavage feeding 93
Gene
    expression 38
    levels of 14
Gestation, period of 33
Gestational age, small for 82, 92, 260
Glandular epithelium, apoptosis of 16
Glandular tissue 16
Global Breastfeeding Collective 245, 246
Global Networking and Promotion of Breastfeeding 241
Glucuronosyltransferase 107
Glutaric acidemia 209, 209t
Glutathione 26
Glycogen storage disease 214
    feeding in 214
Glycoprotein 23
Glycosaminoglycans 23
Glycoside hydrolases 14
Gonadotropin-releasing hormone, secretion of 14
Good complementary feeding, characteristics of 113
Gram-negative bacteria 120, 137
Gross domestic product 272
Group counseling 269
Growth 272
    factors 44
    hormone 14
    spurts 143

Gut
    dysbiosis 120
    microbiota 36, 39

H

H1H1 virus 200, 202
Hand-to-mouth movements 87
Haptocorrin 23
Healthcare
    professionals 132, 277
    providers 250
    system 266
        responsibility of 256
    workers 154
        motivation of 82
Heart
    disease, congenital 166
    rate 80
Hebarman feeder 197, 198f
Hemoglobin 28
Hemolysis, drugs-induced 108
Hemorrhage
    intracranial 166, 169
    postpartum 272
Heparin binding epidermal growth factor 28
Hepatitis
    B 200, 201, 261
    B E antigen 202
    C 200, 202, 261
    transmission of 202
Herpes simplex virus 23, 175, 200, 201
    infection 202
Hind milk 23
Hormone 14, 28, 44
    metabolic 14, 28
    placental 148
    role of 11, 14
Hospital-grade electric pumps 261
Hot air oven 261
Human alpha-lactalbumin 28, 45
Human immunodeficiency virus 23, 37f, 163, 200, 201, 261
    infection, transmission of 200
    maternal 174
Human lactation, basics of 1
Human mammary gland, development of 11
Human milk 23, 25, 28, 29, 42, 219, 264t
    analyzer 262
    bank 260, 261, 263-265, 267
        association 258
        equipment needed for 261
        personnel required for 262
    cells 26

    composition of 22, 26t
    fat components of 24
    fortifiers 93
    microbiota 28
    mucins 24
    oligosaccharides 22, 28, 29, 38, 42, 179
    protein components in 23
    storage
        duration of 263t
        guideline 103t
        temperature of 263t
    supplements 95
    unique features of 28
Human T-cell lymphotropic virus 261
Hunger cues 143
    signs of 87
Hydrocephalus 169
Hydroxymethylglutaryl 38
Hyperbilirubinemia 169
Hypernatremia 165
Hypernatremic dehydration 165
    risk factors of 165b
Hypoglycemia 42, 43, 54, 213
    risk of 92, 174
Hypomania 127
Hypothermia 42, 54, 82

I

Illness 158
    vicious cycle of 158
Immune
    cells 37
    functions, normal 70
    regulatory properties 272
    system 23, 106
        modulate 35
    function 22, 25
Immunoglobulin 27, 37
    A 22, 35, 43
        secretory 23, 28
    G 28, 69
    transcytosis for 15
India Newborn Action Plan 82
Indian Academy of Pediatrics 221, 258
Indian Medical Association 258
Indian National Family Health Survey 98
Induced lactation 234, 235
Infant and young child feeding-emergency tool kit 220
Infant formulae
    composition of 172
    types of 172

Index

Infant gut microbiota 37
Infant Milk Substitute Act 3, 4, 9, 132, 172, 173, 254, 255
   implementation and monitoring of 257
   important provisions of 255
   limitations of 257
   objectives of 255
Infantile colic 117, 224
Infections 43
   maternal 4, 200, 201
   risk of 98
   vicious cycle of 159f
Infectious diseases 158, 266
Inflammatory bowel disease 36
Inflammatory disorders, low-grade 36
Insufficient milk secretion, perception of 4, 147
Insulin 14
   like growth factor 28
Intelligence quotient 9, 49
Interferon
   gamma 28
   synthesis of 25
Interleukin 28
International Baby Food Action Network 245, 267
International Code of Marketing of Breast-Milk Substitutes 242, 267
International Institute for Population Sciences 96
International Labor Organization 268
International Monetary Fund Act 266
Intestinal microbiota 37f
Intestine, small 35
Intrauterine life 11
Intravenous fluids 81
Iodine 60, 64, 66, 70
   deficiency disorder 66
   functions of 66
   primary function of 66
   rich foods 115
Iron 26, 59, 64, 65, 70, 188
   absorption of 23
   deficiency 65
      anemia 65
      effects of 66
   rich foods 115
Isoleucine 211-213
   supplementation of 212
Isoniazid 201, 203
IYCF-E tool kit, overview of 220

J

Jaundice 42, 80
Jaw
   developmental problems 178, 196
   muscles, spasm of 86

K

Kangaroo
   early discharge 79
   father care 81
   feeding 79
      policy 78
   mother care 78, 79f, 80-82, 221, 230, 231f, 261
      benefits of 79, 80b
      components of 78
      effective utilization of 83
      eligibility for 80
      human resource for 81
      immediate 133
      procedures 81
      position 78, 79
Kashin–Beck disease 69
Katori feeding 93
Keshan disease 69
Kidney injury, acute 169
Klebsiella 137

L

La Leche league 250
Labetalol 108
Lactaid supplementer 230f
Lactalbumin 23
Lactase enzyme supplementation 120
Lactation 110, 149
   counselors 250
   early problems in 127
   facilities 101
   failure, primary 149
   management
      centers 268
      units 264
   physiological basis of 227
   physiology of 272
   practical problems of 142
   room 102
   support
      lack of 219
      units 264
   suppression 109
   understanding golden physiology of 148

Lactiferous sinuses 17, 19
Lactobacillus 37, 38
   reuteri 121
Lactoferrin 22, 23, 37, 38
Lactogenesis 14, 15
   delayed 149
Lactoperoxidase 22
Lactose-free infant milk 173
Lamivudine 200
Latch score 86, 87t
Lead 24
Leptin 35
Leucine 213
Lip smacking 87
Lipid soluble drugs 107
Lipopolysaccharides, presence of 120
Lipoprotein lipase 35
Lithium 175
Liver function test 214
Lobes, division of 17f
Local breast, management of 151
Long-chain fatty acid oxidation defect 214
Long-chain polyunsaturated fatty acid 24, 36, 45
Lorazepam 108
Low milk production, prevention of 151
Lumbar puncture 167
Lumen epithelium 12
Luminal cell function 18
Luteal hormones 148
Lycopene 26
Lymphatic drainage 19
Lymphatic vessels 19
Lymphocytes 22
Lysine 209
   age-appropriate requirement of 209t
Lysozyme 22, 23, 37

M

Macromastia 127
Macronutrients 23, 26, 57, 64
Magnesium 26
Maintenance therapy 122
Major childhood illnesses, prevention of 200
Malabsorption 158
Malnutrition 98, 159f, 178, 200, 218
   vicious cycle of 158
Mammary bud 12f
   downward growth of 12f
Mammary epithelial barrier 106
Mammary gland 11, 14, 19
   development of 11, 12

Index

Mammary lobules development 12f
Mammary mesenchyme 11
Mammary nodes, internal 19
Mammary tissue 18
   development, embryonic stages of 12f
   structure of 18f
Mammary tumor growth 36
Mammogenesis 15
Manganese 24, 26
Maple syrup urine disease 174, 212, 213, 213t
   feeding in 212
Mastitis 135, 137
   management of 138
   risk factors of 137
Maternal Benefit Act 100
   eligibility for 100
Maternal fatigue, excessive 149
Maternal health 106
   and lactation 273
Maternal leave policy 101
Maternal literacy and maternal feeding practices 116
Maternity Benefits Act 133, 251
   for working mothers, amendment of 252
Maternity Protection Legislation 268
Mature milk 23, 27, 166
Maxillary processes 195
Mead-Johnson cleft palate nursery bottle 198, 198f
Measles 162
Medium-chain fatty acid oxidation defect 214
Meningitis 166
Menopause 16
Menstrual cycle 224
   phase of 13
Mental
   disorders 184
   health 219
   illness 188
Mesenchymal cells 11
Metabolic disease 179
Metabolism, inborn errors of 166, 206
Methionine 211, 212
Methylmalonic academia 212
Microbiome 36
Microbiota 42
Micronutrients 24, 26, 59, 64, 70
   deficiency 64
      cause of 65
      impact of 65
   importance of 70t
   maternal 59

Micro-ribonucleic acid 26, 33, 35
   potential effects of 35
Midazolam 108
Milk
   and milk products 113
   banking 261
   ejection reflex 15
   expression 264
      method of 94
   hand expression of 231, 231f
   manual expression of 96f
   oversupply of 139
   pH of 107
   production 58
   stasis 137
   synthesis 14
   types of 166
   volume 152
Mineralocorticoid axis abnormality 166
Minerals 25, 26, 29, 59, 174
Minimal enteral nutrition 94
Mitochondria 65
Modern formula milk 156
Modifies syringe technique 129f
Molybdenum 24
Monounsaturated fatty acids 57
Morbidities, anticipation of 78
Moringa oleifera 109
Mother-baby-friendly
   environment 75, 77, 85
   workplace 104
Mothers Absolute Affection Program 5, 244, 252
Mother-to-mother support groups 235
Mucins 28
Multiple births 76, 106
Myoepithelial cells 18
   receptors of 16

N

Nasal
   cavity 93
   obstruction 224
   processes
      lateral 195
      median 195
   regurgitation, recurrent 196
Nasogastric tube 93
National Family Health Survey 3, 53, 92, 99f, 267
National Guidelines on Lactation Management Centers in Public Health Facilities 264, 265

National Health Mission 244, 268
National Health Policy 82
National Neonatology Forum 94, 221
National Tuberculosis Elimination Programme Pediatric guideline 204
Natural killer cells, function of 68
Necrotizing enterocolitis 28, 35, 38, 42, 49, 80, 260, 271
   incidence of 93
Nectarine, sweetness of 7
Neonatal intensive care unit 76, 260, 264
Neural tube defects, development of 67
Neurodegenerative diseases 36
Neuromotor incoordination disorders 86
Neuronal growth factor 28
Neuropeptide Y 16
Nevirapine prophylaxis 202t
Newborn Intensive Care Unit 78
Niacin 30
Nickel 24
Nicotine, maternal use of 155
Night blindness 67
Nipple 18, 155
   abnormally large 127
   anatomical problems of 127
   areolar complex 16
   biting 145
   center of 129
   confusion 179
      increased risk of 178
   cracked 135
   flat 127, 128
   inverted 12f, 127
   long 127
   pain 135
      relieving 136
   problems, management of 151
   pulls inward 128
   shield 128, 129
   short 127
   sore 135
   soreness 149
   stands out 128
   type of 87
Nirmala Kesaree syringe 129
Nitrogen scavengers 210
Noncommunicable diseases 33, 44
Nongovernmental organizations 250
   role of 258
Nose block 144
Not enough milk 147
   management of 150t

Nuclear factor kappa B 38
Nursing strike 86, 224
   causes for 224t
Nutrients 173, 212
   good sources of 115t
Nutrition 218
   enteral 257
   maternal 57, 58
   parenteral 257
   source of 79
Nutritional management, acute 212

O

Obesity 35, 179
   maternal 149
Odd-chain fatty acids 211
Olanzapine 186
Oligosaccharides 28
Omega-3 fatty acids 58
Opioids 175
   analgesics 108
Optimal feeding practices 195, 196
Optimize breastfeeding
      technique 136
Oral thrush 86, 224
Organic acidemias 211, 212t
   feeding in 211
Orogastric tube 93
Oromandibular problems 179
Orthodontics 196
Otitis media 175, 179, 224
   acute 43, 179
   recurrent 196
Otolaryngology 196
Oxazepam 108
Oxytocin 16, 19, 45
   hormones 227
   reflex 17f, 148, 232

P

Paid maternity leaves 4
Pain
   physical 76
   relieving agents 121
Paladai feeding 93
Parkinson's disease 36
Paroxetine 108
Pediatric
   feeding disorder 184
   nutrition, basics of 1
Peripheral oxygen saturation 80
Peroxisome proliferator-activated
      receptor 38
Pharmacokinetics 107, 107t
Phenylalanine 207, 207t
   free milk 174
   intake of 207

Phenylketonuria 174, 206, 207,
      207t, 208t
   management of 207
Phospholipids, synthesis of 25
Phosphorus 25, 26
Pica 188
Picky eating 189
Pigeon nipple 198, 198f
Pinch test 128
Plasma, maternal 106
Plastic surgery 196
Pneumonia 158, 162, 200
Polyethylene glycol 121
Polymastia 127
Polymorphisms, proinflammatory
      36
Polyunsaturated fatty acid 29,
      42, 154
Post-gastrointestinal surgeries 261
Post-pasteurization testing 264
Post-traumatic stress disorder 219
Potassium 25, 26
Pregnancy 14, 110, 273
   physiological change in 107
Prelacteal feed 53, 54
Premenstrual period 13
Prenatal breastfeeding education
      151, 274
Preterm deliveries 260
Preterm milk 23
Progesterone 12, 13
Prolactin 19, 227
   reflex 16f
Prophylaxis therapy 203
Propiogenic amino acids 211
   requirement of 212t
Propranolol 108
Prosthesis 196, 198
Proteins 23, 26, 209, 210, 212
   metabolism 69
   rich foods 115
   synthetic 210
Provitamin A carotenoids 67
Psychomotor skills 58
Psychotherapy 186
Pubertal stage 12
Public health services 275
Pyrexia 43

R

Radioactive drugs 108
Randomized controlled trials 49
Rapid eye movements 87
Rectum reabsorbs water
      content 121
Red blood cells 28
Regurgitation 117

   infant 118
   management for 119
Relactation 226, 230, 232, 234
   complete 226
   concept of 226
   partial 226
   physiological basis of 227
   scope for 227
Respiratory infection 43, 162
Respiratory rate 80
   infection 69, 175
   lower 179
Restrictive food intake disorder 187
Revised ROME IV criteria 118b
Reye syndrome 108
Riboflavin 30
Ribonucleic acid 25, 28, 69
Rubidium 24
Rubus idaeus 109
Rumination
   disorder 117, 188
   syndrome 119

S

Salmonellosis 218
Sanitation 218
Sappey's subareolar plexus 19
Sapropterin dihydrochloride 208
Scissor-hold method 139
Secretory alveoli, mammary cells
      of 227
Seizures 167, 213
Selenium 26, 64, 69, 70
   deficiency 69
Sepsis 44, 82, 166, 260, 261
   neonatal 54
Sertraline 108
Shaker-water bath 261
Sheehan's syndrome 149
Shigella 23
Shock 43
Short gut syndrome 261
Silybum marianum 109
Skin-to-skin
   contact 53
   theory 14
Sleep-wake
   cycle 142
   pattern 142
Smell, change of 224
Sodium 25, 26, 166, 166t
Sotalol 108
Speech problems 196
Spoon feeding 93, 198
Standard Antituberculosis
      Treatment regimen 204

Stanpan Suraksha App 245, 245f
Staphylococcus aureus 43, 137
Stem cells 34
Sterol regulatory element-binding protein 1 35
Straddle method 196
Streptococcus 38
   epidermidis 137
Stress 149
   acute 224
   hormones 33
   psychological 196
   severe 188
Strontium 24
Sucking
   continuous 144
   immature 92
   ineffective 196
   movements 87
   non-nutritive 94
   sounds 87
Sudden infant death 213
   syndrome 42, 49, 180
Superior pectoral fascia 16
Supplementary suckling technique 230, 230f
Surgery, oral 196
Sustaining Workplace Lactation Programme 103
Swallowing reflexes 92
Syphilis 261

T

Teeth
   decay 178
   mineralization 25
Teleconsultation 250
Telephonic helplines 250
Tenofovir 200
Terminal duct lobular unit 12, 13f, 18f
Tetrahydrobiopterin 207, 208
Thoracic
   artery, lateral 18
   veins, internal 18
Threonine 211, 212
Thyroid-stimulating hormone 66
Tin 24
Tissue 25
Tocopherols 26
Transitional milk 23, 27, 166
Trigonella foenum-graecum 109
Trophic feeding 94

Tryptophan 209
   age-appropriate requirement of 209t
Tuberculosis 203
   pulmonary 200
Tubular breast deformity 151
Tumor
   cells 28
   necrosis factor 28
Turnera diffusa 109
Twin babies 156
Tyrosine 207, 208
   intake 207t
Tyrosinemia 209

U

Umbilical lines 80
Umbilicus 93
United Nations International Children's Emergency Fund 3, 8
United Nations International Strategy for Disaster Reduction 217
Urea cycle
   defect, dietary management of 210
   disorders 209
      breastfeeding in 211
      intermediates, replacement of 210
Urinary tract infections 43
Urine osmolality 167

V

Valine 211-213
   supplementation of 212
Varicella 200
   zoster virus infection 203
Vascular endothelial growth factor 28
Venlafaxine 108
Vital agnus-castus 109
Vitamin 24, 29, 60, 154, 174
   A 24, 26, 64, 67, 68, 70, 113
      deficiency 67, 68
      functions of 67
      requirements of 68
      rich foods 115
      supplementation, oral 95
   B 60
   B_1 26

   B_{12} 25, 26, 30
      deficiency 59
   B_2 26
   B_3 26
   B_5 26, 30
   B_6 26, 30, 59, 203
   C 25, 30
      deficiency 59
      rich foods 115
   D 24, 26, 30, 59, 60, 64, 68, 70
      deficiency 68
      functions of 68
      supplementation of 59, 208
   E 26, 59
   K 24-26
      supplementation 59
Vomiting 213

W

Warm compresses 136
Water 218
Witch's milk 11
Workplace Breastfeeding Policies 101t
World Alliance for Breastfeeding Action 245
World Breastfeeding Trends Initiative 245
World Breastfeeding Week 99
World Disaster Report 217
World Health Assembly 254, 266
World Health Organization 53, 113
   International Classification of Disability 184

X

Xerophthalmia 67
Xiphisternum 93

Y

Young child feeding 219

Z

Zinc 24, 26, 59, 64, 68, 70, 273
   absorption of 23
   deficiency 68
   functions of 69
   supplementation 69, 95
   transporter, role of 273
Zoonotic disease transmission 218

EU GSPR Authorised Reprsentative
Logos Europe, 9 rue Nicolas Poussin
1700, La Rochelle, France
Phone: +33 (0) 6 67 93 73 78
E-mail: contact@logoseurope.eu

www.ingramcontent.com/pod-product-compliance
Ingram Content Group UK Ltd.
Pitfield, Milton Keynes, MK11 3LW, UK
UKHW050456150426
5217IPUK00025B/1714